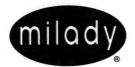

Milady Standard

Cosmetology

14TH EDITION

Workbook

www.milady.com

Milady Standard
Cosmetology
14ᵀᴴ EDITION

Workbook

ISBN: 978-0-357-37892-2

Milady, a part of Cengage Group
200 Pier 4 Boulevard
Boston, MA 02210
USA

Milady hasn't just set the standard for beauty education. We continually raise it with every product and feature release to meet the needs of today's learners, educators, and employers.
Get the full story at *milady.com/about*

Notice to the Reader

Printed in the United States of America

Print Number: 03   Print Year: 2022

Brief Contents

How to Use the Workbook

—

How to Use the Workbook

The *Milady Standard Cosmetology Workbook* strengthens your understanding of essential cosmetology theory and skills by reinforcing material covered in the text. Complete each workbook chapter as the text chapter is covered in class, and you will be one step closer to preparing for your licensure exam and obtaining your license!

This edition includes a wider variety of activities than previous Milady workbooks to engage you and to help you retain the information in each chapter. It contains familiar question types like fill in the blank, true or false, multiple choice, short answer, labeling, matching, collage, and case study activities, as well as head and nail sheets at the end of the workbook for additional practice. It also includes new question types, including reflection, research, draw, sequence, role play, "dos and don'ts," and create exercises for you to take a more hands-on approach to the material covered in your textbook. Some of these activities will recommend you follow a link to answer the question; others may require you to use a separate piece of paper. An Internet connection is required to access the online material.

Many of these activity types will be familiar to you or are self-explanatory; however, directions for the more comprehensive ones are given below.

Case Study

In the Case Study activity, you apply what you have learned to a hypothetical real-world situation. You may be asked to describe a solution or process that you would recommend for the case at hand. Case studies are answered in writing and typically require a paragraph-sized response.

Collage

In a Collage, you create a visual that responds to a given concept or prompt, either digitally through a link or on a separate piece of paper. Find words, phrases, and pictures from magazines or the Internet and bring them together by printing and cutting them out and then taping, gluing, or stapling them to your canvas. Or make a digital collage by copying and pasting together words and images into one image or document. Your instructor will provide guidance on how the class should complete their collages, including whether they will be displayed.

Create

Create exercises ask you to make something, such as designing a set of nail tips or a flyer advertising your salon business. Create exercises can be done digitally, in the workbook, or on a separate sheet of paper, depending on the question.

"Dos and Don'ts"

Much like labeling, "Dos and Don'ts" questions have you determine whether a practice is something that should be done ("Do") or shouldn't be done ("Don't"). You will need to fill in "do" or "don't" in the space provided.

Reflection

Reflection questions ask you to take some time to think about a concept or learning objective, often alongside a life experience, when considering your future career. An example is reflecting on your personal skin care routine and considering how you can improve it based on what you've learned. Reflections require writing a few sentences as a response.

Research

Research questions often include a table and ask you to find more information on a topic, often by finding and selecting different types of products that you may or may not want to use in a salon or recommend to clients. Research questions often include a link to a larger, digital table to complete, but they can be done in the workbook or on a separate sheet of paper, as well.

Role Play

Role Play activities ask students to pair up and enact a scenario where one student is the client and the other the cosmetologist. Some activities may require you to write a short reflection, as well. These exercises are meant to be practice for real-world conversations you will have with your own clients after graduation.

Sequence

Sequence questions require you to put the steps of a procedure in order, from first to last. For longer procedures, some step numbers will be given.

Best of luck to you from the Milady team!

TRACK MY PROGRESS!

Use this simple tracker to record your progress as you work through the activities in each learning objective.

COMPLETED	# OF CORRECT ANSWERS	OBJECTIVE
☐	_____ /6	LO 1 - Explain the benefits of learning cosmetology's history.
☐	_____ /22	LO 2 - Outline how ancient civilization beauty practices influenced modern-day cosmetology.
☐	_____ /5	LO 3 - Describe beauty and grooming during the Middle Ages.
☐	_____ /10	LO 4 - List the Renaissance and Victorian age's beauty developments.
☐	_____ /11	LO 5 - Describe the beauty industry's evolution during the early twentieth century.
☐	_____ /20	LO 6 - Outline the mid- and late twentieth century's major beauty advances.
☐	_____ /7	LO 7 - Describe important trends that defined cosmetology in the twenty-first century.
☐	_____ /5	LO 8 - List career opportunities for licensed cosmetologists.

Why Study Cosmetology History and Career Opportunities?

SHORT ANSWER

1. List three reasons why it's important for cosmetologists to study the cosmetology history and career opportunities.

_____

_____

_____

Indicate whether the statements below are true or false. For any false statements, briefly explain why the statement is false.

2. "Cosmetology" is also referred to as appearance expansion.

   T   F   _____

3. Cosmetology is the art and science of beautifying and improving the skin, nails, and hair, as well as the study of cosmetics and their applications.

   T   F   _____

4. The term *cosmetology* comes from the Spanish word kosmetikos, meaning "skilled in cosmetics use."

   T   F   _____

5. Although procedures, products, and styles have changed over the years, beautification has only recently become important to society.

   T   F   _____

REFLECTION

6. Write three or five sentences explaining what personally interests you about cosmetology and why you would like to become a cosmetologist. Be specific and feel free to share something personal if you wish.

   _____

   _____

   _____

Ancient Cultures

MULTIPLE CHOICE

7. How did people in ancient civilizations use hairstyles and beauty techniques in their societies?

   A) to enhance their appearance

   B) to improve their chances for career advancement

   C) to convey status, wealth, age, and rank

   D) as a way to compete for natural resources

8. Which ancient cultures are credited with many modern beauty practices, according to your text? Select all that apply.

   A) African

   B) Canadian

   C) Egyptian

   D) American

   E) Chinese

   F) Roman

   G) Spanish

   H) Australian

   I) Greek

   J) Mexican

   K) South American

   L) Italian

SHORT ANSWER

9. What are three reasons why braiding was a social art form in ancient African cultures?

   _____

   _____

   _____

Fun fact! The approximate area of each ancient civilization discussed in your text is shown on the map below.

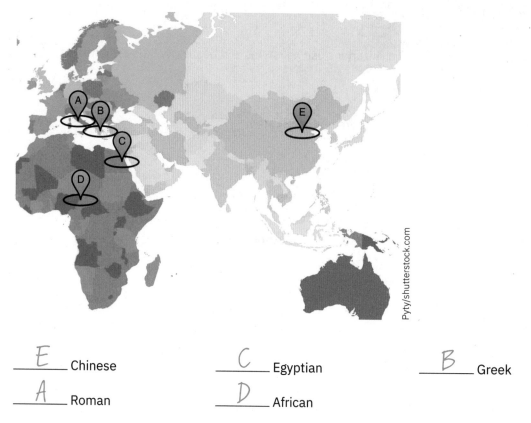

Pyty/shutterstock.com

_E_ Chinese   _C_ Egyptian   _B_ Greek

_A_ Roman   _D_ African

MULTIPLE CHOICE

10. What did many African tribes use to color their hair?

A) yellow earth   C) henna

B) red earth   D) a berry paste

11. In many ancient African tribes, _____ patterns and hairstyles indicated a person's tribe, age, marital status, wealth, power, and religion.

A) curl   C) braid

B) makeup   D) clothing

12. What is another name for Zulu knots?

   A) Himba knots

   B) Bantu knots

   C) Namibia knots

   D) cornrow braids

13. As early as 2630 BCE, Egyptians used all of the following to create makeup for their lips and skin except _____.

   A) bones

   B) insects

   C) berries

   D) minerals

14. Which Egyptian queen had a personal perfume factory?

   A) Nefertiti

   B) Cleopatra

   C) Delilah

   D) Helena

15. _____ was used in ancient Egypt to stain the hair and nails a rich, warm red.

   A) A tincture of essential oils

   B) A paste of palm berries

   C) Henna

   D) Pomegranate juice

16. The Egyptians were the first civilization to use the _____ from plant leaves, bark, and blossoms as perfumes and for purification purposes.

   A) waste products

   B) moisture

   C) essential oils

   D) dry residue

17. Which ancient culture was not known for its use of perfumes?

   A) The Egyptians

   B) The Chinese

   C) The Greeks

   D) The Romans

SHORT ANSWER

18. How did the Ancient Egyptians use kohl makeup?

    _____

    _____

    _____

19. For what three purposes did the Ancient Egyptians use cosmetics?

    _____

    _____

    _____

MULTIPLE CHOICE

20. Throughout the Zhou Dynasty, also known as the Chou Dynasty, _____ were the royal colors.

    A) black and red   C) purple and blue

    B) gold and silver   D) silver and bronze

21. During the Shang Dynasty, what did aristocrats rub onto their nails to turn them crimson or ebony?

    A) a tinted mixture of gum arabic, gelatin, beeswax, and egg whites

    B) a creamy compound of egg whites, paraffin, and essential oils

    C) nothing—colors were for commoners

    D) a paste of crushed walnuts, beeswax, clay, and ash

22. During the Zhou Dynasty, what might have happened to commoners if they wore a royal nail color?

    A) punishment of death   C) banishment for life

    B) banishment for one year   D) there was no royal nail color—all colors were for all statuses

23. Use the word bank below to fill in the blanks.

     Word bank: red, eyes, powder, vermillion, faces, Greece, white, cinnabar, cheeks, kohl

     In 500 BCE, during the Golden Age of _____, hairstyling became a highly developed art. Women

     applied preparations of _____ lead onto their _____, _____ around their _____,

     and _____ on their _____ and lips. Vermillion was a brilliant _____ pigment, made by

     grinding _____, a mineral, into a fine _____.

RESEARCH

24. Use the Internet to search for and identify two or three examples of Ancient Greek or Roman
     sculptures that depict elaborate hairstyles such as crown braids and chignons. Take screenshots
     or print them out. Then search for modern or recent examples of the same (or similar) hairstyles
     that are depicted in the Ancient Greek sculptures you identified, and take screenshots or print
     them out. Write a few sentences explaining why you think these styles have remained popular for
     over 1,000 years.

     _____

     _____

     _____

MULTIPLE CHOICE

25. Roman noblewomen tinted their hair _____; the poor class of ancient Rome wore their
     hair _____.

     A) black; red   C) any color they wished; natural

     B) red; black   D) red; blonde

26. Which of the following was *not* an ingredient used in the facials made by the Romans?

     A) milk   C) honey

     B) fine wine   D) bread

27. Describe Julius Caesar's famous hairstyle in one or two sentences. Then locate two or three modern examples of it in magazines, on celebrity websites, or perhaps in photos of various government officials. What is your impression of the people who sport this style today?

_____

_____

_____

28. Imagine you are a cosmetologist in an ancient civilization. You've decided to create your own signature beauty product (e.g., makeup, essential oils, hand cream, lip balm) using only responsibly sourced natural ingredients. What kind of product would you create? What scent would it have? What ingredients would you use? How would you make it? For inspiration, consider the civilizations above. Then write up a brief description of your product and draw (or use drawing/photoshop tools) a logo or packaging for it.

_____

_____

_____

Middle Ages

29. Why did women in the Middle Ages want to have flaxen hair?

_____

_____

_____

30. Describe the process that women used to achieve flaxen hair in the Middle Ages. And what was the process for darkening their hair?

_____

_____

_____

31. How would you characterize the hairstyles for wealthy women in the Middle Ages?

_____

_____

_____

32. How did men of the early Middle Ages wear their hair? In what way did that change in the later part of the Middle Ages, particularly for noblemen?

_____

_____

_____

33. What innovation did Persian alchemist Avicenna introduce around 1000 CE? Why do you think this was beneficial to beauty and medicine?

_____

_____

_____

Renaissance and Victorian Age

TRUE OR FALSE

Indicate whether each statement is true or false, and for false statements, explain why they are false.

34. The word *hairdresser* made its first appearance in Europe on March 1, 1739, indicating that it was now a recognized profession.

    T   F   _____

35. During the Renaissance, both men and women took great pride in their physical appearance and wore elaborate, elegant clothing.

    T   F   _____

36. Women finally began using a wide variety of very colorful lip, cheek, and eye preparations in the Renaissance period.

    T   F   _____

37. The Van Dyke beard—which consists of a moustache and goatee with shaved cheeks—created an immediate sensation and was adopted by Renaissance men everywhere when it first appeared in a portrait of King Charles I painted by Anthony van Dyck in 1636. Just as quickly, however, the beard style fell out of favor when the king later died.

    T   F   _____

38. During the Age of Extravagance (1755–1793) and the reign of Queen Marie Antionette of France, beauty standards included giant pompadour wigs, face powdering, baths of strawberries and milk, and even the use of crushed geranium petals to color lips and cheeks pink and orange.

    T   F   _____

39. What types of ingredients did Victorian women use in their facial masks to preserve the skin's health and beauty?

    A) natural ingredients such as honey, eggs, and oatmeal

    B) modern concoctions that included specially formulated chemicals

    C) mixtures of exotic herbs and spices

    D) nothing—use of such beauty products was considered unnecessary and vain

40. Women in the Victorian Age—a historic period known for its austerity and restrictiveness—would _____ to induce natural color instead of using cosmetics.

    A) apply warm towels to their faces

    B) pinch their cheeks and bite their lips

    C) gently pat their faces in a circular pattern

    D) hold their breath for 10 seconds at a time as needed

41. In 1880, Franz Ströher founded a German beauty company that has become the longest-lived professional beauty product company still in operation today. What is it called?

    A) Avon   C) Johnson & Johnson

    B) Maybelline   D) Wella Professionals

SHORT ANSWER

42. List three important contributions made to the beauty industry in the later part of the Victorian Age.

    _____

    _____

    _____

43. Your text spotlights Martha Matilda Harper, a pioneering entrepreneur in the beauty industry during the late nineteenth century. Imagine you could go back in time to speak with her about how she got her start in the beauty industry and what advice she might have for you. Jot down a list of three to five questions that you would like to ask her in an interview. Do some research about who she was as a person and cosmetologist, and write what you think her responses would be to your interview questions.

_____

_____

_____

Early Twentieth Century

SHORT ANSWER

44. List two main societal changes that greatly expanded the demand and interest in beauty products and services in the early twentieth century.

_____

_____

_____

MATCHING

45. Match the person associated with their description and contributions to the beauty profession in the first decade of the twentieth century. Some names might be used more than once.

A) Max Factor   D) Gibson Girl   G) Edouard Pinaud
B) Charles Nessler   E) Charles Dana Gibson
C) Garrett Augustus Morgan   F) Eugene Schueller

_____ Immigrated from Lodz, Poland

_____ Created the first commercial hair color; he called the new product Aureole, and it was later changed to L'Oréal

_____ Invented the first perm machine; hair was wrapped around metal rods that were supplied with electrical current, and the heat and current resulted in permanent waves

_____ Created a black oil hair dye and the curved-tooth pressing comb

_____ Created thin greasepaint makeup for motion picture use that wouldn't cake or crack under hot studio lights

_____ Marketed a chemical hair relaxer to African Americans

_____ Sported a pompadour or bouffant

_____ French perfumer

_____ Set the first national beauty standard for American women

_____ Created popular magazine drawings featuring women

_____ Created Brilliantine

SHORT ANSWER

46. The second decade of the twentieth century was characterized by a shift in the definition of femininity, which resulted in the marketing of razors for women. Briefly describe how that happened. Then state what you think the new definition of femininity in the early twentieth century became.

_____

_____

_____

MULTIPLE CHOICE

47. Proline introduced a new product, the first commercial "no lye relaxer," at the first International Beauty Show in 1917. What was its unique ingredient?

    A) hydrogen peroxide   C) potassium extract

    B) potassium hydroxide   D) sodium chloride

48. Which of the following was *not* a feature of the first electromagnetic clipper, invented by Leo J. Wahl?

    A) quiet   C) a direct current (DC) motor

    B) an alternating current (AC) motor   D) lightweight

49. Sarah Breedlove (known as Madam C. J. Walker), a daughter of former slaves and pioneer in the beauty industry of the early twentieth century, achieved which of the following? Select all that apply.

A) organized one of the first national conventions for businesswomen in the United States

B) invented the curling iron

C) pioneered the modern African American hair care and cosmetics industry

D) devised sophisticated sales and marketing strategies for her hair care products

E) invented ammonia-free hair color

F) built a factory, hair salon, and training school in Indianapolis, Indiana

G) developed a best-selling hair tonic

H) became America's first female millionaire

50. The best-known short haircut style for women in the 1920s was the bob. Who typically wore this style?

A) social elites

C) housewives

B) flappers

D) men

51. What accessories accompanied the bob hairstyle?

A) headbands and bobby pins

C) rubber bands

B) barrettes

D) nothing—it was a low maintenance, natural look

52. How did men typically wear their hair in the 1920s?

A) shoulder length, parted on the side

C) slicked-back with a shorter haircut and a center part

B) closely shaved, in a crew cut style

D) wavy with loose curls, parted on the side

53. List the three initial functions of the Associated Master Barbers and Beauticians of America's (AMBBA's) National Education Council and state why it later adopted the Barber Code of Ethics in 1929.

_____

_____

_____

REFLECTION

54. With the rapid growth of the cosmetics industry in the 1920s, its advertising expenditures grew, too. Using the Internet, magazines, or newspapers, identify and collect advertisements for beauty products in the 1920s and the 2020s. Place your findings for each era side by side and take a close look at them. Then write a few sentences about the ways in which the ads are the same and how they differ. What themes or products are popular in each era?

_____

_____

_____

Mid- to Late Twentieth Century

FILL IN THE BLANK

55. Use the words from the word bank to fill in the blanks in the paragraph below.

   Word bank: fade, short, pencil, side, waves, parts, neat and clean, bangs, top, nape

   In the 1930s, the major women's hairstyle trends focused on loose to crisp _____ and

   _____ sweeping to the side or down the middle. Early in the decade, _____ hair

   reigned, but later, shoulder-length hair and _____ also became fashionable. The typical

   1930s men's cut was _____ around the ear, tapered down to nothing at the _____,

   and blended into a longer _____ length with a _____ part—a look that is now

   called the _____ —and was typically paired with a _____ moustache.

56. Which of the following products was *not* invented in the 1930s?

    A) nail lacquer

    B) a machine-free perm method that used heat generated by chemical reaction

    C) permanent haircolor that penetrated the hair shaft

    D) no lye relaxer

57. Who invented and marketed the original pigment-based nail polish?

    A) Lawrence Gelb   C) Max Factor

    B) Charles Revson   D) Ralph L. Evans and Everett G. McDonough

58. Which of the following, invented in 1938, became the precursor to the modern perm?

    A) cold iron   C) electric curling iron

    B) cold wave   D) wave press

TRUE OR FALSE

Indicate whether the statements below are true or false. For any false statements, briefly explain why the statement is false.

59. Aerosol technology, originally developed for military use, was later implemented as a disinfectant spray used in the beauty industry.

    T   F   _____

60. Barbicide is a disinfectant intended for styling tools.

    T   F   _____

61. In 1941, scientists developed a method of permanent waving using waving lotion. It was called a wet wave because it was in liquid form.

    T   F   _____

62. Modern versions of cold waves have been outlawed.

T   F   _____

63. Pedicures and foot massages became salon services in 1941.

T   F   _____

64. The aerosol can was originally invented during World War II to spray troops with insect repellent to prevent malaria.

T   F   _____

SHORT ANSWER

65. In what ways did the activities of World War II influence hairstyles in the 1940s?

_____

_____

_____

LABELING

66. Use the celebrities listed in the word bank to identify the hair color or style that they popularized in the second half of the twentieth century.

Word bank: Farrah Fawcett, Rita Hayworth, Jennifer Aniston, Lucille Ball, Marilyn Monroe

_____ Redhead

_____ Platinum blonde

_____ Redhead

_____ Long-layered look

_____ The "Rachel," a short, layered cut

67. List three celebrities that influenced men's hairstyles in the 1950s.

_____

_____

_____

68. Describe three different hairstyle trends that emerged in the 1960s.

_____

_____

_____

69. What were two developments in hairstyling techniques that marked the 1970s?

_____

_____

_____

70. Compare the makeup trends of the 1970s with those of the 1980s.

_____

_____

_____

71. What were three hairstyle trends that characterized the 1980s?

_____

_____

_____

72. Why did perms go out of fashion in the 1990s?

_____

_____

_____

73. What prompted the popularity of the flat iron in the 1990s?

_____

_____

_____

REFLECTION

74. According to your text, by 1995 men reportedly spent $9.5 million on grooming. Use the Internet to research (1) the reasons for that spending trend, (2) what types of products men were buying, (3) what specific barber services men were spending their money on, and (4) characteristics of the typical consumer of those grooming products and services. Write a short report about your findings, and feel free to include images/photos.

_____

_____

_____

Twenty-First Century

MULTIPLE CHOICE

75. Hairstyle trends of the twenty-first century include _____ lengths, colors, and textures for all hair types.

   A) generic and uniform

   B) a maximum number of

   C) very few distinct

   D) a wide variety of

76. In the early 2000s, what led to a sharp decrease in the use of chemical relaxers?

   A) A crackdown by the Better Government Association resulted in a mass recall of chemicals found in certain hair treatment products.

   B) Hot tools were refined and improved, allowing for blowouts that produced smooth, straight results for even the curliest hair.

   C) The primary companies that manufactured chemical hair relaxers and related products at that time went bankrupt as a result of challenging economic downturns, resulting in very limited inventory.

   D) The use of chemical relaxers never decreased.

77. Which celebrity athlete inspired men to explore a more body-conscious style in 2002, leading to an increase in demand for men's spa services, traditional barber services, and manicures and pedicures for men?

   A) Michael Jordan   C) David Beckham

   B) Tom Brady   D) Alex Rodriguez

78. Which company's success in 2009 resulted in the creation of an entirely new category of beauty products, the treatment oils?

   A) Sephora   C) Moroccanoil

   B) Argan Oil   D) Sally Beauty Supply

79. Early in the second decade of the twenty-first century, how were some of the classic hairstyles commonly reinvented to achieve a more modern look?

   A) "smart" styling tools connected to the Internet

   B) brighter colors, including unicorn-inspired looks

   C) updated hair foil techniques

   D) babylights

80. With cosmetologists focusing specifically on haircolor, texture, or haircutting, and nail technicians now able to offer expertise in artificial nail enhancements, natural nail care, and even pedicures, the beauty industry has entered the _____ age.

   A) specialization   C) retro

   B) YouTube   D) anything-goes

REFLECTION

81. Reflect for a few moments on how the resources and tools of twenty-first technology and social media could be used to bring efficiency, publicity, and wider horizons for you as a cosmetologist embarking on your new career. Partner with a fellow student to create a short two- to three-minute video in which you explain how you plan to use a specific app or tech tool as a cosmetologist. Explain how you would use that technology, how it could benefit your clients and your business, and how it can be improved. Think of yourself as an influencer!

_____

_____

_____

Career Paths for Cosmetologists

82. The table below lists the types of careers available in the beauty industry, with columns for the requirements and recommended skills/qualities for people pursuing those careers, and opportunities offered by those career paths—information that can be found in your text.

     You probably have a lot more questions about cosmetology careers, though. For this activity, you will conduct your own research on each type of career and fill in the table, either in your workbook or by following the website link below for a digital PDF. It's never too early to start thinking about what comes after cosmetology school!

     Be specific. Use the Notes column to record any notes for yourself about your research, for example, a useful job board that you discovered, an interesting continuing education program, or a job title that interests you. When you're finished, you should end up with a comprehensive table and a handy guide to consult as you continue your explorations in the beauty industry.

+ BONUS

Visit: bonus.milady.com/cos-wb/toc

TYPE OF CAREER	REQUIREMENTS AND RECOMMENDED SKILLS/QUALITIES	OPPORTUNITIES AND POSITIONS AVAILABLE
Specialist	Complete additional training and experience in any service type already covered by your license	
Salon trainer	• Experienced salon professional • Training provided by manufacturers and salon chains in areas such as technical training as well as management and interpersonal relationship training	
Manufacturer educator	• Accomplished educator • Good public speaker • Trained by the manufacturer's educator to understand and use the company's hair care, haircolor, and other chemical service products	
Artistic director	• Experience • Confidence • Advanced technique mastery • Excellent communication and presentation skills	

TYPE OF CAREER	REQUIREMENTS AND RECOMMENDED SKILLS/QUALITIES	OPPORTUNITIES AND POSITIONS AVAILABLE
Education director	• Cosmetologists with five or more years of experience • Extensive continuing education • Excellent hairdressing skills • Leadership in prior career roles • Effective communication and presentation skills • Ability to create budgets and work with spreadsheets • Product knowledge of the company's brand and competitors	
Cosmetology instructor	• Robust prior salon career • Meet with your school's instructors to discuss why they went into education	
Film, theatrical, or editorial stylist	• Stamina for fast pace and long workdays • Volunteer to assist • Call agencies • Network with photographers • Ask other hairdressers who work behind the scenes for advice	
Creative director	• 10 or more years of experience in all facets of hairdressing • Executive-level mindset with experience to match • Understanding of how to achieve brand success	

SHORT ANSWER

83. Describe the main business skills that a typical salon manager should have to be successful.

_____

_____

_____

84. Name four types of facilities in which cosmetologists work.

_____

_____

_____

85. What are three suggestions for cosmetologists to be successful in their careers?

_____

_____

_____

86. What will ultimately determine a cosmetologist's success?

_____

_____

_____

DISCOVERIES AND ACCOMPLISHMENTS

In the space below, write notes about key concepts discussed in this chapter. Share your discoveries with some of the other students in your class and ask them if your notes are helpful. You may want to revise your notes based on good ideas shared by your peers.

Discoveries:

_____

_____

_____

_____

_____

_____

_____

_____

List at least three things you have accomplished since you decided to enroll in school.

Accomplishments:

_____

_____

_____

_____

_____

_____

_____

1. Which of the following statements best defines cosmetology?

   A) It is the art and science of beautifying and improving the skin, nails, and hair and includes the study of cosmetics and their application.

   B) It is the medical branch of science that deals with the study of the skin and its nature, structure, functions, diseases, and treatment.

   C) It refers to the objectives, goals, and step-by-step planning developed by cosmetic artists to mold their unique vision into a piece of art.

   D) It is a surgical process that involves restoring, reconstructing, or altering the human body.

2. Cosmetology is also referred to as _____.

   A) dermatology   C) appearance enhancement

   B) plastic surgery   D) cosmetic surgery

3. Cosmetologists should have a thorough understanding of the history of cosmetology because _____.

   A) they are responsible for imparting the history of beauty practices to staff members

   B) many older methods have evolved into techniques still used today

   C) they are required by the professional code of ethics to inform clients about the origins of the beauty services they are providing

   D) cosmetology is the chronological study of beauty practices over many centuries

4. Identify a true statement about the beauty practices in ancient African cultures.

   A) Nail colors were used to indicate social status and promote social disparity.

   B) The Africans were the first civilization to use essential oils from plant leaves, barks, and blossoms as perfumes.

   C) Braid patterns and hairstyles were used to indicate a person's tribe, age, marital status, wealth, power, and religion.

   D) The Africans were the first to cultivate beauty in an extravagant fashion.

5. Ancient Egyptians are credited with creating _____.

   A) haircolors   C) braiding

   B) nail tinting   D) kohl makeup

continued

6. Early Greek sculptures depicted subjects wearing two hairstyles that have remained popular for more than a millennium. These styles are _____.

    A) crown braids and chignons   C) cornrow braids and Bantu knots

    B) Zulu knots and bobs   D) box braids and locs

7. Which of the following statements is true about beauty and grooming during the Middle Ages?

    A) Medieval men wore long hair combed backward.

    B) Medieval women desired brown hair because angels were often depicted as brunette.

    C) Women of wealth wore splendid headwear and a variety of hairstyles.

    D) Male nobility often wore short hair with a side part.

8. Identify an accurate statement about the innovation in beauty and medicine that was introduced by a Persian alchemist named Avicenna around 1000 CE.

    A) He refined the steam distillation process, ushering in the modern era of steam-distilled essential oils used today.

    B) He invented the metal hot comb to temporarily straighten curly hair.

    C) He created the first electromagnetic clipper.

    D) He founded a beauty company called Wella Professionals, which is the longest-lived professional beauty product company still in operation today.

9. Which of the following modern beauty practices originated in the Renaissance period (1450–1837)?

    A) victory rolls   C) the Van Dyke beard

    B) bobs   D) the Fu Manchu moustache

10. Identify a true statement about the beauty practices followed by Victorian women.

    A) They often wore their hair in box braids and locs.

    B) They used beauty masks made from honey, eggs, oatmeal, and other natural ingredients.

    C) They used lavish cosmetic preparations, such as scented face powder made from pulverized starch.

    D) They used lipsticks to induce color on their cheeks and lips.

continued

11. Which of the following is a notable industry contribution from the Victorian Age?

   A) the creation of the first electromagnetic clipper

   B) the creation of the first commercial haircolor

   C) the invention of the first electrical perm machine

   D) the invention of the first curling iron in 1872

12. In the early twentieth century, American beauty applications began to follow trends set by _____.

   A) ancient Greek and Roman civilizations

   B) women in the Victorian Age

   C) celebrities and society figures

   D) working-class women

13. In 1907, French chemist Eugene Schueller took para-phenylenediamine (PPD) and created the first _____.

   A) lipstick   C) pigment-based nail polish

   B) commercial haircolor   D) commercial eyeliner

14. The Associated Master Barbers and Beauticians of America (AMBBA) adopted its Barber Code of Ethics to _____.

   A) promote professional responsibility in the trade

   B) promote equality between barbers and beauticians

   C) set uniform state licensing laws

   D) standardize requirements for barber schools and barber instructor training

15. In 1938, _____ invented the cold wave, the precursor to the modern perm, which used no machines or heat to curl hair.

   A) Arnold F. Willatt   C) Ralph L. Evans

   B) Lawrence Gelb   D) Max Factor

continued

16. _____ were probably the most iconic women's hairstyle in the 1940s.

   A) Afros

   B) Bangs and fringes

   C) Bobs

   D) Victory rolls

17. In the mid-1980s, hairdresser Farouk Shami invented SunGlitz, which is the world's first _____.

   A) electromagnetic clipper

   B) ammonia-free lightener

   C) commercial haircolor

   D) hairstyling tool

18. In 2002, David Beckham inspired men to explore a more body-conscious style. This led to a _____.

   A) sharp increase in the use of chemical relaxers

   B) decrease in the use of grooming services such as manicures and pedicures

   C) growth in men's spa services

   D) decrease in traditional barber services such as chairside shaves

19. Identify a statement that is most likely to be true of the impact of the Internet and social media on stylists' beauty careers.

   A) Social media prevents stylists from building strong interpersonal relationships with their clients.

   B) The Internet provides instant links to other professionals and group pages where one can ask questions.

   C) The Internet drastically reduces the time spent by stylists on catering to each client and providing the requested salon services.

   D) Social media has reduced the available clientele for stylists as people are becoming self-aware about various beauty practices and doing it on their own at home.

20. Which of the following is most likely a career opportunity for licensed cosmetologists?

   A) plastic surgeon

   B) manufacturer educator

   C) dermatologist

   D) physician assistant

continued

21. In the context of the career opportunities for licensed cosmetologists, which of the following positions establishes the standard for a salon or manufacturer's image?

    A) artistic director

    B) manufacturer educator

    C) specialists

    D) salon trainers

22. A licensed cosmetologist with six years of experience is the liaison between a company's brand and hairdresser. The cosmetologist also sets the company's standards by creating education that drives sales. In this context, the cosmetologist is most likely working as a(n) _____.

    A) manufacturer educator

    B) cosmetology instructor

    C) creative director

    D) education director

23. Identify the position that is only obtainable once you have 10 or more years of experience in all facets of hairdressing.

    A) cosmetology instructor

    B) salon trainer

    C) education director

    D) creative director

24. Identify a statement that is most likely true of salon managers.

    A) They should understand advertising, public relations, promotions, and special events.

    B) They seldom need to interact with clients.

    C) They perform high-end services such as haircoloring and hairstyling.

    D) They seldom need to have an aptitude for math and accounting.

25. Which of the following steps should you take to become a successful cosmetologist?

    A) Place your own interests before your clients' interests.

    B) Read trade publications.

    C) Avoid participating in online pro-beauty groups.

    D) Focus on theoretical aspects more than practical application of skills.

finished!

Ch. 02: General Anatomy and Physiology

TRACK MY PROGRESS!

Use this simple tracker to record your progress as you work through the activities in each learning objective.

COMPLETED	# OF CORRECT ANSWERS	OBJECTIVE
☐	_____/5	LO 1 - Explain the importance of anatomy and physiology to cosmetologists.
☐	_____/7	LO 2 - Describe the structure and division of cells.
☐	_____/4	LO 3 - List the four types of tissues in the body.
☐	_____/2	LO 4 - Explain the basic functions of the organs and body systems.
☐	_____/17	LO 5 - Outline the skeletal system's structures and functions.
☐	_____/21	LO 6 - Describe the muscular system's components and supporting structures.
☐	_____/12	LO 7 - Explain the nervous system's divisions and functions.
☐	_____/20	LO 8 - List the functions of the circulatory system's components.
☐	_____/6	LO 9 - Describe the lymphatic system's function.
☐	_____/6	LO 10 - Explain the integumentary system's function.
☐	_____/5	LO 11 - Outline the endocrine system's organs and their functions.

Why Study Anatomy and Physiology?

SHORT ANSWER

1. What is the difference between the study of anatomy and the study of physiology?

_____

_____

_____

2. What are the three parts of the body that cosmetologists focus on? What parts of the body do cosmetology services affect?

_____

_____

_____

3. What are the three reasons that cosmetologists should have a thorough understanding of anatomy and physiology?

_____

_____

_____

4. When it comes to observing possible illnesses or infections in a client, what is always outside of a cosmetologist's scope of practice?

_____

_____

_____

LABELING

5. Label each image of an organism and its components below.

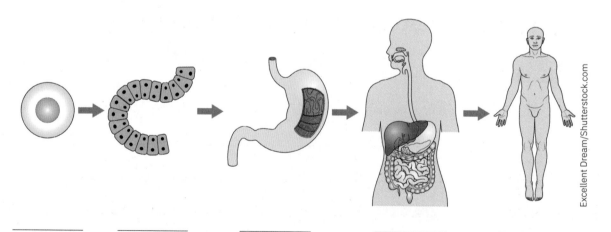

Excellent Dream/Shutterstock.com

_____   _____   _____   _____   _____

Cell Structure and Functions

6. Match the part of the cell with its description/function. Each cell part will be used three times.

   a. Nucleus   b. Cytoplasm   c. Cell membrane

   Cell Part   **Description/Function**

   _____ Controls the growth and reproduction of the cell

   _____ Provides a structure for the cell parts so they can move freely

   _____ Protects the interior of the cell from its surroundings

   _____ Thin layer of tissue that surrounds the cell

   _____ The watery fluid that surrounds the nucleus

   _____ Contains the cell's genetic material

   _____ Semipermeable, meaning it allows certain substances to enter the cell

   _____ Specialized structure in the center of the cell

   _____ Contains enzymes that help digest and break down other molecules for food

7. Complete the sentences below using words form the word bank. Not all words will be used.

   Word bank: three, grow, temperatures, special, mitosis, eliminate, daughter, consume, divides, food, child, reproduction, two, favorable

   The process of cell _____ is called _____. It occurs when the cell

   _____ into _____ identical _____ cells. Cells require _____

   conditions to _____ and reproduce. These conditions include adequate _____

   supply, oxygen, water, suitable _____, and the ability to _____ waste.

8. Label each part of the cell.

    a. Cytoplasm   b. Nucleus   c. Cell membrane

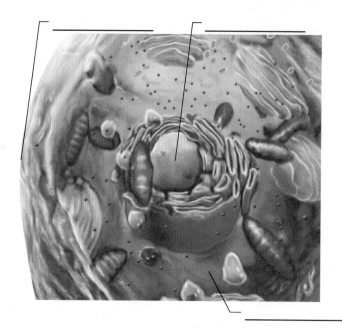

9. Cells are the basic units for all what?

    _____

    _____

    _____

10. What does the protoplasm of a cell contain?

    _____

    _____

    _____

11. Describe the two types of metabolism, the chemical process in which cells convert nutrients to energy.

_____

_____

_____

12. Why is it important for a cosmetologist to understand cell structure?

_____

_____

_____

Tissues

SHORT ANSWER

13. Define tissue.

_____

_____

_____

MATCHING

14. Match the type of tissue with its description. Some types will be used more than once.

   a. Connective   c. Nerve
   b. Epithelial   d. Muscle

Type of Tissue Description

_____ Found within many parts of the body such as skin, mucous membranes, digestive and respiratory organs, the lining of the mouth, the lining of the heart, and the glands

_____ Binds and supports other body tissues and organs

_____ Controls and coordinates all bodily functions

_____ Fibrous

_____ Provides a covering that protects the body

_____ Contracts and moves various parts of the body

_____ Carries messages to and from the brain

LABELING

15. Label each type of tissue shown below.

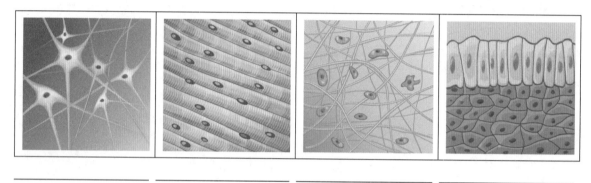

_____   _____   _____   _____

RESEARCH

16. Use the textbook, Internet, or magazines to find three examples of each type of tissue and list them in the table below. (Examples for epithelial tissue have already been provided.)

TYPE OF TISSUE	EXAMPLE 1	EXAMPLE 2	EXAMPLE 3
Connective			
Epithelial	Skin	The lining of the mouth	Mucous membranes
Nerve			
Muscle			

Based on the examples you found, write one or two sentences explaining why you think it is important for cosmetologists to be familiar with the different types of tissues.

Organs and Body Systems

SHORT ANSWER

17. What are organs? What are body systems? Describe the relationship between organs and body systems.

   _____

   _____

   _____

FILL IN THE BLANK

18. Complete the chart below. The function of each body system and an image have been provided for you.

NAME OF BODY SYSTEM	FUNCTION	WHY IS IT IMPORTANT FOR COSMETOLOGISTS TO KNOW THIS?	MAJOR ORGANS, TISSUES, AND RELATED STRUCTURES	IMAGE
	Makes blood and oxygen available to body; eliminates carbon dioxide			
	Coordinates all other body systems, causes body to react to the environment			

NAME OF BODY SYSTEM	FUNCTION	WHY IS IT IMPORTANT FOR COSMETOLOGISTS TO KNOW THIS?	MAJOR ORGANS, TISSUES, AND RELATED STRUCTURES	IMAGE
	Provides protective covering and regulates body temperature			
	Forms the physical foundation of the body; comprised of 206 bones			
	Eliminates waste from the body, reducing the buildup of toxins			
	Controls blood movement throughout the body			
	Produces offspring and differentiates males from females as assigned at birth			
	Protects the body from disease and destroys pathogens			

NAME OF BODY SYSTEM	FUNCTION	WHY IS IT IMPORTANT FOR COSMETOLOGISTS TO KNOW THIS?	MAJOR ORGANS, TISSUES, AND RELATED STRUCTURES	IMAGE
	Breaks food down into nutrients or waste for nutrition or excretion			
	Controls hormone levels within the body; determines growth, development, reproduction			
	Covers, shapes, and holds the skeletal system in place; allows for movement of body structures			

Skeletal System

SHORT ANSWER

19. What is a joint?

_____

_____

_____

20. Describe the two types of joints: movable and immovable.

_____

_____

_____

21. Define osteology.

_____

_____

_____

22. What is an exception among the immovable joints?

_____

_____

_____

23. What is the composition of bone?

_____

_____

_____

24. List the five primary functions of the skeletal system.

_____

_____

_____

25. In your own words, explain why it is important for cosmetologists to understand the workings of the skeletal system, both for themselves and for their clients.

_____

_____

_____

26. What in the body is the only tissue that is harder than bone?

_____

_____

_____

27. Complete the sentences below using the words from the word bank. Some words will be used more than once, and some words will not be used.

   Word bank: eight, three, brain, skull, facial, 12, cranium, 14, two

   The _____ is the head's skeleton and is divided into _____ parts: the

   _____ and the _____ skeleton. The _____ is an oval, bony case

   consisting of _____ bones that protect the _____. The _____ skeleton

   forms the framework of the face and is composed of _____ bones.

LABELING

28. Identify the bones of the cranium.

   a. Temporal bone   c. Parietal bone   e. Ethmoid bone
   b. Sphenoid bone   d. Frontal bone   f. Occipital bone

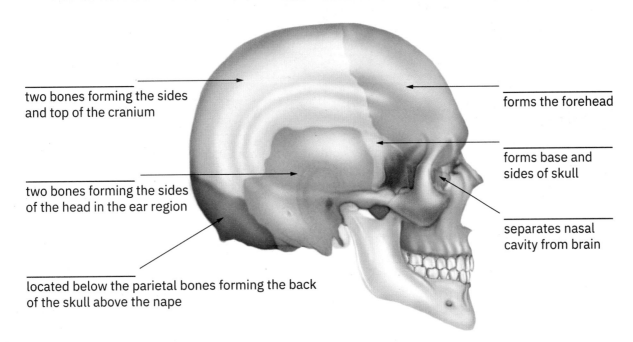

_____
two bones forming the sides
and top of the cranium

_____
two bones forming the sides
of the head in the ear region

_____
located below the parietal bones forming the back
of the skull above the nape

_____
forms the forehead

_____
forms base and
sides of skull

_____
separates nasal
cavity from brain

29. Identify the facial bones.

a. Nasal bones   c. Mandible   e. Zygomatic bones
b. Maxillae bones   d. Lacrimal bones

_____
also known as *cheekbones* or
malar bones, they form the
prominence of the cheeks and
outer part of the eye socket

_____
two small, thin bones located
in the front inside wall of the
eye sockets (orbits)

_____
two bones that form
the bridge of the nose

_____
two bones that form
the upper jaw

_____
largest and strongest
bone of the face that
forms the lower jaw

FILL IN THE BLANK

30. Complete the sentences below using the words from the word bank. Some words will be used more than once, and others will not be used.

Word bank: seven, throat, neck, hyoid, face, skull, tongue, cervical, four

The U-shaped bone at the base of the _____ is the _____. It supports the _____ and

its muscles. It's the only bone of the _____.

The _____ vertebrae are _____ bones located below the _____. They provide support,

structure, and flexibility to the _____.

31. Identify the neck bones.

    a. Cervical vertebrae

                                        b. Hyoid bone

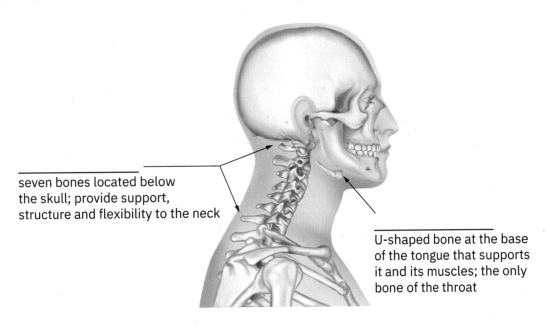

_____
seven bones located below
the skull; provide support,
structure and flexibility to the neck

_____
U-shaped bone at the base
of the tongue that supports
it and its muscles; the only
bone of the throat

FILL IN THE BLANK

32. Complete the sentences below.

Word bank: wraps, injury, landmarks, shoulder, massage

The bones of the chest and _____ are important in cosmetology when performing full-body

treatments, such as body _____. It's also useful to learn about these bones as reference

_____ for use in performing _____—and more importantly, to prevent _____ to these

areas.

33. Identify the bones of the chest and shoulder.

a. Scapula   b. Clavicle

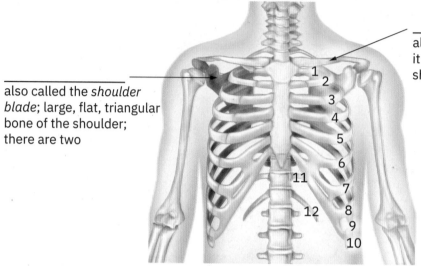

also called the *shoulder blade*; large, flat, triangular bone of the shoulder; there are two

also known as *collarbone*, it joins the sternum to a shoulder bone

34. Identify the bones of the arm and hand.

a. Phalanges   c. Carpus   e. Humerus
b. Ulna   d. Radius   f. Metacarpus

five bones of the palm located between the carpus and phalanges

also known as the *wrist*; flexible joint composed of eight small, irregular bones

also known as *digits*; bones of the fingers or toes; three in each finger and two in each thumb

uppermost and largest bone in the arm, extending from the elbow to the shoulder

smaller bone in the forearm on the same side as the thumb

inner and larger bone in the forearm located on the side of the little finger

35. Identify the bones of the leg, ankle, and foot.

a. Tarsals
b. Fibula
c. Metatarsals

d. Tibia
e. Phalanges
f. Talus

g. Patella

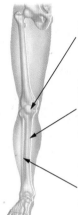

_____
also called the *kneecap*;
forms the kneecap joint

_____
also called the *shinbone*,
it's the larger of the two leg
bones below the knee on the
big toe side that supports
most of the body's weight

_____
located on the little-toe
side of the lower leg;
smaller of the two leg
bones below the knee

_____
seven irregularly shaped
bones in the ankle area
including the talus,
calcaneus (heel),
navicular, cuboid,
and three cuneiform
bones

_____
five long, slender
bones similar to the
metacarpal bones of
the hand

_____
also called the *ankle bone*;
between the heel bone,
tibia, and fibula

_____
also known as *digits*;
there are fourteen
total with two in each
big toe and three in
each smaller toe

Muscular System

SHORT ANSWER

36. How does the muscular system work with the skeletal system?

_____

_____

_____

37. Describe the muscle's tissue and how muscles move.

_____

_____

_____

38. What is myology?

_____

_____

_____

39. How many muscles are in the body?

_____

_____

_____

40. List the seven ways that you can stimulate muscles.

_____

_____

_____

41. Match the type of muscle with its description. Each type of muscle will be used more than once; a description might have more than one answer.

    a. Cardiac   b. Involuntary   c. Voluntary

Type of Muscle Description

_____ Type of nonstriated muscle

_____ Control body functions such as breathing and digestion

_____ Muscles that we control at will

_____ Type of striated muscle

_____ Controlled by the autonomic nervous system

_____ Found only in the heart

42. Complete the sentences below.

   Word bank: voluntary, fatigued/sore, pain, control, cosmetologists, nerve, negative, locations, improper, nail

   For _____, it is important to know about _____ muscles and what they _____,

   as these muscles can become _____ from excessive work or injury. Knowing

   the _____ of muscles will also help you avoid using _____ massaging during skin and

   _____ services, which could result in _____ effects for the client, such as residual

   _____ or _____ inflammation.

LABELING

43. Label the parts of the muscle indicated below and write a brief description of each one.

   a. Belly   b. Origin   c. Insertion

   Part of Muscle   Description

   _____ Part of the muscle that does not move and is anchored to the bone; attached closest to the skeleton

   _____ Movable part of the muscle anchored to the bone; attached farthest from the skeleton

   _____ Middle part of the muscle

44. What is the recommended direction and location for exerting massage pressure?

_____

_____

_____

LABELING

45. Identify each scalp and neck muscle shown below.

   a. Occipitalis
   b. Epicranial aponeurosis

   c. Frontalis
   d. Platysma

   e. Sternocleidomastoideus
   f. Epicranius

_____
broad muscle that covers the top of the skull and consists
of the occipitalis and frontalis; also called *occipitofrontalis*

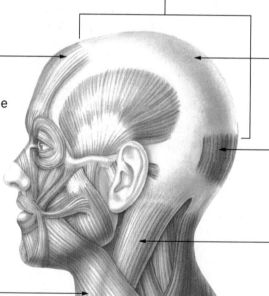

_____
front (anterior) portion of the
epicranius; scalp muscle that
raises the eyebrows, draws the
scalp forward, and causes
wrinkles across the forehead

_____
tendon that connects
the occipitalis and
frontalis muscles

_____
back (posterior) portion of
the epicranius; muscle that
draws the scalp backward

_____
neck muscle that lowers and
rotates the head; originates
at the clavicle and inserts at
the temporal bone near
the ear

_____
broad muscle extending from the pectoral
and deltoid muscles to the side of the chin;
responsible for lowering the lower jaw and lip

46. Identify the muscles of the face, mouth, and nose depicted below.

a. Orbicularis oculi
b. Levator labii superioris
c. Buccinator
d. Mentalis
e. Masseter
f. Corrugator
g. Zygomaticus minor

h. Orbicularis oris
i. Temporalis
j. Risorius
k. Triangularis
l. Levator palpebrae superioris
m. Zygomaticus major

n. Depressor labii inferioris
o. Levator anguli oris
p. Procerus

_____ small muscle located between the eyebrows below the frontalis; draws the eyebrow down and wrinkles the forehead vertically

_____ located near the temple, it opens and closes the jaw

_____ ring muscle of the eye socket that closes the eyelids and assists in pumping tears

_____ muscle that surrounds and elevates the upper lip and dilates the nostrils, as when expressing distaste

_____ originates at the lower part of the zygomatic; moves the mandible, causing the mouth to close

_____ muscle of the cheek between the upper and lower jaw that compresses the cheeks and expels air between the lips

_____ muscle at the corner of the lip that extends over the chin and pulls down the corners of the mouth when frowning

_____ muscle that surrounds and lowers the lower lip and draws it to one side, as when expressing sarcasm

_____ muscle that covers the bridge of the nose, lowers the eyebrows, and causes wrinkles across the bridge of the nose

_____ thin muscle that controls the movement of the eyelid

_____ muscle that raises the angle of the mouth and draws it inward

_____ muscle that works with the zygomaticus major to make facial expressions

_____ muscle that extends from the zygomatic bone to the angle of the mouth; directs the lip outward and upward when laughing or smiling

_____ muscle at the corner of the mouth that draws it out and back, as when grinning

_____ muscle that circles the mouth and contracts, puckers, and wrinkles the lips

_____ muscle at the tip of the chin that elevates the lower lip and raises and wrinkles the skin of the chin

47. For each picture below, identify the muscles responsible for making those expressions:

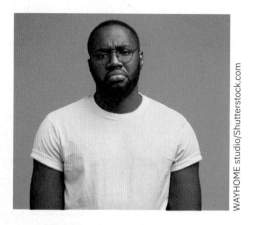

WAYHOME studio/Shutterstock.com

_____

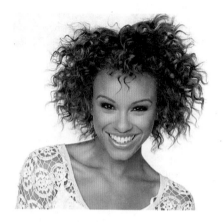

_____

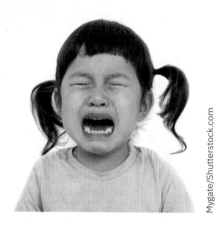

Mygate/Shutterstock.com

_____

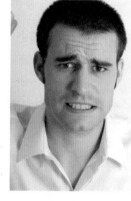

Photick/Shutterstock.com

_____

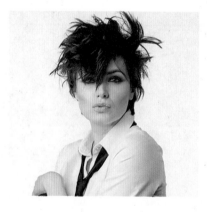

_____

48. What are the three principal shoulder and upper arm muscles?

_____

_____

_____

49. As a cosmetologist, which part of the shoulders or arms will you mostly focus on and use?

_____

_____

_____

LABELING

50. Identify the shoulder and arm muscles shown below.

a. Extensors
b. Supinator
c. Flexor

d. Trapezius
e. Bicep
f. Tricep

g. Pronator
h. Deltoid

_____
covers the back of the neck as well as the upper and middle regions of the back; lifts and turns the head; raises the shoulders; controls swinging movements of the arm

_____
large, triangular muscle covering the shoulder joint that allows the arm to extend outward and to the side of the body

_____
large muscle covering the entire back of the upper arm that extends the forearm and straightens the elbow

_____
front of the upper arm; produces the contour of the front and inner side of the upper arm; lifts the forearm and flexes the elbow

_____
muscle that turns the hand inward so the palm faces downward

_____
muscles that extend and straighten joints such as the wrist, hand, and fingers to form a straight line

_____
forearm muscle that rotates the radius outward and the palm upward

_____
extensor muscle of the wrist involved in flexing or bending it

Anterior or front

Posterior or back

51. Describe what makes the hand one of the most complex body parts.

_____

_____

_____

MATCHING

52. Match the type of hand muscle with its description. Each hand muscle type will be used at least once.

   a. Adductors   b. Abductors   c. Opponens

   Type of Hand Muscle   **Description**

   _____ Draw the fingers together in the hand

   _____ Muscles that draw a body part away from the midline of the body

   _____ Muscles that draw a body part toward the midline of the body

   _____ Muscle that allows the thumb to be moved toward a finger of the same hand

   _____ Separate the fingers in the hand

FUN FACT

Did you know that many words used today are a combination of root words from the Latin language? For example, the Latin prefix *ab* means "away from," *ad* means "toward" or "to," and *de* means "down" or "down from." The root word *duct* (sometimes appearing in the form *duce*) means "to lead." So, for example, "deduct" = "de" + "duct" and can be translated to mean "lead down from" (deduct 10 percent off the cost; deduce what happened based on clues, etc.).

53. Identify the types of hand muscles shown below.

    a. Opponens   b. Adductors   c. Abductors

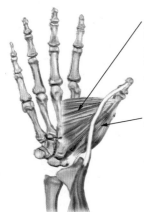

_____
muscles that draw a body part toward the midline of the body; draw the fingers together in the hand

_____
muscles that draw a body part away from the midline of the body; separate the fingers in the hand

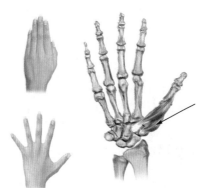

_____
muscle that allows the thumb to be moved toward a finger of the same hand

SHORT ANSWER

54. What is the function of the lower leg and foot muscles?

_____

_____

_____

55. For which cosmetology service is it helpful to understand the lower leg and foot muscles? Based on your knowledge of muscles more broadly, why do you think that is?

_____

_____

_____

FUN FACT

The Latin word *brevis* means "brief" or "short," and the Latin word *flex* means "to bend" (e.g., reflex, reflect, flexible, deflect).

Other common Latin root words are *ante* (which means "before") and *post* (which means "after" or "behind"). *Ante up!* directs players to place their bets *before* a game begins, and *antique* refers to an earlier period—one that came before. *Postpone* means to move an event to a time *after* the original date, while a *postscript* (abbreviated *P.S.*) is a note that appears *after* the main message. How many words do you use on a regular basis that include these Latin roots? Probably more than you realized!

56. Identify the lower leg and foot muscles that are shown below.

a. Flexor digitorum brevis
b. Soleus
c. Extensor digitorum longus
d. Peroneus longus
e. Peroneus brevis
f. Extensor hallucis longus
g. Gastrocnemius
h. Abductor hallucis
i. Abductor digiti minimi
j. Tibialis anterior
k. Flexor digiti minimi

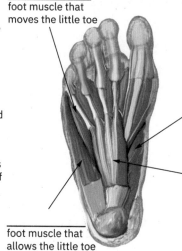

muscle that covers the outer side of the calf, inverts the foot, and turns it outward _____

muscle that originates on the lower surface of the fibula and bends the foot down and out _____

muscle that bends the foot up and extends the toes _____

muscle that extends the big toe and flexes the foot _____

muscle attached to the lower rear surface of the heel that pulls the foot down _____

muscle covering the front of the shin that bends the foot upward and inward _____

muscle that originates at the upper portion of the fibula and bends the foot down _____

foot muscle that moves the little toe _____

foot muscle that moves the big toe away from the other toes _____

foot muscle that flexes the toes and helps maintain balance while walking and standing _____

foot muscle that allows the little toe to flex and move _____

Nervous System

SHORT ANSWER

57. What is neurology?

_____

_____

_____

58. What are the three main subdivisions of the nervous system?

_____

_____

_____

59. Describe the nervous system, and list the three body parts that are included in it. What does the nervous system do?

_____

_____

_____

60. From a safety perspective, which services are most likely to affect the nervous system of a client? Explain why and provide a specific example involving a client's nervous system that might occur in the salon.

_____

_____

_____

61. Why is it important to know whether your clients have chronic conditions such as diabetes? Describe two adjustments you can make to certain services to safely and comfortably treat clients who have chronic conditions such as diabetes.

_____

_____

_____

MATCHING

62. Match each subdivision of the nervous system with its description. Each nervous system subdivision will be used twice.

a. Peripheral   b. Autonomic   c. Central

Subdivisions of the Nervous System   **Description**

_____   Regulates the action of the smooth muscles, glands, blood vessels, the heart, and breathing

_____   Carries impulses to and from the central nervous system

_____   Consists of the brain, spinal cord, spinal nerves, and cranial nerves

_____   Has both sensory and motor nerves

_____   Controls voluntary muscle actions

_____   Controls involuntary muscle actions

63. Label each subdivision of the nervous system shown below.

a. Central nervous
    system (CNS)

b. Peripheral nervous
    system (PNS)

c. Autonomic nervous
    systems (ANS)

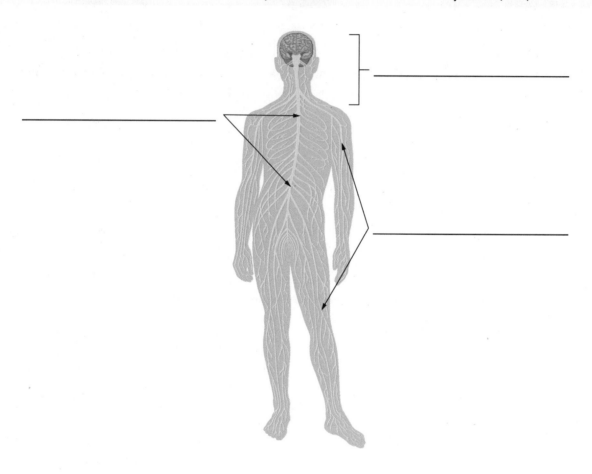

64. Describe the spinal cord and specify what protects it.

_____

_____

_____

65. Describe the brain and specify which bones protect it.

_____

_____

_____

66. How many pairs of nerves extend from the spinal cord? What three types of body parts do they connect to?

_____

_____

_____

FILL IN THE BLANK

67. Complete the sentences below using words from the word bank. Some words will be used twice.

Word bank: receptor, neuron, fibers, stimulus, nerve, motor, impulse, spinal cord, muscle, sensory, reaction, reflex, brain

The simplest form of nervous activity that includes a _____ and a _____ nerve

is called a _____. A _____ reaction to an outside _____,

for instance, is an automatic _____ that involves sending an _____ from

a sensory _____ along the sensory _____ to the spinal cord. In response,

an _____ is sent along a motor _____ to a _____, causing a

_____ (e.g., removing your hand from a hot object quickly).

Nerves are whitish bundles of nerve _____ that transmit impulses. They originate in the

_____ and _____ and send their branches to all parts of the body.

68. Match the two types of nerves with their descriptions.

a. Sensory nerves   b. Motor nerves

Cell Part   **Description/Function**

_____ Carry messages from the sense organs (heat, cold, sight, sound, smell, taste) to the brain and spinal cord

_____ These nerve endings (receptors) are located close to the skin's surface

_____ Also known as efferent nerves

_____ Also known as afferent nerves

_____ Pass impulses to the brain and back through the motor nerves to the muscles, which causes movement

_____ Carry impulses from the brain to the muscles or glands and these transmitted impulses produce movement

Circulatory System

SHORT ANSWER

69. What is another term for the circulatory system?

_____

_____

_____

70. What does the circulatory system do?

_____

_____

_____

71. What are the four main components of the circulatory system?

_____

_____

_____

72. What are some possible effects that clients might experience if they have an impaired circulatory system?

_____

_____

_____

73. How can you help prevent a client from experiencing a sudden drop in blood pressure (and possibly fainting)? How can you assist your client after a service?

_____

_____

_____

74. Why should you acknowledge and discuss any medical conditions that your client has listed as part of your consultation? What are three conditions that might contraindicate massage?

_____

_____

_____

75. Which service should be skipped if a client has impaired foot or leg circulation, or loss of feeling in their feet or legs?

_____

_____

_____

76. What should you do if you determine that your client with a medical condition has not discussed massage with their physician?

_____

_____

_____

77. What is an overall good rule of thumb when it comes to deciding whether to perform a service such as massage on a client who has a medical condition?

_____

_____

_____

FILL IN THE BLANK

78. Complete the sentences below using the words from the word bank. Not all the words will be used.

Word bank: lungs, blood, filter, motion, oval, organs, circulation, heart, muscles, nitrogen, kidneys, circulatory, dilute, cone, nervous, oxygen

The _____ is a muscular,_____-shaped organ that keeps the blood moving

within the _____ system. Blood is in constant _____ from the time that it

leaves the heart. It travels throughout the body to deliver nutrients and _____, and it

takes waste products to the _____ that will _____ them (_____, liver,

_____).

79. Match the two types of circulation systems with their descriptions.

    a. Pulmonary   b. Systemic

Type of Circulation System	Description
_____	Returns oxygen-poor blood back to the heart
_____	Carries oxygen-poor blood to the lungs for oxygenation
_____	Carries oxygen-rich blood from the heart throughout the body
_____	Returns clean, oxygenated blood to the heart (left atrium) so that it can be delivered to the body
_____	Carries oxygen-poor blood to the lungs for waste removal
_____	Also known as general circulation

FILL IN THE BLANK

80. Complete the chart below.

TYPE OF BLOOD VESSEL	DESCRIPTION	IMAGE
	Largest artery in the body	
Arteries		
	Small veins that connect capillaries to larger veins	

TYPE OF BLOOD VESSEL	DESCRIPTION	IMAGE
	Tiny blood vessels that connect the smaller arteries to the venules, bring nutrients to the cells, and carry away waste materials	
Veins		
Arterioles		

SHORT ANSWER

81. What is blood?

_____

_____

_____

82. What are the five main functions of blood?

_____

_____

_____

83. Why is it important as a cosmetologist to know about arteries and their locations?

_____

_____

_____

84. How does the blood flow when returning to the heart from the head, face, and neck?

_____

_____

_____

85. Describe the location of the face and neck veins in relation to the arteries.

_____

_____

_____

MATCHING

86. Match the types of arteries with their descriptions.

    a. External carotid   b. Internal carotid   c. Common carotid

Type of Artery   **Description**

_____ Artery that supplies blood to the brain, eyes, eyelids, forehead, nose, and internal ear

_____ Artery that supplies blood to the anterior (front) parts of the scalp, ear, face, neck, and sides of the head

_____ Main arteries on both sides of the neck that supply blood to the head, face, and neck

87. Match the type of vein with its description. Some descriptions might include both types of veins.

a. External jugular   b. Internal jugular

Type of Vein   **Description**

_____   Collects blood from the brain and parts of the face and neck

_____   Located at the side of the neck

_____   Carries blood returning to the heart from the head, face, and neck

LABELING

88. Identify the types of arteries and veins in the images below.

a. Internal carotid artery   c. Common carotid arteries   e. External carotid artery
b. External jugular   d. Internal jugular

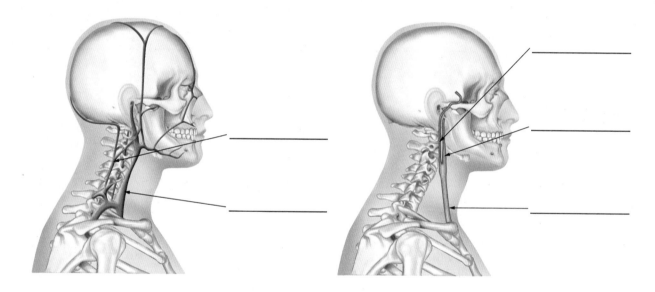

Lymphatic System

89. Complete the sentences below using words from the word bank. Some words will be used more than once, and others will not be used.

    Word bank: red, cells, yellow, bacteria, lymph, white, viruses, vessels, nodes, green

    Lymph _____ are glandlike structures that filter _____, _____, and

    cancer _____ and are connected by lymph _____.

    _____ is a clear or pale_____ fluid that contains _____ blood

    _____ and travels through lymph _____.

SHORT ANSWER

90. Which system includes the lymphatic system?

    _____

    _____

    _____

91. What does the lymph system do to protect the body?

    _____

    _____

    _____

92. What are the five main components of the lymphatic system?

    _____

    _____

    _____

93. What are the four primary functions of the lymphatic system?

_____

_____

_____

94. How will understanding the lymphatic and immune systems help you and your clients?

_____

_____

_____

Integumentary System

SHORT ANSWER

95. What does the word *integument* mean?

_____

_____

_____

96. In addition to skin, what are the accessory organs that complete the integumentary system?

_____

_____

_____

97. What is the largest organ in the body?

_____

_____

_____

98. What might the appearance or condition of your client's skin tell you as a cosmetologist?

_____

_____

_____

99. What are three outside elements that the skin protects the body against?

_____

_____

_____

100. How does skin affect body temperature?

_____

_____

_____

Endocrine System

MATCHING

101. Match the type of gland with its description. The types of glands will be used more than once.

   a. Endocrine   b. Exocrine

Type of Gland   **Description**

_____ Include the pituitary, thyroid, and adrenal glands, among others

_____ Produce a substance that travels through small tubelike ducts

_____ Include the sebaceous and sudoriferous glands, among others

_____ Release hormones directly into the bloodstream

_____ Also known as *ductless glands*

_____ Also known as *duct glands*

102. Define endocrine system.

_____

_____

_____

103. What is the function of glands? What are three examples of glands?

_____

_____

_____

104. What are hormones? What are three examples of hormones?

_____

_____

_____

105. What might changes in nail or hair growth indicate about a client's endocrine system?

_____

_____

_____

DISCOVERIES AND ACCOMPLISHMENTS

In the space below, write notes about key concepts discussed in this chapter. Share your discoveries with some of the other students in your class and ask them if your notes are helpful. You may want to revise your notes based on good ideas shared by your peers.

Discoveries:

_____

_____

_____

_____

_____

_____

_____

List at least three things you have accomplished since you decided to enroll in school.

Accomplishments:

_____

_____

_____

_____

_____

_____

_____

1. Why should cosmetologists have a thorough knowledge of anatomy and physiology?

   A) because cosmetologists are required to differentiate between mild and serious physical conditions in order to treat such conditions

   B) because cosmetologists are required to perform procedures that are listed under a medical license or podiatry license

   C) because working with the bones of the face and skull adds to flattering haircuts, hairstyles, and makeup applications

   D) because learning about anatomy and physiology helps cosmetologists inform a client that a specific disease is present and explain the disease

2. Epithelial tissue in the body _____.

   A) carries messages to and from the brain

   B) is fibrous tissue that binds and supports other body tissues and organs

   C) contracts and moves various parts of the body

   D) is seen within many body parts such as mucous membranes and the skin

3. Which of the following types of tissue in the body controls as well as coordinates all functions of the body?

   A) connective tissue   C) muscle tissue

   B) nerve tissue   D) epithelial tissue

4. What are organs?

   A) They are specialized structures in the center of a cell.

   B) They are the basic units of all living things.

   C) They are groups of specialized tissues that carry out specific functions.

   D) They are thin layers of tissue that surrounds a cell.

5. What is the function of the circulatory system?

   A) to break food down into nutrients or waste for nutrition or excretion

   B) to control hormone levels within the body that determine the growth, development, reproduction, and health of the entire body

   C) to regulate blood movement throughout the body

   D) to coordinate with all other body systems, allowing them to work efficiently and react to the environment

continued

6. Understanding how nerves work will most likely help cosmetologists _____.

    A) protect their own body by using proper body mechanics when they work

    B) perform services such as massages, shampoos, and facial and nail services in a more safe and proficient way

    C) determine the placement of makeup during application

    D) influence haircutting and hairstyling options according to a client's facial bone structure

7. Which of the following body systems provides a protective covering and controls body temperature?

    A) the immune system

    C) the integumentary system

    B) the skeletal system

    D) the respiratory system

8. Which of the following statements about the muscular system is true?

    A) It protects the body from illness.

    B) It eliminates toxic substances that can affect other body system functions.

    C) It coordinates with all other body systems.

    D) It is affected by massages performed during cosmetology services.

9. One of the primary functions of the skeletal system is to _____.

    A) provide a protective covering and regulate body temperature

    B) protect the body from disease by developing immunities

    C) help in the production of red and white blood cells

    D) control hormone levels within the body

10. A cosmetologist should have an understanding of the skeletal system because _____.

    A) the skeletal system is the body's messaging system

    B) the main function of the skeletal system is to nourish and oxygenate all the systems at the cellular level

    C) it helps protect the cosmetologist and clients from exposure to infection and disease

    D) it helps protect the cosmetologist's own body by using proper body mechanics while working

continued

11. _____ are two bones that form the sides and top of the skull's cranium.

   A) Occipital bones   C) Parietal bones

   B) Frontal bones   D) Temporal bones

12. _____ bones, also called cheekbones or malar bones, form the prominence of the cheeks and outer parts of the eye sockets.

   A) Lacrimal   C) Zygomatic

   B) Temporal   D) Maxillae

13. The uppermost and largest bone in the arm, extending from the elbow to the shoulder, is called the _____.

   A) radius   C) humerus

   B) ulna   D) phalanges

14. Voluntary muscles (striated) are _____.

   A) muscles found only in the heart

   B) controlled by the autonomic nervous system

   C) muscles that a person can control at will

   D) responsible for controlling body functions such as digestion

15. Identify a true statement about origin, which is one of the three parts of a muscle.

   A) It is the movable part of the muscle anchored to the bone.

   B) It is attached farthest from the skeleton.

   C) It is the middle part of the muscle.

   D) It is anchored to the bone.

16. The broad muscle that extends from the pectoral and deltoid muscles to the side of the chin and is responsible for lowering the lower jaw and lip is called the _____.

   A) occipitalis   C) sternocleidomastoideus

   B) platysma   D) frontalis

continued

17. Muscles that draw a body part toward the midline of the body and draw the fingers together in the hand are called _____.

   A) deltoids

   B) extensors

   C) adductors

   D) abductors

18. Which of the following is the foot muscle that flexes the toes and helps with the maintenance of balance while standing and walking?

   A) abductor digiti minimi

   B) flexor digitorum brevis

   C) flexor digiti minimi

   D) abductor hallucis

19. The _____ controls involuntary muscle action and the action of the smooth muscles, glands, blood vessels, heart, and breathing.

   A) integumentary system

   B) skeletal system

   C) autonomic nervous system (ANS)

   D) peripheral nervous system (PNS)

20. Motor nerves _____.

   A) carry messages from the sense organs to the brain and spinal cord

   B) are also known as afferent nerves

   C) carry impulses from the brain to the glands or muscles

   D) pass impulses to the brain and back through the sensory nerves to the muscles

21. The external carotid artery _____.

   A) supplies blood to the anterior parts of the face, neck, scalp, ear, and sides of the head

   B) supplies blood to the brain, eyes, eyelids, forehead, nose, and internal ear

   C) is on both sides of the neck

   D) divides into an internal and external branch

22. The _____ system is a significant part of the immune system, which helps defend against infection.

   A) endocrine

   B) lymphatic

   C) integumentary

   D) circulatory

continued

23. The integumentary system includes the _____ and its accessory organs.

    A) thymus gland   C) heart

    B) pituitary gland   D) skin

24. Identify a true statement about the skin.

    A) It is part of the endocrine system.

    B) It protects the body from outside elements, such as chemicals, germs, and sun exposure.

    C) Its primary function is to transport waste material from the body cells to the blood.

    D) It supplies oxygen and nutrients to cells.

25. Which of the following statements associated with the endocrine system is true?

    A) The endocrine system includes skin, oil glands, sweat glands, hair, and nails.

    B) The endocrine system coordinates with all other body systems, allowing them to work efficiently and react to the environment.

    C) Hormones secreted by the endocrine glands seldom influence the body.

    D) Hormones secreted by the endocrine glands are chemical substances such as estrogen, insulin, and adrenaline, which stimulate activities in the body.

finished!

ch. 03: Skin Structure and Growth

Why Study Skin Structure and Growth?

TRUE OR FALSE

Indicate whether the statements below are true or false. For any false statements, explain why they are false.

1. Young clients want their beauty providers to inspire them to have healthy-looking hair and skin and a radiant appearance.

   T   F   _____

2. It is acceptable—and sometimes even expected—for licensed cosmetologists to diagnose, prescribe medications for, and provide treatment for irregular skin conditions, illnesses, or diseases.

   T   F   _____

3. Dermatology is a medical branch of science that involves the study of skin and its nature, structure, functions, diseases, and treatment.

   T   F   _____

4. Other than providing excellent skin care to clients, why else is it crucial that cosmetologists study skin structure and growth?

    _____

    _____

    _____

REFLECTION

5. Take a few moments to think about your own skin care routine (whether you practice it on a regular basis or just as needed) and list three or four procedures and/or products that you use on you face, feet, hands, and so on. Are you satisfied with the results? What might convince you to change a component of your skin care routine? As you work through this chapter, keep your skin care routine in mind and think about adjustments you might want to make based on what you learn about skin—applying what you learn will not only help you but is also likely to be useful for your clients!

    _____

    _____

    _____

Skin Layers and Their Functions

FILL IN THE BLANK

6. Complete the sentences below using words from the word bank.

    Word bank: sudoriferous, texture, organ, surface, infection, acidic, touch, sebaceous, visible, appendages, moist, immune

    Healthy skin is free of any _____ signs of disease, _____, or injury. It is slightly

    _____ and soft, and has a smooth, fine-grained _____ (feel and appearance).

    The _____ of healthy skin is slightly _____, and its _____ responses

    react quickly to organisms that _____ or try to enter it. _____ of the skin include

    hair, nails, and _____ (sweat) and _____ (oil) glands. Skin is the body's largest

    _____.

7. Match each layer of the epidermis, provided in the word bank below, with its features. Each stratum will be used more than once.

    Word bank: Stratum corneum, Stratum lucidum, Stratum granulosum, Stratum spinosum, Stratum germinativum

    (Study Tip: After you have correctly matched each stratum, you might find it helpful to convert this list to flash cards for more practice.)

    _____ The largest layer of the epidermis

    _____ What we see when we look at the skin

    _____ The living layer that produces new epidermal skin cells; responsible for "germinating" the epidermis's growth

    _____ Contains special cells called melanocytes, which produce skin pigment called melanin

    _____ Forms a barrier to protect underlying tissues from infection, dehydration, chemicals, and mechanical stress

    _____ Composed of cells that look like granules and are filled with keratin

    _____ Clear, translucent layer that consists of small cells through which light can pass

    _____ Has overlapping skin cells and is made up of keratin, a fibrous protein

    _____ Where the process of skin cell shedding begins

    _____ Has cells that combine with lipids (fats) to help make it a protective, water-resistant layer; the cells are continually being shed and replaced by cells rising to the surface from the skin's sublayers

    _____ Located only on the palms of the hands, soles of the feet, and digits; forms our unique fingerprints and footprints

    _____ Its cells die as they are pushed to the surface to replace dead cells shed from the top layer of skin

8. Label each stratum of the epidermis in the illustration below. Be sure to include other names for the layers if they have them (spiny layer, horny layer, basal cell layer, and granular layer).

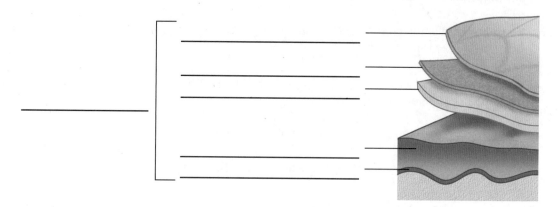

9. The highly sensitive dermis layer of connective tissue is about _____ times thicker than the epidermis.

   A) 2

   B) 2.5

   C) 25

   D) 10

10. The dermis, also known as _____, is the skin's underlying or inner layer, extending to form the subcutaneous tissue.

   A) epiderma, corium, cutis, or true skin

   B) derma, corium, cutis, or true skin

   C) media, corium, cutis, or true skin

   D) derma, corium, cutis, or actual skin

11. The dermis is made up of which two layers?

   A) the papillary layer and superficial layer

   B) the reticular layer and deeper layer

   C) the papillary layer and subcutaneous layer

   D) the papillary layer and reticular layer

12. The reticular layer of the dermis includes which two glands?

    A) sudoriferous and sweat

    C) sudoriferous and sebaceous

    B) sebaceous and oil

    D) sulphurous and sebaceous

13. Some papillae contain small epidermal structures called_____, with nerve endings that are sensitive to touch, pain, heat, cold, and pressure.

    A) tactile corpuscles

    C) tensile corpuscles

    B) red corpuscles

    D) tactile capillaries

SHORT ANSWER

14. Describe the arrector pili muscles—where they are located and what they do.

_____

_____

_____

FILL IN THE BLANK

15. Fill in the blanks with the terms provided in the word bank below.

Word bank: protective, dermis, gender, thickness, fats, age, subcutaneous, epidermis, tissue, superficial, health

The _____ layer, also known as hypodermis or _____ fascia, is the fatty

_____ below the _____ layer (which is found just below the _____

layer). It gives the body smoothness and contour, contains _____ for energy, and acts

as a _____ cushion for the skin. It varies in _____ according to an individual's

_____, _____, and general _____.

16. Circle the parts of the diagram below (seven items) that make up the reticular layer of the dermis.

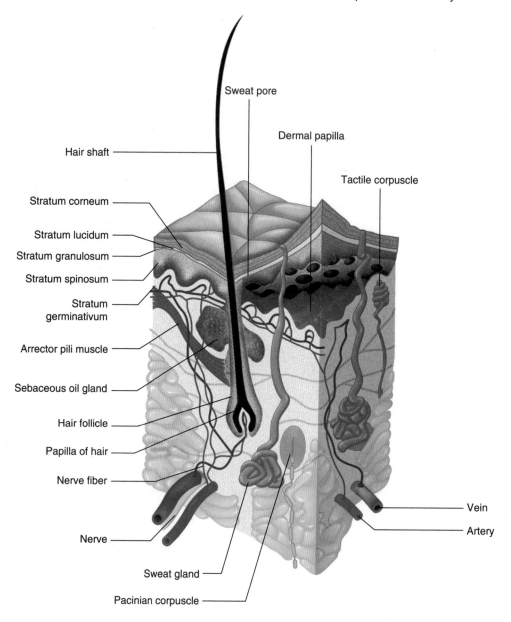

Sweat pore

Dermal papilla

Tactile corpuscle

Hair shaft

Stratum corneum

Stratum lucidum

Stratum granulosum

Stratum spinosum

Stratum germinativum

Arrector pili muscle

Sebaceous oil gland

Hair follicle

Papilla of hair

Nerve fiber

Vein

Artery

Nerve

Sweat gland

Pacinian corpuscle

17. Draw the three main components of skin.

18. Using various household items or food products, create a model cross-section of the following layers of the skin:

    • Stratum germinativum (basal cell layer)

    • Stratum spinosum

    • Stratum granulosum

    • Stratum lucidum

    • Stratum corneum

    • Papillary layer

    • Reticular layer

    • Subcutaneous tissue

You can use food like cereal, a slice of bread or tortilla, or honey, as well as items like aluminium foil or a sponge. You can even bake a cake! Once you have built your model, compare it to Figure 3–2 on page 64 in your textbook.

Nerves That Affect the Skin

CROSSWORD

19. Complete the crossword below:

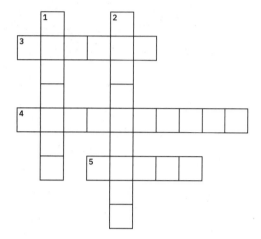

Across

3. These form a network of pathways for conducting information throughout the body.
4. What your nerve fibers cause related to your skin when you are cold or afraid
5. Nerve fibers that convey impulses to the muscles or glands to stimulate muscles, including arrector pili muscles

Down

1. Nerve fibers that send messages to the central nervous system and brain to react to heat, cold, touch, pressure, and pain
2. These nerve fibers are attached to your sweat and oil glands.

EXPERIMENT

20. Use a toothpick to do a touch test on one or two partners to determine the skin's sensitivity. Take a toothpick and poke the areas of the body in the table below, using the same pressure each time. For each poke, ask your partner to rate their sensitivity on a scale from 1 to 5—with 1 being "What poke?" to 5 being "Ouch!"—and record their answers below. What areas seemed most sensitive? Was there a difference if your partner knew they were going to be poked? Finally, consider how this experiment will influence how you approach clients when performing services such as manicures, facials, and hair treatments.

AREA	PARTNER 1 (EYES OPEN)	PARTNER 1 (EYES CLOSED)	PARTNER 2 (EYES OPEN)	PARTNER 2 (EYES CLOSED)
Tip of finger				
Palm of hand				
Upper arm				
Scalp				
Cheek				

Skin Pigments

TRUE OR FALSE

Indicate whether each statement below is true or false. If a statement is false, explain why.

21. Melanin, the tiny grains of pigment (coloring matter), is produced by melanocytes and then deposited into cells in the stratum spinosum layer of the epidermis and the reticular layers of the dermis.

    T   F   _____

22. One person's melanocytes (pigment-producing cells) may make more melanin than another person's do.

    T   F   _____

23. An example of an internal factor that affects melanin activation and production is found in people who have less activity in their melanocytes, resulting in darker skin.

    T   F   _____

24. An external factor influencing melanin production is sun exposure.

    T   F   _____

25. Every person has the same number of melanocytes, or pigment-producing cells.

    T   F   _____

26. Individuals with lighter skin and melanin have more activity in their melanocytes.

    T   F   _____

27. The size, number, and makeup of the pigment granules have nothing to do with the depth and tone of an individual's skin, hair, and eye color.

    T   F   _____

28. The body produces two types of melanin: eumelanin, which is red to yellow, and pheomelanin, which is dark brown to black.

    T   F   _____

29. People who have a pheomelanin dominance tend to have rosy skin, with red or neutral hair tones.

    T   F   _____

30. People with a eumelanin dominance likely have cooler hair and skin tones.

    T   F   _____

Strength and Flexibility of the Skin

MATCHING

31. While collagen and elastin both give skin strength and flexibility, there are some specific differences between them. Look at each item below, and mark E if it is a trait of elastin, C if it is a trait of collagen, B for both, or N if it is for neither of them.

    _____ A fibrous, connective tissue

    _____ Gives skin flexibility

    _____ Is not affected by the sun

    _____ Helps skin retain its shape after stretching

    _____ Gives skin strength and form

    _____ Weakens with age and UV light

    _____ Important for the skin's overall health and appearance

    _____ Provides structural support to the dermis

CASE STUDY

32. Imagine that you are specializing in facial services for a large salon and want to help clients improve the look and feel of their skin. You won't be able to do this without knowing more about their skin care routine and lifestyle, but know that this can be a sensitive subject. Using a software program or pen/marker/magazine cutouts and paper, design a flyer that you could post at your station to comfortably and kindly prompt this discussion with clients. Your flyer should serve as a checklist of 5 to 10 key questions about their skin care routine and lifestyle, and it should include any appropriate images or visual examples and a statement that encourages them to talk with you. Compare your flyer with a fellow student's and give each other feedback on what might be missing or even what could be stated more sensitively or humorously if appropriate.

Skin Glands

33. What do the sebaceous and sudoriferous duct glands in the skin extract materials from to form new substances?

    A) papillae

    C) keratin

    B) blood

    D) fat cells

34. What do the sebaceous glands secrete?

    A) sweat

    C) hormones

    B) oil

    D) odors

35. What do the sudoriferous glands excrete?

    A) sweat

    C) hormones

    B) oil

    D) odors

36. What is the *main* function of the sweat glands?

    A) cool down the body

    B) detoxify the body by excreting excess salt and unwanted chemicals

    C) provide moisture

    D) protect the skin from diseases

37. What happens when sweat evaporates from the skin?

    A) The skin dries out and can become cracked from the salt left behind.

    B) The body warms up to room temperature.

    C) The body cools down.

    D) The sweat cycle begins again.

38. What significantly increases activity in the sudoriferous gland? Select all that apply.

Heat

Greasy food

Strong winds

Exercise

Certain drugs

Noisy crowds

Antiperspirants

Certain insects

Emotions

Large quantities of water

39. How much fluid is typically excreted by sweat pores on a daily basis?

A) 1 to 2 liters

B) 1 to 2 cups (¼ to ½ liter)

C) 1 to 2 pints (½ to 1 liter)

D) 1 to 2 teaspoons

40. Sweat contains trace amounts of minerals such as _____, potassium, and magnesium.

A) iron

B) sodium

C) selenium

D) zinc

41. All body parts have sudoriferous glands, but they are _____ on the palms of the hands, the soles of the feet, the forehead, and the underarm (armpit).

A) never found

B) rarely found

C) smaller

D) more numerous

TRUE OR FALSE

Identify whether the statements below are true or false. If a statement is false, explain why it is false.

42. Sebaceous glands secrete sebum, a fatty or oily substance that lubricates the skin and preserves hair's softness.

T   F   _____

43. Sebaceous glands, also known as sweat glands, are connected to the hair follicles.

T   F   _____

44. With the exception of the scalp and face, the sebaceous glands are found in all body parts.

T   F   _____

45. Sebaceous glands in the scalp and face are larger than those found in other body parts.

T   F   _____

46. In the illustration below, the sebaceous gland is correctly identified (circled in blue).

T   F   _____

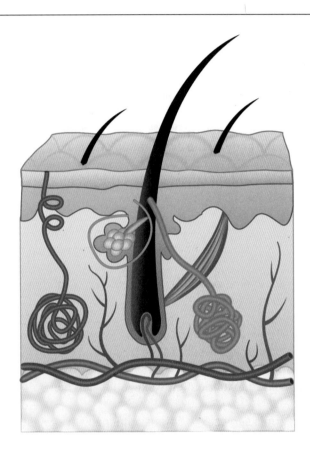

Skin Functions

REFLECTION

47. Take some time to jot down the internal and external factors in your daily life that might affect the elements of your own skin. Next, recall your responses from the start of this chapter where you were asked to examine your skin care routine and the products you use. Identify areas in your routine—and your lifestyle—that you could change to improve the health and appearance of your skin. What will you change? Why? Do you see any challenges to making these changes? How do you hope to overcome them? Be specific.

48. Match the six functions of the skin, listed in the word bank, with the descriptions of their features and how they perform their role. Some functions will be used more than once.

Word bank: Protection, Sensation, Heat regulation, Excretion, Secretion, Absorption

_____ Guards against external factors, such as bacteria invasion

_____ Pulling away if you touch something hot

_____ The perspiration emitted by sudoriferous glands

_____ Adjustments made by the skin's blood and sudoriferous glands to help cool down the body by the evaporation of sweat

_____ Small amounts of fatty materials can penetrate the epidermis via hair follicles and sebaceous gland openings.

_____ An acid mantle made up of sebum, lipids, sweat, and water, which form a hydrolipidic film and prevent the skin from drying out

_____ The water emitted through perspiration, including salt and other trace minerals and chemicals

_____ When the nerve endings are stimulated by heat, cold, touch, pressure, and pain, a message is sent to the brain.

_____ Oil emitted to lubricate the skin and keep hair soft

_____ Epidermis serves as a defense mechanism against injury to the body.

_____ Scratching if your skin itches

_____ Maintains the body's internal temperature of about 98.6 degrees Fahrenheit (37 degrees Celsius)

_____ Sebum emanating from sebaceous glands

_____ An acid mantle with an average pH of 5.5, which reduces the entry of pathogens into the body

DISCOVERIES AND ACCOMPLISHMENTS

In the space below, write notes about key concepts discussed in this chapter. Share your discoveries with some of the other students in your class and ask them if your notes are helpful. You may want to revise your notes based on good ideas shared by your peers.

Discoveries:

_____

_____

_____

_____

_____

_____

List at least three things you have accomplished since you decided to enroll in school.

Accomplishments:

_____

_____

_____

_____

_____

_____

1. Cosmetologists should have a thorough understanding of skin structure and growth because _____.

   A) knowing the skin's underlying structure and needs is crucial to providing excellent skin care for clients

   B) cosmetologists are physicians specialized in a medical branch of science that involves the study of the skin and its nature, structure, and functions

   C) cosmetologists are responsible for informing clients about the skin structure that will be modified as a result of the services availed by them

   D) it will help them diagnose, prescribe medications for, and provide treatment for irregular skin conditions, illnesses, or diseases

2. A physician who specializes in diseases and disorders of the skin, hair, and nails is known as a _____.

   A) dermatologist   C) rheumatologist

   B) cosmetologist   D) hematologist

3. The _____ is the outermost and thinnest layer of the skin and is made up of five layers—stratum corneum, stratum lucidum, stratum granulosum, stratum spinosum, and stratum germinativum.

   A) subcutaneous layer   C) hypodermis

   B) dermis   D) epidermis

4. Which of the following roles does the barrier function play in the skin?

   A) It contains nerve endings that make the skin sensitive to touch and pressure.

   B) It protects sensitive cells in the skin from the destructive effects of the sun's ultraviolet light.

   C) It supplies the skin with oxygen and nutrients.

   D) It keeps the skin moist by preventing water evaporation.

5. Which of the following statements is true of the dermis?

   A) It contains special cells that produce a dark skin pigment called melanin.

   B) It contains no blood vessels, but it does have many small nerve endings.

   C) It is the skin's underlying layer and extends to form the subcutaneous tissue.

   D) It is made up of five layers called strata.

continued

6. Which of the following is a function of subcutaneous tissue?

   A) It produces new epidermal skin cells.

   B) It helps guard against irritants penetrating the skin surface.

   C) It gives the body smoothness and contour.

   D) It helps regulate the pH of the skin.

7. Which of the following statements is true of secretory nerve fibers?

   A) They are sensory nerves attached to sweat and oil glands.

   B) They send messages to the central nervous system to react to pain.

   C) They send messages to the brain to react to cold and heat.

   D) They control the flow of sebum to the surface of the skin.

8. Which of the following nerve fibers send messages to the central nervous system and brain to react to heat, cold, touch, pressure, and pain?

   A) efferent nerve fibers   C) sensory nerve fibers

   B) secretory nerve fibers   D) motor nerve fibers

9. _____ refers to the tiny grains of pigment deposited into cells in the stratum germinativum layer of the epidermis and papillary layers of the dermis.

   A) Melanin   C) Elastin

   B) Keratin   D) Collagen

10. Differences in genetic skin color among people are due to _____.

   A) the amount of melanin activated in the skin and the way it is distributed

   B) an overabundance of elastin and collagen in the dermis

   C) the different number of melanocytes in each person

   D) a dominance of keratin in the skin and hair

continued

11. Which of the following is a function of melanin?

   A) It protects skin cells by absorbing and blocking ultraviolet radiation.

   B) It supplies the skin with oxygen and nutrients.

   C) It keeps the skin moist by preventing water evaporation.

   D) It helps guard against irritants penetrating the skin surface.

12. Daily use of a broad-spectrum sunscreen with a sun protection factor (SPF) of 15 or higher can _____.

   A) reduce the keratin present in the outermost layer of the epidermis

   B) help the melanin protect the skin from burning, skin cancer, and premature aging

   C) enable the skin to freely absorb UVA and UVB radiation from the sun

   D) help reduce collagen and elastin in the skin

13. _____ is a type of melanin that is red to yellow in color.

   A) Eumelanin   C) Pheomelanin

   B) Pyomelanin   D) Allomelanin

14. The skin gets its strength, form, and flexibility from two protein fibers found within the _____.

   A) epidermis   C) dermis

   B) hypodermis   D) subcutaneous layer

15. _____ is a fibrous, connective tissue made from protein that gives the skin form and strength.

   A) Elastin   C) Sebum

   B) Collagen   D) Keratin

16. Identify a factor that weakens collagen.

   A) infrequent weight changes   C) the use of a broad-spectrum sunscreen

   B) moisture   D) age

continued

17. Which of the following statements is true of elastin?

    A) It gives the skin its flexibility and elasticity.

    B) It is never affected by age.

    C) It exists separately from collagen fibers.

    D) It is found within the stratum corneum.

18. Which of the following actions is most likely to slow the weakening of collagen and elastin fibers and help the skin look younger longer?

    A) keeping the skin free of disease

    B) refraining from adding moisture to the skin

    C) using a daily broad-spectrum sunscreen with an SPF of 10 or lower

    D) letting the skin freely absorb the UVA and UVB radiation from the sun

19. Which of the following statements is true of sudoriferous glands?

    A) They consist of little sacs with ducts that open into the hair follicles.

    B) They consist of a secretory coil and a tube-like sweat duct that ends at the skin's surface to form the sweat pore.

    C) They secrete a fatty or oily substance that lubricates the skin and preserves the hair's softness.

    D) Their activity is significantly reduced by heat, exercise, emotions, and certain drugs.

20. Glands that are connected to the hair follicles and secrete sebum are called _____.

    A) ceruminous glands   C) sweat glands

    B) sudoriferous glands   D) sebaceous glands

21. Which of the following is a fatty or oily secretion that lubricates the skin and preserves the softness of the hair?

    A) pheomelanin   C) sebum

    B) collagen   D) keratin

continued

22. Which of the following is one of the six principal functions of the skin?

    A) cell differentiation   C) digestion

    B) sensation   D) neurogenesis

23. When the environmental temperature changes and the skin's blood and sudoriferous glands make necessary adjustments to help cool down the body by the evaporation of sweat, the skin is most likely performing the function of _____.

    A) sensation   C) nutrient absorption

    B) heat regulation   D) protection

24. Perspiration from the sudoriferous glands is expelled through the skin. Which of the following functions of the skin does this information most closely relate to?

    A) sensation   C) secretion

    B) excretion   D) protection

25. Which of the following factors is most likely to increase the flow of sebum?

    A) decreased consumption of fats and carbohydrates

    B) low levels of androgens in the body

    C) stimulation of sudoriferous glands

    D) emotional stress and hormone imbalances

finished!

TRACK MY PROGRESS!

Use this simple tracker to record your progress as you work through the activities in each learning objective.

COMPLETED	# OF CORRECT ANSWERS	OBJECTIVE
☐	_____/6	**LO 1** - Explain why cosmetologists need to understand skin disorders and diseases.
☐	_____/11	**LO 2** - Identify and describe common skin lesions, differentiating between primary and secondary lesions.
☐	_____/12	**LO 3** - List and describe common sebaceous and sudoriferous gland disorders.
☐	_____/21	**LO 4** - List and describe common skin inflammations and infections.
☐	_____/2	**LO 5** - Identify skin hypertrophies.
☐	_____/20	**LO 6** - List and describe common skin pigmentation changes.
☐	_____/10	**LO 7** - Identify and describe major acne causes and current treatments.
☐	_____/10	**LO 8** - List contributing factors to skin aging.
☐	_____/17	**LO 9** - Explain the effects of sun exposure on the skin.
☐	_____/8	**LO 10** - Identify forms of skin cancer, including symptoms and survival rates.
☐	_____/16	**LO 11** - Describe contact dermatitis and prevention measures for cosmetologists.

Why Study Skin Disorders and Diseases?

FILL IN THE BLANK

1. Fill in the blanks in the paragraph below using the word bank.

   Word bank: regulate, defense, disorders, protection, skin, minimal, assaults, life-threatening, temperature

   The _____ is the body's largest organ. It offers _____ from harmful organisms; it is the first

   _____ against environmental _____; and it helps _____ body _____. Skin _____

   and infections can either be a _____ medical concern or present _____ situations.

2. What are three unique perspectives that a cosmetologist can offer by studying skin irregularities?

_____

_____

_____

3. As a cosmetologist, what should you always do when you are uncertain about a client's skin condition?

_____

_____

_____

4. What would be an advantage or benefit of splitting your work between skin care and haircutting?

_____

_____

_____

5. Are cosmetologists required to choose between skin care and hair? Why or why not?

_____

_____

_____

MULTIPLE CHOICE

6. Cosmetologists need a thorough understanding of skin disorders and diseases because cosmetologists need to _____. Select all that apply.

A) diagnose disease

B) understand skin structure and common skin problems

C) make appropriate skin care recommendations to clients

D) know when to send a client to a healthcare provider

E) treat skin cancer

F) know what salon services can be safely performed

G) know how to use skin care services to hide skin disorders they do not recognize

Common Skin Disorders and Diseases

TRUE OR FALSE

Indicate whether the statements below are true or false. For any false statements, explain why they are false.

7. If your client has inflamed skin, whether it's infectious or not, you can serve them, as long as they provide you with a physician's note that permits them to receive services.

    T   F   _____

8. Inflammation, a skin issue that typically presents as swelling and redness, is one of the most difficult to detect.

    T   F   _____

9. Sunburn is a good example of short-term skin inflammation.

    T   F   _____

10. Cosmetologists should not be concerned by long-term inflammation in their clients because it only causes short-term tissue damage.

    T   F   _____

11. When clients have long-term skin inflammation, the cosmetologist should refer them to a radiologist to determine the cause and discuss possible treatments.

    T   F   _____

12. Solve the crossword based on the clues below about primary and secondary lesions.

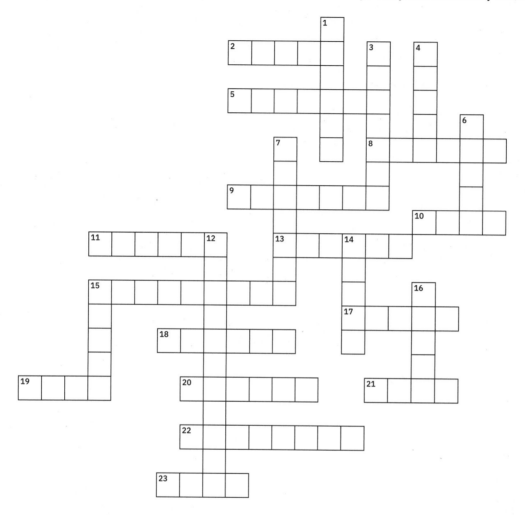

Across

2. Large blister containing a watery fluid; similar to a vesicle; requires medical referral

5. Crack in the skin that penetrates the dermis

8. Thick scar resulting from excessive growth of fibrous tissue

9. Raised, inflamed papule with a white or yellow center containing pus in the top of the lesion

10. Closed, irregularly developed sac that contains pus, semifluid, or morbid matter, above or below the skin; requires medical referral

11. Solid bump larger than 0.4 inch (1 centimeter) that is easily felt; requires medical referral

13. Type of tumor

15. A cyst that cannot be drained

17. Thin, dry, or oily plate of epidermal flakes

18. Type of ulcer

19. Slightly raised or depressed skin area formed as a result of the healing process related to an injury or lesion

20. Flat spot or discoloration on the skin

21. Example of a papule

22. Another name for a scar

23. Kind of pustule

Down

1. Small skin elevation that contains no fluid but may develop pus
3. Type of macule
4. Itchy, swollen lesion caused by a blow, scratch, insect bite, urticaria (skin allergy), or nettle sting
6. Kind of wheal
7. Small blister or sac containing clear fluid, lying within or just beneath the epidermis; requires medical referral if cause is unknown or untreatable with over-the-counter products
12. Skin sore or abrasion produced by scratching or scraping
14. Dead cells that form over a wound or blemish while healing
15. Any type of irregular mass varying in size, shape, and color; requires medical referral
16. Open skin lesion or mucous membrane of the body, accompanied by loss of skin depth and possibly weeping of fluids or pus

MULTIPLE CHOICE

13. A lesion can be any mark, wound, or irregularity, as indicated by structural changes in the tissues that have been caused by _____.

   A) genetics

   B) a poor diet

   C) damage or injury

   D) the environment

14. What are the three main types of lesions?

   A) primary, secondary, tertiary

   B) primary, tertiary, sextile

   C) ordinary, secondary, tertiary

   D) ordinary, tertiary, sextile

SHORT ANSWER

15. What is a primary lesion?

   _____

   _____

   _____

16. Which two characteristics can help you differentiate among the types of primary lesions?

   _____

   _____

   _____

17. What is a secondary lesion?

_____

_____

_____

Sebaceous and Sudoriferous Gland Disorders

18. What is sebum? What happens if too much sebum is produced?

_____

_____

_____

19. What are two potential outcomes for people who experience disorders with their sebaceous or sudoriferous glands?

_____

_____

_____

MATCHING

20. Match the type of sebaceous gland disorder with its description. Some words from the word bank might be used more than once.

    Word bank: epidermoid cyst, comedones, rosacea, seborrheic dermatitis, acne vulgaris, milia, telangiectasia

    _____ Usually found around the eyes, cheeks, and forehead, this condition appears as tiny benign (harmless), keratin-filled cysts that appear just under the epidermis and have no visible opening

_____ Chronic condition that appears primarily on the cheeks and nose and is characterized by flushing (redness); in some cases, symptoms can progress to pustular-type breakouts that can be confused with acne

_____ Characterized by chronic inflammation of the sebaceous glands from retained secretions and bacteria

_____ A large protruding pocketlike lesion filled with keratin

_____ A cosmetic irregularity, not a medical condition

_____ One of its causes is thought to be the colonization of lipophilic yeast

_____ Commonly associated with newborn babies but can appear at any age; in many states, only physicians can remove them (by piercing the skin with a sharp instrument called a lance)

_____ "Open" version of this sebaceous gland disorder; a hair follicle filled with keratin and sebum that oxidizes and turns black.

_____ Often appears in eyebrows, beard, scalp, hairline, middle of the forehead, and sides of the nose

_____ Commonly called a *sebaceous cyst*

_____ Involves visible capillaries, 0.02 to 0.04 inch (0.5 to 1.0 millimeter) in diameter, commonly found on the face, particularly around the nose, cheeks, and chin

_____ Develop when skin flakes become trapped in small pockets near the skin's surface

_____ A noninflamed buildup of cells, sebum, and other debris inside hair follicles

_____ Caused by chronic inflammation of the sebaceous glands and is often characterized by redness, dry or oily scaling, stubborn dandruff, crusting, and/or itchiness

_____ Creates a ruddy complexion called couperose skin

_____ Often thought to be a teenage skin disorder, but can affect people of all ages

_____ Frequently seen on the scalp and back and may be surgically removed by a dermatologist

_____ "Closed" version of this sebaceous gland disorder; a bump just under the skin's surface that appears as a whitish or cream color

21. Which of the following is *not* a component of sweat?

    A) fatty acids

    C) minerals

    B) sebum

    D) fluids

22. Bacteria and _____ are two common causes of disorders of the sudoriferous glands.

    A) heat

    C) nerve damage

    B) nervousness

    D) discomfort

23. What is the scientific name for prickly heat, an acute inflammatory disorder of the sweat glands that is caused by excessive heat exposure but usually clears in a short time without treatment?

    A) maxima rosacea

    C) miliaria rubra

    B) militaria rubella

    D) telangiectasia

24. _____ is characterized by a deficiency in perspiration or the inability to sweat.

    A) Bromhidrosis

    C) Dehydrosis

    B) Hyperhidrosis

    D) Anhidrosis

25. Anhidrosis is often a result of damage to the _____. This condition can be life threatening and requires medical attention.

    A) underarms

    C) autonomic nerves

    B) sweat glands

    D) milia

26. _____ is characterized by foul-smelling perspiration and is usually noticeable in the armpits or on the feet.

    A) Bromhidrosis

    C) Dehydrosis

    B) Hyperhidrosis

    D) Anhidrosis

27. Bromhidrosis is generally caused by _____, and treatments can include over-the-counter preparations, Botox injections, and lasers.

    A) bacteria

    C) synthetic clothing

    B) nerve damage

    D) clothing made of natural fibers

28. _____ is excessive sweating caused by heat, genetics, stress, medications, or general body weakness. It requires a medical diagnosis and treatment.

A) Bromhidrosis

C) Dehydrosis

B) Hyperhidrosis

D) Anhidrosis

RESEARCH

29. What is the difference between deodorant and antiperspirant? Which one is "better" for you? Why? Conduct some research to identify and explain the different approaches that people take to manage the excretions from their sudoriferous glands. Write one to two paragraphs about your findings and be sure to include a fun fact that was interesting or that surprised you.

_____

_____

_____

Skin Inflammations and Infections

TRUE OR FALSE

Indicate whether the statements below are true or false. For any false statements, explain why they are false.

30. Infection is a defense mechanism that occurs when something harmful or irritating affects a part of the body.

    T   F   _____

31. Inflammation is intended to remove or eliminate the offending object or organism.

    T   F   _____

32. Inflammation symptoms can be uncomfortable, indicating that the body is weakening.

    T   F   _____

33. Skin inflammation does not necessarily indicate there is a skin infection, but a skin infection can cause skin inflammation.

    T   F   _____

34. Most skin infections are not contagious.

T   F   _____

35. Eczema is not contagious.

T   F   _____

36. Bacteria enter the body through a break in the skin, while viral infections are typically transferred through mucous membranes, saliva, or fluid oozing from a sore.

T   F   _____

37. It is recommended that you always throw away any products that have touched infected eyes to avoid spreading the infection.

T   F   _____

SHORT ANSWER

38. Describe the characteristics of eczema.

_____

_____

_____

39. What should you do if you suspect a client has dermatitis or eczema?

_____

_____

_____

40. How do bacteria enter the body? How are viral infections typically transmitted?

_____

_____

_____

41. In addition to parasites, what are the other three causes of skin infections?

_____

_____

_____

42. What is another name for conjunctivitis?

_____

_____

_____

43. What should you do if your client arrives for an appointment with obviously irritated eyes, even if they are just scheduled for a pedicure?

_____

_____

_____

44. Where does impetigo typically occur on the body? How does it manifest?

_____

_____

_____

45. What usually causes impetigo?

_____

_____

_____

46. If your client arrives for an appointment and you notice weeping skin or open facial lesions, what should you do?

_____

_____

_____

47. Describe how the herpes simplex 1 virus appears.

_____

_____

_____

48. How long do the sores from herpes simplex 1 last?

_____

_____

_____

49. What is the difference between herpes simplex 1 and herpes simplex 2?

_____

_____

_____

CROSSWORD PUZZLE

50. Solve the crossword based on the clues below about skin inflammations and infections.

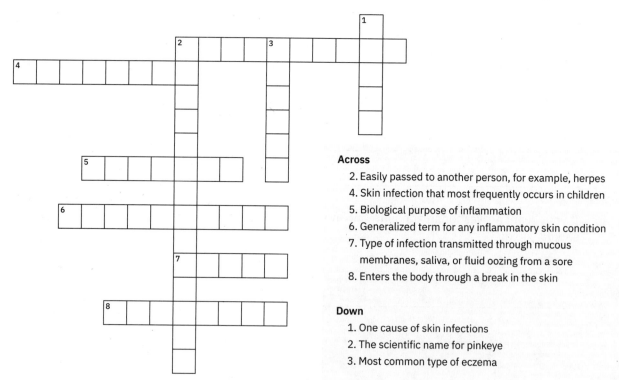

Across

2. Easily passed to another person, for example, herpes
4. Skin infection that most frequently occurs in children
5. Biological purpose of inflammation
6. Generalized term for any inflammatory skin condition
7. Type of infection transmitted through mucous membranes, saliva, or fluid oozing from a sore
8. Enters the body through a break in the skin

Down

1. One cause of skin infections
2. The scientific name for pinkeye
3. Most common type of eczema

Skin Hypertrophies

51. Use the word bank to match each term with its definition or description. Some terms will be used more than once.

    Word bank: hypertrophy, skin tag, mole, keratoma, psoriasis, benign, verruca

    _____ Characterized by red patches covered with silver-white scales and is usually found on the scalp, elbows, knees, chest, and lower back

    _____ Ranges in color from pale tan to brown or bluish black; might be small and flat (resembling freckles) or raised and darker in color

    _____ In general terms, any irregular growth of the skin

    _____ Also known as a wart

    _____ Examples: calluses and corns

    _____ Most hypertrophies

    _____ Small outgrowth of skin that occurs most frequently on the neck and chest

    _____ Not advised to remove one, or even a hair growing out of one, because it could irritate or alter the structure; only a physician should remove a hair from it

    _____ Caused by a virus and is infectious, spreading from one location to another, particularly along a scratch in the skin.

    _____ Not contagious; treatable but not curable

    _____ Caused by repeated pressure or friction, usually formed on the hands and feet

    _____ A hypertrophy of the papillae and epidermis

52. Identify the following hypertrophies.

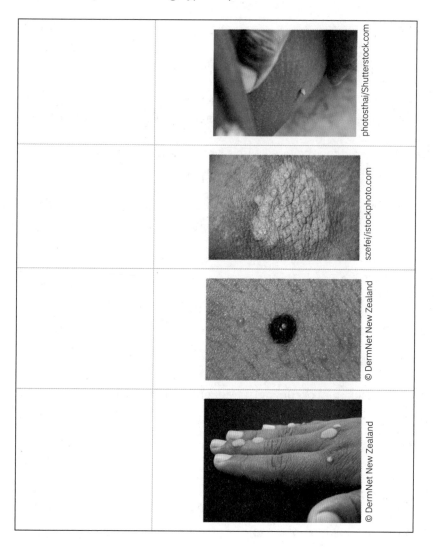

Pigment Disorders

SHORT ANSWER

53. Pigmentation disorders do not usually have a cure. What are three possible things you can do, as a cosmetologist, to assist a client who may have such a disorder?

_____

_____

_____

54. What is the difference between hyperpigmentation and hypopigmentation disorders?

_____

_____

_____

55. What internal factor influences pigmentation disorders?

_____

_____

_____

MATCHING

56. The sentences below include pairs of words and phrases, but only one of the items in each pair is correct. Circle the correct word or phrase in each pair so that the resulting sentence is true and makes sense.

There are six forms of **hyperpigmentation/hypopigmentation**: chloasma, **vitiligo/lentigines**, **melasma/melanoma**, nevus, stain, and tan. Of the six forms, melasma and **chloasma/rosacea** are similar. Lentigines is another term for mask of **pregnancy/freckles**. Various internal and **genetic/external** factors, such as sun exposure and **medications/psoriasis**, can, however, cause **irregular/uniform** pigmentation, referred to as dyschromia.

MULTIPLE CHOICE

57. What causes chloasma?

A) cumulative sun exposure or aging

B) genetics

C) allergies

D) burns or scars

58. Lentigines are small yellow to brown spots on skin exposed to sunlight and air; in older adults they are commonly referred to as _____.

A) chloasma

C) liver spots

B) gray areas

D) freckles

59. Melasma, also known as the mask of pregnancy, is a type of _____ hyperpigmentation disorder that appears during pregnancy or with the use of birth control pills.

A) hormonal

C) external

B) genetic

D) internal

60. Where does melasma most often occur on the body?

A) feet

C) neck and back

B) forehead, cheeks, upper lip, and chin

D) abdominal region

61. What is another name for a nevus?

A) watermark

C) birthmark

B) mask

D) stain

62. A nevus is a malformation of the skin due to irregular pigmentation or _____.

A) dilated capillaries

C) a skin inflammation

B) sun exposure

D) certain medications

SHORT ANSWER

63. Describe the hyperpigmentation disorder known as a stain.

_____

_____

_____

64. What causes a stain on the skin?

_____

_____

_____

65. List three hyperpigmentation disorders that are either caused or exacerbated by exposure to the sun.

_____

_____

_____

TRUE OR FALSE

Indicate whether the statements below are true or false. For any false statements, explain why they are false.

66. Albinism and vitiligo are examples of leukoderma.

    T   F   _____

67. Hypopigmentation has three forms: albinism, leukoderma, and vitiligo.

    T   F   _____

68. Hypopigmentation is more common than hyperpigmentation disorders.

    T   F   _____

69. Vitiligo is a skin disorder characterized by light or white irregular patches (hypopigmentation) caused by a burn, a scar, inflammation, or a congenital disease.

    T   F   _____

70. Albinism is a rare genetic condition characterized by absence of melanin pigment in the body, including the skin, hair, and eyes.

    T   F   _____

71. Although albinism is characterized by the absence of melanin, people who have it will still tan.

    T   F   _____

72. Match the type of hypopigmentation disorder (albinism, leukoderma, vitiligo) with its description. Each type will be used twice.

a. leukoderma   b. albinism   c. vitiligo

_____ Skin ages prematurely; is sensitive to light

_____ Characterized by light or white irregular patches

_____ Caused by a burn, a scar, inflammation, or a congenital disease; example: albinism

_____ Rare genetic condition

_____ Appears as hypopigmented spots and splotches on the skin that often appear milky white

_____ Part of an autoimmune disease

Acne and Problem Skin

73. What two factors cause a predisposition to acne?

_____

_____

_____

74. What are two hereditary traits that specifically affect the tendency to develop acne?

_____

_____

_____

75. How do hormones specifically influence the potential for acne?

_____

_____

_____

76. Describe retention hyperkeratosis.

_____

_____

_____

77. How does an overproduction of sebum contribute to acne development?

_____

_____

_____

MULTIPLE CHOICE

78. Acne bacteria (*Propionibacterium acne* or *P. acnes*) are anaerobic. What does *anaerobic* mean?

    A) healthy (or "good")   C) cannot survive in the presence of oxygen

    B) requires oxygen to thrive   D) unhealthy (or "bad")

79. What happens when follicles are blocked?

    A) Oxygen is blocked from the bottom of the follicles, allowing acne bacteria to multiply.

    B) Oxygen is blocked from the bottom of the follicles, allowing acne bacteria to die.

    C) Sunlight is blocked from the bottom of the follicles, allowing acne bacteria to multiply.

    D) Sunlight is blocked from the bottom of the follicles, allowing acne bacteria to die.

80. Acne bacteria's main food source are fatty acids, which are easily obtained from the abundance of _____ in the follicle.

    A) blood   C) sebum

    B) oxygen   D) serotonin

81. The following events take place after acne bacteria begin to multiply in the follicle. Number them from 1 to 8, first to last.

_____ Redness appears in the acne lesion.

_____ The acne bacteria rupture the follicle wall.

_____ An acne pustule forms.

_____ The immune system is alerted.

_____ An acne papule forms.

_____ Blood rushes to the ruptured follicle wall.

_____ Inflammation and swelling occur in the follicle.

_____ Blood (carrying white blood cells to fight bacteria) surrounds and engulfs the follicle.

DOS AND DON'TS

82. What are three to four dos and don'ts that you would share with a client who has a mild case of acne?

Dos:

_____

_____

_____

Don'ts:

_____

_____

_____

Aging Skin Issues

SHORT ANSWER

83. What are the two types of factors that influence the aging of skin? Briefly describe each one.

_____

_____

_____

84. What are the three categories of intrinsic factors that affect the aging of the skin?

_____

_____

_____

FILL IN THE BLANK

85. Use the words in the word bank to complete the paragraph below. Each word will only be used once.

   Word bank: hormonal, pigmentation, radicals, ethnicity, cumulative, atrophy, aging, collagen, repair, degenerative, epidermal, firmness

   The genetically determined _____ process occurs naturally and is affected by the

   _____ effects of free _____, _____ shifts, and the body's inability to

   perfectly _____ skin damage. Intrinsically aged skin shows _____ and dermal

   _____; a reduced number of fibroblasts; and less _____ production, which

   affects _____ and elasticity. _____ also influences skin aging, primarily because

   of the differences in pigmentation among different ethnic groups. High levels of _____

   help protect the skin from the _____ effects of photoaging over the years.

Indicate whether each statement is true or false. For any false statements, explain why they are false.

86. Gravitational pull is the irregular pulling downward on our skin and bodies.

T   F   _____

87. Gravitational pull is a consistent skin-aging factor for everyone.

T   F   _____

88. When the skin becomes more elastic, gravity makes eyebrows and eyelids droop and creates looseness and fullness under the cheeks and jaw, resulting in jowls and a double chin.

T   F   _____

89. Gravity has been known to have the power to lengthen ear lobes.

T   F   _____

SHORT ANSWER

90. What are three examples of how repetitive facial expressions can affect the aging of skin?

_____

_____

_____

91. What are the six categories of extrinsic factors that influence the aging of skin?

_____

_____

_____

92. Each row in the table below relates to one of the six extrinsic factors that affect skin aging and includes a description of it. Complete the table by (1) specifying each extrinsic factor and (2) finding and pasting (or drawing) images to represent a method for preventing or treating the effects of that extrinsic aging factor.

EXTRINSIC AGING FACTOR	DESCRIPTION OF AGING EFFECT	SUGGESTED PREVENTION OR TREATMENT OF THE EFFECT
	Tanning and sunbathing are significant contributors to both aging and skin cancer and should always be discouraged by skin care professionals.	
	Significantly damages the skin as well as the lungs. It produces free radicals and has a devastating effect on the body, causing skin wrinkling and sagging, particularly on the face and neck.	
	Inhibits the body from repairing itself and interferes with proper nutrition distribution to the skin and body tissues	
	Causes biochemical changes at the cellular level, leading to the tissue damage we call aging.	
	Deprives the skin of nutrients required to maintain, protect, and repair itself.	
	Produces free radicals, interferes with proper oxygen consumption, and affects the lungs and other internal organs as well as the skin.	

Sun Damage

TRUE OR FALSE

Indicate whether the statements below are true or false. For any false statements, explain why they are false.

93. UV light, also known as a UV ray, is just a shorter way of saying that it is a form of radiation.

    T   F   _____

94. The skin's collagen and elastin fibers naturally weaken as we age, but this weakening happens at a much slower rate if unprotected skin is only occasionally exposed to UV light.

   T   F   _____

95. A sunburn will only result in first-degree burns.

   T   F   _____

96. Of all the extrinsic aging factors, the sun and its ultraviolet (UV) light have a barely noticeable impact on skin aging.

   T   F   _____

97. Approximately 80 to 85 percent of aging skin symptoms are caused by the cumulative effects of damaging rays from the sun.

   T   F   _____

SHORT ANSWER

98. What is the most common form of sun protection?

   _____

   _____

   _____

99. What does SPF stand for, and what does it tell you?

   _____

   _____

   _____

100. What are four factors that can affect the amount of time that a sunscreen product will offer protection?

   _____

   _____

   _____

101. What is an example of a barrier SPF?

_____

_____

_____

102. What two things should be combined for ideal sun protection, according to the Skin Cancer Foundation?

_____

_____

_____

103. What is another name for UVA rays? For UVB rays?

_____

_____

_____

104. Which two terms are no longer allowed to appear on the labels of sunscreen products? What is now allowed in their place?

_____

_____

_____

CASE STUDY

105. Think about some of your favorite outfits that you wear outside in the summer. Make a list of four or five pieces of clothing (different colors, types of fabric), and then go to the Skin Cancer Foundation's website to find out the estimated UPF (ultraviolet protection factor) for each one. Based on your findings, write a few sentences describing what changes, if any, you might make to your sun protection plan the next time you head outside.

Fill in the blanks to complete each sentence about recommended precautions to take when you will be exposed to the sun.

106. It is important to avoid prolonged exposure to the sun during peak hours, usually between _____.

107. You should apply sunscreen at least _____ before sun exposure, to allow time for absorption and to prevent irritation from the sunscreen's chemicals on inflamed skin.

108. If your skin is exposed to hours of sun, such as a day at the beach, you should _____ throughout the day as a precaution.

CASE STUDY

109. Imagine that you have a client who comes to see you for facial treatments on a regular basis. During their last appointment with you, your client mentioned that they're planning a hiking trip. You recommend they bring a broad-spectrum sunscreen to protect themselves from UV rays that can cause skin damage and cancer, but your client worries that sunscreen will bother their sensitive skin or reactive negatively to their sweat while hiking. Do some research at a local drug store, online, or in magazines to identify three to four sunscreen products for your client. Take pictures of the products, note their specific features (e.g., waterproof, moisturizing, SPF number, hypoallergenic), and write a brief description explaining why each sunscreen might benefit your client's sensitive skin and active lifestyle.

Skin Cancer

SHORT ANSWER

110. What is one of the most common forms of cancer that cosmetologists should be able to recognize?

_____

_____

_____

111. Label each of the images below. Then match the type of skin cancer or skin condition with the correct image. Some types will be used more than once.

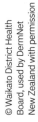
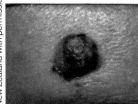
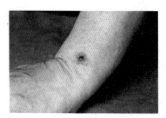
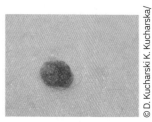
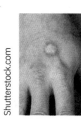

© Waikato District Health Board, used by DermNet New Zealand with permission

© D. Kucharski K. Kucharska/Shutterstock.com

_____   _____   _____   _____

_____ More serious than basal cell carcinoma; characterized by scaly red or pink papules or nodules; also appear as open sores or crusty areas

_____ 100 percent fatal if left untreated

_____ Characterized by light or pearly nodules

_____ Small spot on the skin ranging in color from pale tan to brown or bluish black

_____ Can spread to other parts of the body

_____ Least common, but most dangerous, form of skin cancer; characterized by black or dark brown patches on the skin that may appear uneven in texture, jagged, or raised

_____ Survival rates depend on the stage at diagnosis

_____ Most common and least severe skin cancer

_____ Not a type of cancer

_____ Early detection and treatment may result in a 99 percent five-year survival rate for the localized stage, but that drops drastically (66 percent) once it spreads to local lymph nodes

_____ Has an 85 to 95 percent recurrence-free rate with early diagnosis and treatment

_____ Characterized by black or dark brown patches on the skin that may appear uneven in texture, jagged, or raised

112. Complete the paragraph below with words from the word bank. Some words will be used more than once.

   Word bank: scalp, unique, hands, skin, new, changes, preventable, scaly, melanomas, ears, early, dark, unexpected, neck

   _____ cancer is _____, and _____ detection is possible if you

   know what to look for. Because of a cosmetologist's ability to see a client's _____,

   _____, and _____, cosmetologists are in a _____ position to help their

   clients detect _____ cancer. Be aware of the following as you service your clients:

   - Unusual lesions on the skin or the scalp or _____ in color, size, or shape of an existing

     lesion or mole

   - Irregularly shaped _____ spots (_____) on the _____ and _____; often first

     detected by cosmetologists

   - A(n) _____ lesion or discoloration on the skin or scalp

   - Client complaints about sores that do not heal or _____ skin bleeding

   - Recurrent _____ areas that may be rough to the touch, especially in sun-exposed areas

     such as the face, arms, or _____

113. What are two reasons that skin cancer is one of the most common causes of cancer-related deaths, particularly in young people?

   _____

   _____

   _____

114. What are the three types of skin cancer?

   _____

   _____

   _____

115. What should cosmetologists do when they recognize signs of potential skin cancer in a client—even in a client who is young or in good health? What attitude should help motivate the cosmetologist to speak up?

_____

_____

_____

ROLE PLAY

116. You have a young, physically active client who arrives for their regular hair appointment. The last few appointments, you noticed several brown spots on their ears. Although the spots are faint on their dark skin, today you notice that they are not uniform in color. You mention them, since early detection of skin cancer is key. Your client does not seem worried. What can you recommend to your client to convince them to take the spots seriously? Jot down the points you would make to your client and find a partner in class to role play a scenario discussing skin cancer, taking turns as the client and the cosmetologist. What persuasive techniques and facts did you use? What did you learn from your partner? To make this conversation easier to have with a client in the future, be sure to write down what works.

MATCHING

117. Identify and match the ABCDEs of melanoma detection with their description.

a. Border irregularity   c. Diameter   e. Evolution
b. Asymmetry   d. Color

_____ The mole might be shades of tan, brown, or black, and sometimes have red, blue, or white patches.

_____ One half of the mole does not match the other half.

_____ The mole changes. This process may include darkening or variations in color and changes in shape or growth; the mole may also itch or hurt.

_____ The mole is ragged or notched around the edges.

_____ The mole is wider than about 0.25 inch (0.5 centimeter) (although doctors are now finding smaller melanomas).

Contact Dermatitis

118. What is the most common work-related skin disorder for cosmetology professionals? What causes it?

_____

_____

_____

119. What are the two types of contact dermatitis?

_____

_____

_____

TRUE OR FALSE

Indicate whether each statement is true or false. For any false statements, explain why they are false.

120. Once a product allergy is established, the person affected by the allergy (cosmetologist or client) must stop using that particular product until the allergic symptoms clear; in severe or chronic cases, affected people should see a dermatologist for allergy testing.

    T   F   _____

121. Water, monomer liquids, haircolor, and chemical texture solutions are all common causes of allergic reactions with repeated exposure.

    T   F   _____

122. Sensitization is an allergic reaction created by repeated exposure to a chemical or a substance.

    T   F   _____

123. Allergic contact dermatitis (ACD) occurs when a person develops an allergy to an ingredient or a chemical; it is usually caused by just a single skin contact with the chemical.

    T   F   _____

124. Common places for allergic contact dermatitis include the fingers, palms, back of the hands, scalp, hairline, forehead, and neckline, but it's rarely seen on the face and cheeks.

T   F   _____

SHORT ANSWER

125. What is irritant contact dermatitis (ICD)? How does it differ from allergic contact dermatitis (ACD)?

_____

_____

_____

126. What types of products have the potential to cause irritant contact dermatitis?

_____

_____

_____

127. Describe the symptoms of contact dermatitis.

_____

_____

_____

MULTIPLE CHOICE

128. Using gloves or _____ when working with irritating chemicals is the best way to prevent both occupational types of contact dermatitis.

A) a hazmat suit   C) mitts

B) implements   D) a face shield

129. Who is more likely to get contact dermatitis from exfoliation products and drying agents?

A) nail technicians   C) estheticians

B) cosmetologists   D) No one, as the chemicals in those products will not cause contact dermatitis.

130. Who is more likely to get contact dermatitis from chemicals such as haircolor, straighteners, and permanent wave solutions?

A) nail technicians

B) cosmetologists

C) estheticians

D) No one, as the chemicals in those products will not cause contact dermatitis.

131. Who is more likely to get contact dermatitis from products such as monomer liquids and polymer powders?

A) nail technicians

B) cosmetologists

C) estheticians

D) No one, as the chemicals in those products will not cause contact dermatitis.

132. Although hand washing is important to prevent the spread of disease, it can dry out hands and crack the skin, allowing the penetration of irritating chemicals and causing further irritation. What is one way to balance hand washing with the need to keep your hands in good condition?

A) limit your hand washing between clients

B) use cold water when you wash your hands

C) apply protective hand creams afterward

D) soak your hands in Epsom salts once a day

133. What is a possible consequence if you fail to keep brush handles, containers, and tabletops clean and free from product, dust, and residue?

A) Repeatedly handling such items in that condition could result in the suspension of your cosmetology license.

B) Repeatedly handling these items will cause overexposure and skin reactions that, in some cases, could end your beauty career.

C) You are not likely to handle dirty items very frequently, so this is not a concern.

D) Simply wear gloves all the time, and everything will remain clean and dust-free.

DISCOVERIES AND ACCOMPLISHMENTS

In the space below, write notes about key concepts discussed in this chapter. Share your discoveries with some of the other students in your class and ask them if your notes are helpful. You may want to revise your notes based on good ideas shared by your peers.

Discoveries:

_____

_____

_____

_____

_____

_____

_____

List at least three things you have accomplished since you decided to enroll in school.

Accomplishments:

_____

_____

_____

_____

_____

_____

_____

1. The body's largest organ is the _____.

   A) heart

   C) liver

   B) skin

   D) brain

2. Which of the following statements is true about the skin?

   A) It is the last defense against environmental assaults.

   B) It is the body's smallest organ.

   C) It protects the body from harmful organisms.

   D) It seldom helps control body temperature.

3. Cosmetologists need a thorough understanding of skin disorders and diseases because _____.

   A) skin disorders and infections always present life-threatening situations and require a lot of attention

   B) cosmetologists are required to dedicate their entire workday to skin care services instead of hair care services

   C) recommending suitable skin care preparations to clients requires complete knowledge of the skin and potential disorders

   D) providing skin care services seldom requires the knowledge of the skin's structure and common skin problems

4. Identify a true statement about practicing cosmetology in the context of studying skin conditions, disorders, and diseases.

   A) Cosmetologists need to avoid referring a client to a healthcare provider if they are unsure about the severity of the client's skin condition.

   B) Cosmetologists are required to choose between hair and skin care services as the focus of their practice.

   C) Recognizing when salon services can be safely performed, and when the skin condition requires a healthcare provider referral, is crucial to managing a safe practice.

   D) Recommending suitable skin care preparations to clients seldom requires thorough knowledge of the skin and potential disorders.

5. Structural alterations in the tissues that are caused by injury or damage are known as _____.

   A) moles

   C) comedones

   B) milia

   D) lesions

continued

6. Lesions that are in the initial stages of development or change are called _____.

    A) secondary lesions   C) vascular lesions

    B) primary lesions   D) tertiary lesions

7. Which of the following is an example of a primary lesion?

    A) a fissure

    B) an ulcer

    C) a crust

    D) a wheal

8. Postoperative repair is an example of secondary lesions called _____.

    A) macules   C) cicatrix

    B) crust   D) scale

9. A closed comedo is _____.

    A) also known as a blackhead

    B) a bump just under the surface of the skin that appears when the follicle is not exposed
       to the environment

    C) a hair follicle filled with keratin and sebum

    D) usually brown in color and appears most frequently in the T-zone, which is the center
       of the face

10. Identify a characteristic of the skin disorder called milia.

    A) They are medically known as acne vulgaris or acne simplex.

    B) They are big, jutting, pocketlike lesions filled with keratin.

    C) They develop when skin flakes get trapped in small pockets near the surface of
       the skin.

    D) They can usually be found on the eyebrows, beard, scalp, hairline, and sides
       of the nose.

continued

11. _____ is a chronic condition that mainly appears on the cheeks and nose and is characterized by flushing (redness); in some cases, symptoms may progress to pustular-type breakouts that may look like acne.

   A) Milia

   B) Anhidrosis

   C) Telangiectasia

   D) Rosacea

12. Identify an accurate statement about seborrheic dermatitis.

   A) It is usually characterized by redness, dry or oily scaling, stubborn dandruff, crusting, and/or itchiness.

   B) It produces red, flaky skin that appears behind the ears and on the elbows and knees.

   C) It can be cured by applying fatty skin care products.

   D) It is extremely contagious.

13. Which of the following is a generalized term for any inflammatory skin condition?

   A) anhidrosis

   B) rosacea

   C) dermatitis

   D) milia

14. Which of the following is a characteristic of eczema?

   A) It is characterized by weeping lesions.

   B) It is extremely contagious.

   C) It is an eye infection and may be caused by a virus or a bacterium.

   D) It involves moderate to severe inflammation, scaling, and, occasionally, severe itching.

15. Conjunctivitis is _____.

   A) a contagious bacterial skin infection characterized by weeping lesions

   B) characterized by the eruption of a single vesicle or group of vesicles on a red swollen base

   C) an eye infection and may be caused by a virus or a bacterium

   D) characterized by moderate to severe inflammation, scaling, and, occasionally, severe itching

continued

16. Identify a characteristic of psoriasis.

   A) It is extremely contagious.

   B) It is typically curable.

   C) It typically occurs on the scalp, knees, chest, elbows, and lower back.

   D) It is a keratoma caused by repeated pressure or friction on any part of the skin.

17. A verruca, or a wart, is a _____.

   A) thickening of the skin that forms on pressure areas of the foot

   B) small spot or blemish on the skin

   C) condition caused by *staphylococcus* bacteria

   D) hypertrophy of the papillae and epidermis

18. _____, a hereditary skin condition, causes hypopigmented skin splotches and spots that are often milky white in appearance.

   A) Keratoma   C) Impetigo

   B) Psoriasis   D) Vitiligo

19. The fundamentals of mild acne treatment involve the use of _____.

   A) makeup and skin care products that are comedogenic

   B) skin care products without benzoyl peroxide

   C) harsh facial cleansers that help remove oil from the skin

   D) mild exfoliation treatments that gently remove dead skin cells

20. Which of the following statements associated with the extrinsic factors that influence skin aging is true?

   A) Smoking reduces the number of free radicals, which are unstable molecules that cause biochemical aging.

   B) Extrinsic factors are skin-aging factors that cannot be controlled.

   C) Tanning and sunbathing, which contribute significantly to skin cancer and aging, should always be discouraged by skin care professionals.

   D) Alcohol facilitates the distribution of nutrition distribution to the skin and body tissues.

continued

21. To reduce sun damage to the skin, _____.

    A) wear cotton shirts that offer less than Ultraviolet Protection Factor (UPF) 7

    B) avoid using sunscreens labeled *broad spectrum*

    C) use only sunscreens labeled *waterproof* or *sweat proof*

    D) apply sunscreen on the body and wear protective clothing

22. Identify a true statement about squamous cell carcinoma.

    A) It is less serious than basal cell carcinoma.

    B) It is the most dangerous form of skin cancer.

    C) It is characterized by uneven, black patches on the skin.

    D) It is characterized by scaly red or pink papules or nodules.

23. Suggest that a client consult a dermatologist for diagnosis and treatment when you notice that the client has _____.

    A) sores that heal quickly without any treatment

    B) recurrent scaly areas that may be rough to touch

    C) lentigines

    D) a nevus

24. According to the American Cancer Society, professionals should use the ABCDE Cancer Checklist to spot signs of change in an existing mole. Which of the following is a sign included in this checklist?

    A) One half of the mole matches the other half.

    B) The mole's color is the same all over.

    C) The mole's edges are ragged or notched.

    D) The mole is wider than about 0.1 inch.

25. To prevent contact dermatitis, _____.

    A) create sensitization by repeatedly using containers with products in them

    B) avoid moisturizing your hands frequently

    C) wash your hands frequently without using hand creams after the wash

    D) use implements or gloves when you need to work with irritating chemicals

finished!

TRACK MY PROGRESS!

Use this simple tracker to record your progress as you work through the activities in each learning objective.

COMPLETED	# OF CORRECT ANSWERS	OBJECTIVE
☐	_____/3	**LO 1** - Explain why cosmetologists need to understand nail structure and growth.
☐	_____/7	**LO 2** - Define the natural nail unit.
☐	_____/42	**LO 3** - Label nail structures.
☐	_____/17	**LO 4** - Describe the factors that affect nail growth.

Why Study Nail Structure and Growth?

SHORT ANSWER

1. What can the appearance of a client's nails tell you?

   _____

   _____

   _____

2. What is the overall goal of all nail services?

   _____

   _____

   _____

3. What are three reasons for cosmetologists to have a thorough understanding of nail structure and growth?

_____

_____

_____

The Natural Nail Unit

TRUE OR FALSE

Indicate whether each statement is true or false. For any false statements, explain why they are false.

4. A healthy nail is firm and flexible, shiny, and slightly pink. Its surface is usually smooth and unspotted, with no splits or deep grooves.

   T   F   _____

5. An unhealthy nail is translucent, with the nail bed's pinkish or beige color showing through.

   T   F   _____

6. The natural nail is technically referred to as the granite.

   T   F   _____

7. The natural nail is composed mainly of keratin, the fiber-shaped protein found in skin and hair.

   T   F   _____

8. The keratin in natural nails is less durable than the keratin in hair and skin.

   T   F   _____

9. The natural nail unit includes all parts of the finger from the tip to the wrist.

   T   F   _____

10. In your own words, describe the characteristics of a healthy natural nail.

_____

_____

_____

Nail Structures

SHORT ANSWER

11. List the nine major parts of the natural nail unit.

_____

_____

_____

12. Which parts of the natural nail unit make up the perionychium?

_____

_____

_____

MATCHING

13. Match the terms in the word bank with their description. Some words will be used more than once.

    Word bank: nail folds, nail plate, lateral nail fold

    _____ Skin folds that surround the nail plate

    _____ Also known as the sidewall

    _____ The nail itself

    _____ Skin fold that overlaps the nail's side

    _____ Form the nail grooves on the nail's sides

14. Draw a simple picture of a finger or toe and include the nail. Label the hyponychium, paronychium (lateral nail folds), and nail grooves.

MULTIPLE CHOICE

15. What is PNF, the skin flap that extends from the edge of the visible nail plate's edge to the first joint of the finger (or toe)?

    A) partial new fold

    B) proximal nail foundation

    C) proximal nail fold

    D) primary nearest fold

16. What area does the PNF cover?

    A) the matrix

    B) the keratin

    C) the grid

    D) the shield

17. The tissue of the PNF folds back underneath itself to create a _____ flap that covers and protects the matrix, a sensitive area.

    A) tissue

    B) keratinized

    C) stretchy

    D) thin

18. The nail matrix exists in the keratinized proximal nail tissue, and this is where cells proliferate and keratinize to form the _____.

    A) nail grooves

    B) sidewalls

    C) nail plate

    D) nail bed

19. Make a simple sketch of a finger or toe and include the nail. On your drawing, indicate where the PNF is in relation to the matrix.

FILL IN THE BLANK

20. Complete the following three sections based on the word bank. Some words will be used more than once.

    Word bank: bed, matrix, tip, grows, nail, 100, keratin, free, visible, unit

    a. The _____ plate is hardened _____ and sits on top of the nail _____ . The _____ cells create the nail plate cells. This is the most _____ and functional part of the natural nail _____.

    b. Although the nail plate appears to be one solid piece, it is constructed of approximately _____ nail cell layers. As it _____, the nail plate slowly slides across the nail _____.

    c. The part of the nail plate that extends over the _____ of the finger or toe as it grows is known as the _____ edge.

SHORT ANSWER

21. The nail plate is relatively porous to water. What does that mean?

    _____

    _____

    _____

22. Although a healthy nail may look dry and hard, it contains approximately how much water content?

_____

_____

_____

23. Describe how water and the humidity of the surrounding environment can affect the nail.

_____

_____

_____

24. What are two ways that a cosmetologist can help their clients manage water content of the nails?

_____

_____

_____

25. What causes the area under the nail plate to have a pinkish color? Where on the nail plate can the pinkish color be seen?

_____

_____

_____

26. As the portion of living skin in the nail structure, what is the role of the nail bed?

_____

_____

_____

27. What is the name of the thin tissue layer that helps guide the nail plate along the nail bed as it grows?

_____

_____

_____

28. Describe the physical characteristics of the nail bed in relation to the nail plate.

_____

_____

_____

29. Is nail polish applied to the nail plate or to the nail bed?

_____

_____

_____

MULTIPLE CHOICE

30. What is the term for what the matrix cells do to become specialized so that they can perform specific tasks and ultimately keratinize to form the nail plate?

    A) differentiate   C) divide

    B) procreate   D) double up

31. What is the role of the nerves, lymph, and blood vessels contained in the matrix area?

    A) control the rate of nail plate formation

    B) nourish the matrix cells so that they stay healthy

    C) support the nail bed

    D) help shed excess or malformed matrix cells

32. What is the term for the light-colored visible part of the matrix that extends from underneath the living skin to the nail plate's base?

   A) uvula

   B) lunar tip

   C) lunula

   D) the bridge

33. If a client has suffered an injury to their matrix, how will this affect their nails?

   A) delayed growth of the nail bed

   B) no effect because the nail plate is keratinized

   C) yellowish bruise on the lunula

   D) a stunted free edge

SHORT ANSWER

34. What is the cuticle's critical function?

   _____

   _____

   _____

35. Describe the cuticle's physical appearance and state where it originates.

   _____

   _____

   _____

36. How does the cuticle form the seal between the PNF and the nail plate?

   _____

   _____

   _____

37. What is the difference between the cuticle products that are marketed to consumers and those that are intended for professional cosmetologists?

_____

_____

_____

TRUE OR FALSE

Indicate whether these statements are true or false. For any false statements, explain why they are false.

38. The eponychium is the dead skin underneath the PNF found at the nail plate's base covering the matrix area; the cuticle is the living tissue adhered to the nail plate.

   T   F   _____

39. The eponychium is a thin section of tissue found on the bottom side of the PNF. It is approximately 0.004 to 0.006 inch (0.1 to 0.15 mm) thick.

   T   F   _____

40. Only two layers of stem cells make up the eponychium.

   T   F   _____

41. The eponychium extends from the front edge of the proximal nail fold and stops at the nail matrix.

   T   F   _____

42. The section of skin over the eponychium that covers the nail matrix and the nail plate is the PNF.

   T   F   _____

43. Cosmetologists can gently push back the PNF and are allowed to cut or trim living tissue, including the PNF, even if this skin appears dry and hardened. Cutting any part of the PNF or other living skin is within the scope of cosmetology nail services.

   T   F   _____

44. Draw a close-up picture of a finger or toe, and include the nail plate. On your drawing, indicate where the eponychium is in relation to the matrix area, the cuticle, and the nail plate.

SHORT ANSWER

45. List two or three questions that you can ask yourself to determine the difference between a client's cuticle and their eponychium.

_____

_____

_____

46. Describe the hyponychium and state where it can be found.

_____

_____

_____

47. Why is it especially important to treat the hyponychium carefully when performing nail services for clients?

_____

_____

_____

DRAW

48. Draw a simple picture of the finger and nail and indicate where the hyponychium is located. (*Hint:* You might want to draw this in such a way that the viewer is looking at the finger and nail from the side, not the top.)

SHORT ANSWER

49. What is a ligament?

_____

_____

_____

50. What two parts of the nail structure are connected to the underlying bone by the specialized ligaments?

_____

_____

_____

51. Where are the specialized ligaments located in the nail structure?

_____

_____

_____

LABELING

52. Use the word list below to label the parts of the natural nail unit.

Lunula   Hyponychium (used twice)   Eponychium
Nail plate (used twice)   Nail bed (used twice)   PNF
Free edge   Matrix (used twice)   True cuticle

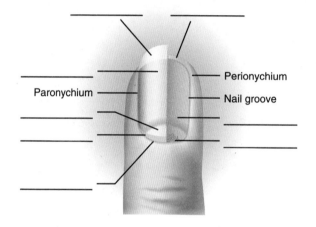

Paronychium

Perionychium

Nail groove

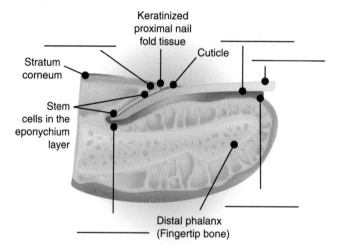

Keratinized
proximal nail
fold tissue

Cuticle

Stratum
corneum

Stem
cells in the
eponychium
layer

Distal phalanx
(Fingertip bone)

Nail Growth

Complete the sentences below.

53. The nail plate's growth is affected by _____, exercise, and overall health.

54. A healthy nail plate will grow in various shapes, depending on the _____ of the matrix.

55. The matrix's length determines the plate's _____. For example, a longer matrix produces a _____ nail plate.

56. A highly _____ matrix creates a highly curved _____ edge.

57. Nothing can make the nail plate grow _____ because this would require the matrix to also grow _____.

SHORT ANSWER

58. Which finger's nail on the hand grows the fastest? The slowest?

    _____

    _____

    _____

59. During what time of year does the nail plate grow more quickly? More slowly?

    _____

    _____

    _____

60. What happens to nail growth rates in older people?

    _____

    _____

    _____

61. How does the growth of toenail plates differ from that of fingernail plates?

_____

_____

_____

62. What is the average nail plate growth rate per month for the typical adult?

_____

_____

_____

63. How does pregnancy affect nail growth? What role do prenatal vitamins play?

_____

_____

_____

MULTIPLE CHOICE

64. What can cause the nail plate's shape or thickness to change?

   A) damage or infection of the matrix   C) the time of year

   B) overexposure to sunlight   D) a weakening lunula

65. How long does it typically take to completely replace a fingernail plate?

   A) 2 to 3 months   C) 4 to 6 months

   B) 4 to 6 weeks   D) 9 to 12 months

66. How long does it typically take to completely replace a toenail plate?

   A) 2 to 3 months   C) 4 to 6 months

   B) 4 to 6 weeks   D) 9 to 12 months

67. If nail cells are produced more quickly, the plate grows more _____. The reverse is also true.

    A) evenly

    B) unevenly

    C) quickly

    D) slowly

68. What happens if a small portion of the matrix stops making new cells?

    A) The nail plate becomes thinner and develops a narrow groove.

    B) The nail plate becomes thicker and develops a narrow groove.

    C) The nail plate becomes thinner and develops a yellowish color.

    D) The lunula disappears.

MATCHING

69. Match the following terms to their definition by adding the correct number to the table

_____ Cuticle	1. The dead colorless tissue attached to the nail plate
_____ Hyponychium	2. The living skin at the base of the nail plate covering the matrix area
_____ Nail grooves	3. The most visible and functional part of the nail
_____ Lunula	4. Where the nail plate cells are formed
_____ Nail folds	5. A tough band of fibrous tissue that connects bones or holds an organ in place
_____ Free edge	6. The lighter color shows the true color of the matrix
_____ Nail malformation	7. Slits or furrows at either side of the nail upon which the nail moves as it grows
_____ Eponychium	8. A thin layer of tissue that attaches the nail plate and the nail bed
_____ Matrix	9. Normal skin that surrounds the nail plate
_____ Nail bed	10. The part of the nail plate that extends over the tip of the finger
_____ Ligament	11. The portion of the living skin on which the nail plate sits
_____ Nail plate	12. The slightly thickened layer of skin that lies underneath the free edge of the nail plate
_____ Bed epithelium	13. When the nail is abnormal in shape or form

DISCOVERIES AND ACCOMPLISHMENTS

In the space below, write notes about key concepts discussed in this chapter. Share your discoveries with some of the other students in your class and ask them if your notes are helpful. You may want to revise your notes based on good ideas shared by your peers.

Discoveries:

_____

_____

_____

_____

_____

_____

_____

List at least three things you have accomplished since you decided to enroll in school.

Accomplishments:

_____

_____

_____

_____

_____

_____

_____

1. Cosmetologists should have a thorough understanding of nail structure and growth because _____.

    A) they are physicians specialized in a medical branch of science that involves the study of nails and their structure

    B) they must be able to differentiate between the nail cuticle and the eponychium before performing nail services

    C) they are responsible for informing clients about the parts of the nails that will be affected as a result of the nail services offered by them

    D) it will help them diagnose, prescribe medications for, and provide treatment for nail diseases

2. Identify a reason why cosmetologists should be knowledgeable about nail structure and growth.

    A) Understanding nail structure helps cosmetologists diagnose and treat irregular nail conditions.

    B) Cosmetologists are responsible for imparting the biological aspects of nail structure to staff members.

    C) Understanding natural nail structure and growth cycles prepares cosmetologists for advanced nail services.

    D) Cosmetology is the branch of medicine dealing with the natural nail unit and its major parts.

3. The natural nail unit includes _____.

    A) all parts of the finger from the tip to the second knuckle

    B) all parts of the finger from the tip to the first knuckle

    C) the nail plate and the nail bed but excludes the cuticle

    D) only the tip of the finger

4. The natural nail is technically called the _____.

    A) hyponychium   C) lunula

    B) cuticle   D) onyx

5. The natural nail unit is mainly made up of _____, which is the fiber-shaped protein found in skin and hair.

    A) collagen   C) melanin

    B) elastin   D) keratin

continued

6. Identify a characteristic of a healthy nail.

   A) It is soft but inflexible.

   B) It has 50 to 75 percent water content.

   C) Its surface is generally spotted and has deep grooves.

   D) It is translucent, and the beige or pinkish color of the nail bed shows through.

7. The nail bed, nail fold, eponychium, paronychium, and hyponychium are collectively referred to as the _____.

   A) cuticle   C) perionychium

   B) bed epithelium   D) lunula

8. The _____ is the whole skin flap that covers the matrix, from the visible nail plate's edge to the first joint of the finger or toe.

   A) proximal nail fold   C) perionychium

   B) bed epithelium   D) lateral nail fold

9. The _____ is the section of living skin that supports the nail plate as it extends toward the free edge.

   A) cuticle   C) nail matrix

   B) eponychium   D) nail bed

10. Which of the following statements is true of the nail plate?

    A) It is the hardened keratin plate that rests on top of the nail bed.

    B) It is the least visible and functional part of the nail unit.

    C) It is formed by melanocytes.

    D) It is water-resistant.

11. The _____ is part of the natural nail that contains nerves, blood vessels, and lymph to nourish cells that differentiate and become keratinized to form the nail plate.

    A) cuticle   C) hyponychium

    B) matrix   D) eponychium

continued

12. Which of the following statements best describes the lunula?

    A) It is the thin tissue layer between the nail plate and the nail bed.

    B) It is the nonliving colorless tissue attached to the nail plate.

    C) It is the section of living skin that supports the nail plate as it extends toward the free edge.

    D) It is the whitish, half-moon shape under the nail plate's base.

13. Identify a difference between the cuticle and the eponychium.

    A) The cuticle contains nerves, blood vessels, and lymph, whereas the eponychium does not.

    B) The cuticle is approximately 0.004 to 0.006 inch thick, whereas the eponychium is approximately 0.5 inch thick.

    C) The cuticle is the dead tissue stuck to the nail plate, whereas the eponychium is the living skin under the proximal nail fold found at the nail plate's base covering the matrix area.

    D) The cuticle is the visible matrix part that extends from underneath the living skin, whereas the eponychium is the slightly thickened skin layer between the fingertip and the nail plate's free edge.

14. Identify a function of the hyponychium.

    A) It forms a protective barrier that keeps microorganisms from infecting the nail bed.

    B) It helps guide the nail plate along the nail bed as it grows.

    C) It forms an important seal between the proximal nail fold and nail plate.

    D) It attaches the nail bed and matrix to the underlying bone.

15. A tough band of fibrous tissue that links bones or keeps an organ in place is called _____.

    A) the stratum corneum   C) collagen

    B) a ligament   D) the dermis

continued

16. Which of the following statements is true of the growth of the nail plate?

    A) The nail plate's growth is affected by nutrition, exercise, and overall health.

    B) The nail plate's width, thickness, and curvature are independent of the matrix's width, length, and curvature.

    C) A healthy nail plate begins from the lunula and ends slightly before the tip of the finger.

    D) The nail plate grows only in an almond shape.

17. Which of the following grows the fastest?

    A) the nail of the middle finger   C) the nail of the little finger

    B) the thumbnail   D) the nail of the index finger

18. Which of the following statements is true of nail growth rates?

    A) Nail growth rates generally decrease with age.

    B) Nail plates grow quicker in the winter than in the summer.

    C) Toenail plates grow quicker than fingernail plates.

    D) Nail growth rates decrease significantly during the last trimester of pregnancy.

19. Ordinarily, complete nail plate replacement for a fingernail takes about _____.

    A) two to six weeks   C) a year

    B) four to six months   D) eight months

20. The nail matrix causes the nail plate to develop a series of slender grooves because _____.

    A) the rate of production of new matrix cells improves with age

    B) the eponychium, which is the dead tissue adhered to the nail plate, increases with age and collects on the nail plate

    C) parts of the nail matrix begin to permanently reduce production of new cells as a result of aging

    D) the nail matrix grows ridges in the nail plate, which inadvertently leads to the formation of grooves

continued

21. What is the water content of a healthy nail?

    A) 5 to 10 percent   C) 15 and 25 percent

    B) 10 and 20 percent   D) 20 and 30 percent

22. The average rate of nail plate growth in an adult is about _____.

    A) ¹⁄₁₀ to ⅛ inches (0.25 to 0.32 cm) per month.

    B) ¼ to ½ inch (1.3 to 1.9 cm) per month

    C) ½ to ¾ inches (1.3 to 1.9 cm) per week

    D) ⅛ to ⅙ (0.32 to 0.42 cm) inch per week.

23. Which of the following is NOT part of the perionychium?

    A) the eponychium   C) the hyponychium

    B) the distal phalanx   D) the paronychium

24. What does a longer matrix lead to?

    A) a thinner nail plate   C) faster nail growth

    B) nail grooves   D) a thicker nail plate

25. Which of the following is NOT a natural nail shape?

    A) acorn   C) olive

    B) almond   D) date

finished!

ch. 06: Nail Disorders and Diseases

Why Study Nail Disorders and Diseases?

SHORT ANSWER

1. What are the three main reasons that cosmetologists should study nail disorders and diseases?

_____

_____

_____

2. What are two examples of conditions that can be easily addressed by a cosmetologist in the salon?

_____

_____

_____

3. Cosmetologists are expected to do what three things that require a thorough understanding of nail disorders and diseases?

_____

_____

_____

Unhealthy Nails

SHORT ANSWER

4. What four medical practice activities are you, as a licensed cosmetologist, prohibited from engaging in?

_____

_____

_____

5. Are cosmetologists allowed to identify whether a client has an unhealthy condition that precludes receiving salon services?

_____

_____

_____

6. Are cosmetologists allowed to identify the specific disease or disorder that appears to be present in a particular client?

_____

_____

_____

7. Each row represents a nail disorder. Each row is missing information. Complete the missing items for each row, and then indicate either Y (yes, you are allowed to provide service for this disorder at the salon) or N (no, you are not allowed to provide salon service).

NAIL DISORDER	DESCRIPTION	CAUSE	SALON SERVICE (Y/N)
a. Beau's lines			
b. _____ DD Images /Shutterstock.com	Dark purplish spots		
c. _____ Pradit.Ph/Shutterstock .com	Nails turn a variety of colors		
d. Eggshell nail			
_____ FCG/Shutterstock.com		Dry skin and small cuts	
f. Leukonychia			
g. _____ Dermatology11 /Shutterstock.com		Caused by increased pigment cells (melanocytes)	

NAIL DISORDER	DESCRIPTION	CAUSE	SALON SERVICE (Y/N)
h. Nail pterygium			
i. Onychophagy			
j. _____		Potentially caused by heredity, matrix injury, excessive exposure to cuticle removers, harsh cleaning agents, or aggressive filing techniques	
k. _____	A form of dramatically increased nail curvature of the free edge, whereby the nail can curl in upon itself or may be deformed only on one sidewall		
l. Plicatured nail, also known as a folded nail			
m. _____ Toa55/Shutterstock.com	Lengthwise grooves in the plate		
n. _____	Appearance of a lengthwise small splinter underneath the nail plate		

Indicate whether the statements below are true or false. If any statement is false, explain why.

8. A nail disorder is an unhealthy nail condition that is hereditary or caused by injury or disease of the nail unit.

   T   F   _____

9. It is rare for people to experience one of any number of common nail disorders.

   T   F   _____

10. You may help your clients with nail disorders by telling them you observed what may be an unhealthy condition and refer them to a healthcare provider.

    T   F   _____

11. You are not allowed to improve the appearance of certain conditions you observe in your clients' nails, even if the problem is cosmetic and not a medical condition or disorder.

    T   F   _____

12. It is your professional responsibility and a requirement of your license to know which nails can and cannot be safely worked on in a salon.

    T   F   _____

13. A client whose nail or skin is infected, inflamed, broken, or swollen should not receive salon services, unless the issue involves ingrown toenails.

    T   F   _____

14. What general practice can reduce the spread of nail infections between clients?

   _____

   _____

   _____

15. What should you do if you find that your clients' nails are repeatedly infected?

   _____

   _____

   _____

16. How often should you change your disinfectant solution?

   _____

   _____

   _____

17. To avoid infections, how should you handle metal implements, reusable implements, and single-use items? What are two examples of single-use items?

   _____

   _____

   _____

18. How should towels and table surfaces be handled for each procedure?

   _____

   _____

   _____

Indicate whether each statement is true or false. For any false statements, explain why they are false.

19. It is unlikely that you will encounter nail diseases in the salon.

    T   F   _____

20. Signs of infection or inflammation include broken skin, redness, pain, swelling, or pus.

    T   F   _____

21. Clients whose nail conditions or diseases show signs of infection or inflammation can be treated or diagnosed in the salon.

    T   F   _____

22. If your client has a physician's note explaining your client's nail disease, you are permitted to provide nail services to them.

    T   F   _____

23. While it is not critical that you know the names of all nail diseases, it is vital that you be able to identify whether an unhealthy condition exists.

    T   F   _____

24. Onychosis refers to any natural nail deformity or disease.

    T   F   _____

ROLE PLAY

25. It is important for all cosmetologists to be able to identify nail diseases that cannot be treated at a salon. For this activity, first you will find images of the different nail diseases and disorders from your textbook (Tables 6-1 and 6-2). On the back of each image or a separate sheet of paper, write the condition and whether a cosmetologist is able to perform a service. Then pair with a partner and alternate roles, playing a client who has a nail condition from one of their images and a cosmetologist who needs to decide whether to accept or refuse service. What tips can help you remember which nail conditions are safe and which are not, especially if they look similar?

26. What does frequent exposure to soaps, solvents, and similar substances do to the skin?

    A) keeps it clean

    B) removes the natural oils

    C) irritates it

    D) builds up its strength

27. What type of gloves are recommended to be worn to protect your hands while working as a licensed cosmetologist?

    A) latex

    B) rubber

    C) nitrile

    D) polyester

28. If you are unsure how to safely handle and use a specific product, contact the product manufacturer. You also might want to look up or obtain the SDS for the product. What does SDS stand for?

    A) Safety Design Sheet

    B) Single Data Source

    C) Safety Data Sheet

    D) Safety Data Supplement

Hand, Nail, and Skin Analysis

SHORT ANSWER

29. What are the goals of performing a hand, nail, and skin analysis on your clients?

    _____

    _____

    _____

30. What are three signs of infection?

    _____

    _____

    _____

31. What is the first step of any hand, nail, and skin analysis?

_____

_____

_____

32. What five things should you observe with sight and touch during the hand, nail, and skin analysis?

_____

_____

_____

33. When you are examining the skin's moisture level, what are you looking for?

_____

_____

_____

34. What will the skin's temperature tell you?

_____

_____

_____

35. If the condition of the skin is red, what might that indicate?

_____

_____

_____

36. When examining for tenderness to touch, what are you trying to determine?

_____

_____

_____

37. What specific areas of the nail unit should you look at during the analysis?

_____

_____

_____

38. Once you've completed your analysis, what four pieces of information do you share with your client?

_____

_____

_____

ROLE PLAY

39. For this activity, you and a partner will perform a hand, nail, and skin analysis on each other.

    Before you meet with your partner, review the steps recommended for the analysis in your text and sketch out a list of specific questions that you plan to ask your "client" (partner) during the analysis. Your questions should be designed to gain specific information about your client, such as lifestyle habits; any recent changes in their skin; use of medications; and any home care they perform on their hands, nails, skin, and soon. Be sure to wear gloves when doing the analysis, as you would with any client.

    As you perform the analysis, jot down your observations and your client's responses. Use your observations and notes to prepare for the final part of the analysis in which you share your findings with your client.

    After you've shared your findings with each other and completed the analysis, take a few moments to reflect on what you learned from your partner's technique; what went well; what was challenging; and any changes you think you should make to your approach for future hand, nail, and skin analyses.

Scope of Practice

RESEARCH

40. Search online for your license's scope of practice, found in your state's cosmetology laws or statutes under Definitions. Review it very carefully, and while you do so, think about where you live, if you're planning to move to another state, which cosmetology services you are interested in performing once you're licensed, and how the scope of practice for your state might affect the direction of your studies. Then, write four to five sentences that summarize the specific scope of practice that applies to your situation.

DISCOVERIES AND ACCOMPLISHMENTS

In the space below, write notes about key concepts discussed in this chapter. Share your discoveries with some of the other students in your class and ask them if your notes are helpful. You may want to revise your notes based on good ideas shared by your peers.

Discoveries:

_____

_____

_____

_____

_____

_____

_____

List at least three things you have accomplished since you decided to enroll in school.

Accomplishments:

_____

_____

_____

_____

_____

_____

_____

1. Why should cosmetologists have a thorough understanding of nail disorders and diseases?

   A) Cosmetologists need to ignore medical conditions that require a healthcare provider's attention.

   B) Cosmetologists need to identify any unhealthy conditions on clients' nails and determine if they can be treated in the salon.

   C) Cosmetologists are required to tell a client that a specific nail disease or disorder is present.

   D) Cosmetologists are licensed to diagnose, treat, prescribe, or work on unhealthy skin or nails.

2. As a cosmetologist, you should _____.

   A) be licensed to diagnose, treat, prescribe, or work on unhealthy skin or nails

   B) be able to tell a client that a specific nail disease or disorder is present

   C) identify whether a client has an unhealthy condition that prevents the client from receiving salon services

   D) improve the appearance of certain nail conditions if the problem is a medical condition or disorder

3. Which of the following is a symptom of a nail disorder called Beau's lines?

   A) dark purplish spots, usually due to a small nail bed injury

   B) a noticeably thin white nail plate that is more flexible than usual

   C) depressions running across the nail plate's width due to a slowing production of matrix cells

   D) damaged skin around the nail plate, which is often on the eponychium, that splits or tears

4. Which of the following refers to a noticeably thin white nail plate that is more flexible than usual and is typically caused by poor diet, heredity, medication, internal disease, or overfiling with an abrasive?

   A) hangnail   C) nail psoriasis

   B) eggshell nail   D) onychophagy

5. Which of the following terms refers to irregular split or brittle nails appearing as nail plate surface roughness, potentially a result of heredity, excessive exposure to cuticle removers, matrix injuries, harsh cleaning agents, or aggressive filing techniques?

   A) nail psoriasis   C) onychophagy

   B) splinter hemorrhage   D) onychorrhexis

continued

6. Lengthwise grooves in the nail plate that are typically the result of aging are referred to as a(n) _____.

A) plicatured nail   C) pincer nail

B) ridged nail   D) eggshell nail

7. Which of the following is most likely a sign of onychophagy?

A) irregular split or brittle nails appearing as nail plate surface roughness

B) bitten nails

C) increased nail curvature of the free edge

D) nail surface pitting

8. Which of the following is most likely a symptom of nail psoriasis?

A) whitish discolored spots on the nails, usually caused by a minor injury to the nail matrix

B) nail surface pitting, onycholysis, roughness, and randomly or evenly spaced bed discolorations

C) depressions running across the nail plate's width due to a slowing production of matrix cells

D) a noticeably thin white nail plate that is more flexible than usual

9. Identify a true statement about the nail disorder called nail pterygium.

A) Nail pterygium refers to bitten nails and can be cured by frequent manicures.

B) Cosmetologists should never attempt to treat or push back nail pterygium with any instrument.

C) The symptoms of nail pterygium include nail surface pitting, roughness, and onycholysis.

D) Nail pterygium refers to significant nail darkening caused by increased pigment cells.

10. Damage to the capillaries under the nail, caused by physical trauma or nail bed injury, is typically a sign of _____.

A) onychorrhexis   C) nail pterygium

B) splinter hemorrhage   D) nail psoriasis

continued

11. What should cosmetologists do to reduce the risk of spreading nail infections between clients?

   A) They should utilize shortcuts when cleaning and disinfecting to save time.

   B) They should reuse items such as buffers, nail files, and wooden pusher sticks.

   C) They should tell clients that a specific nail disease is present if they find associated symptoms.

   D) They should always mix disinfectants according to the product label, use them correctly, and follow the steps of implementation and disinfection of the work station.

12. Any natural nail disease or deformity is known as _____.

   A) dermatitis   C) onychosis

   B) eczema   D) impetigo

13. Matrix inflammation and nail shedding, resulting from injury or infection, is known as _____.

   A) impetigo   C) onychomycosis

   B) onychia   D) paronychia

14. Paronychia refers to _____.

   A) bacterial inflammation of the tissues around the nail plate, causing pus, swelling, and redness

   B) fungal infections of the feet, seen as red patches or scaling of the skin on the bottom of feet

   C) separation of the nail plate and nail bed, often due to injury or allergic reactions

   D) ingrown nails, wherein the nail grows into the sides of the tissue around the nail

15. Which of the following is most likely a symptom of a nail infection caused by *Pseudomonas aeruginosa*?

   A) whitish patches that can be scraped off the nail's surface

   B) a yellow–green spot that becomes darker in its advanced stage

   C) matrix inflammation and nail shedding

   D) lengthwise grooves in the nail plate

continued

16. Severe nail inflammation, in which a lump of red tissue grows up from the nail bed to the nail plate, is known as _____.

    A) tinea pedis

    B) splinter hemorrhage

    C) pyogenic granuloma

    D) nail pterygium

17. Tinea pedis _____.

    A) refers to the bacterial inflammation of the tissues around the nail plate

    B) is the medical term for fungal infections of the feet

    C) is also known as an eggshell nail

    D) refers to ingrown nails, wherein the nail grows into the sides of the tissue around the nail

18. A nail plate fungal infection, consisting of whitish patches that can be scraped off the nail's surface or long whitish or pale yellowish streaks within the nail plate, is referred to as _____.

    A) tinea pedis

    B) onychocryptosis

    C) pyogenic granuloma

    D) onychomycosis

19. Identify a point that cosmetologists should keep in mind.

    A) Frequent exposure to soaps, solvents, and similar substances replenishes the skin's natural oils.

    B) Nitrile gloves are more likely to cause allergic reactions than latex or rubber gloves.

    C) When the skin is broken or cut, germs can enter the body and cause infection.

    D) Leukonychia is a nail disorder that indicates a serious nail disease.

20. Identify the first step in performing a hand, nail, and skin analysis.

    A) examining the condition and length of the client's nails

    B) cleaning the hands of both the cosmetologist and the client

    C) feeling the client's hands and asking if there is any pain

    D) checking the skin's moisture level

continued

21. Which of the following should be ensured by a cosmetologist when performing a hand, nail, and skin analysis?

    A) The skin should be either cold or warm.

    B) The nails should have whitish spots, which indicate that the nails are healthy.

    C) The skin should be soft and supple and have no signs of dehydration or flaking.

    D) The nails should have depressions that run across the nail plate's width.

22. In the context of skin analysis, cold skin most likely indicates _____.

    A) infection   C) inflammation

    B) poor blood circulation   D) increased blood flow

23. Which of the following should be asked or stated by a cosmetologist when analyzing a client's hand, nail, and skin?

    A) Have you been diagnosed with leukonychia?

    B) You have a nail disease called onychomadesis that is caused by infection.

    C) Do you take medication for diabetes, high blood pressure, or chemotherapy?

    D) You have an infected finger, but you can avail nail services.

24. In the United States, nail services are governed under _____.

    A) personal injury laws   C) cosmetology laws

    B) entertainment laws   D) health laws

25. In the context of cosmetology laws in the United States, which of the following statements is true?

    A) In most states, the definition of manicuring includes removing hair.

    B) Anyone licensed under cosmetology can perform a procedure that is listed under any medical license or podiatry license.

    C) Beauty services and cosmetics affect the body rather than enhancing one's appearance.

    D) In some states, an individual licensed under cosmetology cannot perform acts listed in the definition of any other license in that state unless otherwise licensed.

finished!

Ch. 07: Hair and Scalp Properties

Why Study Hair and Scalp Properties?

SHORT ANSWER

1. What is the first step in providing services that maintain the health and integrity of your clients' hair and scalp?

    _____

    _____

    _____

2. Why is it important to understand how the hair structure is formed and how hairstyling and chemical services alter hair?

    _____

    _____

    _____

3. What will help you, as a cosmetologist, make better recommendations for your clients' hair loss treatments?

_____

_____

_____

4. In your own words, why do you think it's important for a cosmetologist to study the properties of the hair and scalp? What excites you most about gaining an understanding of the properties of the hair and scalp?

_____

_____

_____

Hair Root Structure

MULTIPLE CHOICE

5. What does the Greek root word in *trichology* (*trichos*) mean?

   A) worm

   B) hair

   C) strand

   D) root

6. Where is the hair root located?

   A) above the epidermis

   B) below the epidermis

   C) on the palms of the hands and soles of the feet

   D) only in the scalp

7. Where is the hair shaft located?

   A) above the epidermis

   B) below the epidermis

   C) on the palms of the hands and soles of the feet

   D) only in the scalp

8. Which body system do hair, skin, and nails belong to?

    A) circulatory   C) integumentary

    B) nervous   D) glandular

9. Although hair is no longer needed for warmth and protection, it still impacts our _____ in significant ways.

    A) personality   B) body temperature

    C) defenses   D) psychology

MATCHING

10. Use the word bank to match the five main structures of the hair root with their descriptions. Each structure will be used twice.

Word bank: hair bulb, hair follicle, sebaceous glands, arrector pili muscle, dermal papillae

_____ Contraction of this structure causes the hair to stand up, resulting in "goose bumps"

_____ Found at the base of the hair follicle

_____ Contains blood vessels that supply nutrients that allow the hair to grow

_____ Tube-like structure that surrounds the hair root and anchors the hair in the skin or scalp

_____ Produces a substance called sebum, also known as oil, which lubricates the hair and skin

_____ Involuntary muscle in the dermis that attaches to the hair follicle

_____ Cone-shaped elevation at the base of the hair bulb

_____ Attached to the hair follicle

_____ Bulb-shaped; contains living cells that will form the hair strand

_____ Not found on the palms of the hands or the soles of the feet

11. Label the numbered parts in the illustration below.

1. Hair root
2. Hair follicle

3. Hair shaft
4. Hair bulb

5. Epidermis

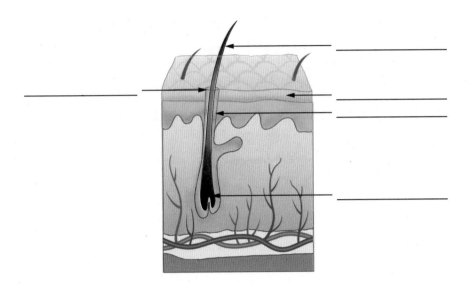

Hair Shaft Structure

TRUE OR FALSE

Indicate whether the statements below are true or false. For any false statements, explain why they are false.

12. Beard hair always contains a medulla.

    T   F   _____

13. All hair types have a medulla.

    T   F   _____

14. The hair cuticle is responsible for hair's strength, elasticity, and color.

    T   F   _____

15. The cortex is the fibrous protein layer of the hair and contributes to about 20 percent of hair's weight.

    T   F   _____

16. The hair cuticle is the hair's outermost layer and is formed from cells that overlap, similar to shingles on a roof.

    T   F   _____

17. The cortex is also known as the hair's pith or core.

    T   F   _____

18. The hair cuticle protects the cortex.

    T   F   _____

19. In healthy hair, the cuticle lies flat, but during chemical services, it will shrink, making it difficult for the chemicals to penetrate the cortex.

    T   F   _____

20. The hair shaft, also known as the hair strand or hair fiber, is the living portion of hair that extends beyond the skin or scalp.

    T   F   _____

21. Label the numbered parts of the hair shaft illustrated below.

    1. Medulla   2. Cortex   3. Cuticle

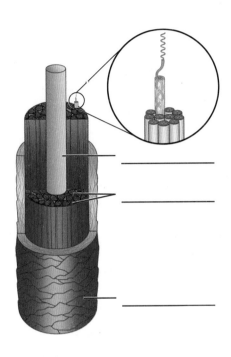

Chemical Composition of Hair

SHORT ANSWER

22. What is the name of the fibrous protein that makes up 90 percent of hair? What is the composition of the remaining 10 percent of hair?

    _____

    _____

    _____

23. Where are the living cells that keratinize to form hair located?

    _____

    _____

    _____

24. What are the five COHNS elements that make up human hair? List the percentage of each element that is found in a typical hair strand.

_____

_____

_____

25. What are the protein building blocks that comprise hair called?

_____

_____

_____

26. What is the name of the very strong chemical bond that links amino acids end to end?

_____

_____

_____

27. Describe a polypeptide chain.

_____

_____

_____

SEQUENCE

28. Number the following steps of the keratinization process from beginning to end.

_____ The hair strand emerges from the scalp.

_____ The cells move upward, lose their nucleus, and die.

_____ Cells mature and fill up with keratin.

_____ The hair strand's cells are completely keratinized.

_____ The hair strand's cells are dead.

29. The side bonds that link across the polypeptide chains in the cortex are responsible for hair's strength and _____.

    A) pigment

    B) elasticity

    C) life cycle

    D) direction

30. What are the three types of side bonds?

    A) hydrogen, carbon, and disulfide

    B) hydrogen, salt, and nitrogen

    C) hydrogen, salt, and disulfide

    D) helix, salt, and disulfide

31. The side bonds account for about _____ of hair's overall strength.

    A) 1/2

    B) 1/3

    C) 1/4

    D) 1/10

32. Which of the following is a weak physical bond?

    A) hydrogen

    B) disulfide

    C) side

    D) end-to-end

33. How can a hydrogen bond be broken?

    A) during vigorous brushing

    B) by a change in pH, such as from the application of strong alkaline or acidic solutions

    C) by water or heat, such as during wet and thermal styling

    D) It cannot be broken.

34. How can a salt bond be broken?

    A) during vigorous brushing

    B) by a change in pH, such as from the application of strong alkaline or acidic solutions

    C) by water or heat, such as during wet and thermal styling

    D) It cannot be broken.

35. A disulfide bond is a strong _____ side bond.

   A) chemical   C) physical

   B) salt   D) end-to-end

36. What will alter disulfide bonds?

   A) hair spray   C) thermal conditioners

   B) hair relaxers   D) water

37. Which of the following is *not* a recommended precaution to take before using thermal styling tools, to ensure that hair is protected?

   A) use heat protectant styling products

   B) choose the correct thermal tools and use the tool's recommended settings

   C) test the tools out on your own hair first

   D) conduct research on curling and flat irons before purchasing them

CREATE

38. Create a set of flashcards from the two lists below—front and back of card—to test yourself on the characteristics of the different side bonds. Make sure that you include the correct characteristic with the correct side bond, then test yourself with a partner. If you wish to make the flash cards more challenging for either you or your partner, feel free to add more characteristics beyond what's on the list.

Front of Card TYPE OF BOND
disulfide peptide hydrogen salt

Back of Card CHARACTERISTIC
• Broken by permanent wave solutions • Broken by chemical depilatories • Weak physical bond • Strong chemical bond • Broken by alkaline or acidic solutions • When broken, can be reformed by drying or cooling • Very strong chemical bond • When broken, cannot be reformed • When broken, can be reformed by balancing the pH

39. Describe melanin, the pigment that creates natural hair color. Be sure to specify its location and the name of the cells from which it forms.

_____

_____

_____

40. What are the two types of melanin? Describe their pigments and identify the hair colors in which they are each predominant.

_____

_____

_____

41. How does the beauty industry distinguish between the terms *hair color* and *haircolor*?

_____

_____

_____

42. What causes gray hair? How does gray hair grow compared to pigmented hair?

_____

_____

_____

WORD SCRAMBLE

43. Unscramble the answer to each clue below.

_____	YLOCI	The four types of wave patterns are straight, wavy, curly, and _____.
_____	VPEWTRTNEA	Refers to the amount of movement or shape of the hair strand. (2 words)
_____	LTTFRAE; IURCLRE	The _____ the hair follicle is, the _____ the hair will be.

_____	ENGECTIS	Influences wave patterns
_____	NURDO	Shape of the cross-section of hair that results in straight hair
_____	AOLV	Shape of the cross-section of hair that results in wavy or curly hair
_____	ILILPTCLAE	Shape of the cross-section of hair that results in coily hair
_____	RMHNEOOS	Can affect the wave pattern over someone's lifetime
_____	INZGRMIOSIUT	One type of product recommended for very curly (coily) hair, to prevent breakage between the twists and coils
_____	UEBMS	Substance whose ability to lubricate and moisturize the hair and scalp is affected by the shape of the hair follicle
_____	TLDGENRLAE	Another type of solution recommended for very curly (coily) hair, to prevent breakage between the twists and coils
_____	LFICELOL	The part of the hair structure that determines the shape of the hair strand
_____	YCLRU	Type of wave pattern in hair that tends to be drier

TRUE OR FALSE

Indicate whether the statements below are true or false. For any false statements, explain why they are false.

44. Analyzing a client's wave pattern is an important component of haircutting and hairstyling.

    T   F   _____

45. Wave pattern is the only area of a hair analysis that looks at the strength and condition of the hair.

    T   F   _____

46. Wave pattern remains uniform throughout a person's head.

    T   F   _____

47. All wave patterns are possible in anyone, regardless of genetics.

    T   F   _____

Scalp and Hair Analysis

48. Match the type of hair texture with its description and styling recommendations. Each texture will be used three times.

   a. fine   b. medium   c. coarse

   Cell Part   **Description/Function**

   _____ Largest diameter

   _____ Does not present problems or concerns in styling

   _____ Can be dry and/or frizzy

   _____ May feel limp or flat

   _____ The standard to which other hair textures are compared

   _____ May process faster during chemical services; requires lower heat during thermal services

   _____ Average diameter

   _____ May require stronger chemicals; requires higher temperatures during thermal services

   _____ Smallest diameter

SHORT ANSWER

49. What are three goals of the scalp and hair analysis?

   _____

   _____

   _____

50. List three conditions of the hair and scalp that might prevent you from performing services on a client's hair.

   _____

   _____

   _____

51. What are the six items that a cosmetologist will examine during a hair and scalp analysis?

_____

_____

_____

52. Describe the process for analyzing the texture of a client's hair. In your description, explain how you can determine whether the client's hair has a fine, medium, or coarse texture.

_____

_____

_____

MULTIPLE CHOICE

53. What does hair density measure?

    A) the number of individual hair strands per 1 square centimeter of scalp

    B) the number of individual hair strands per 1 square inch of scalp

    C) the average number of individual hair strands per 1 square centimeter of scalp, based on samples taken from four locations on the head

    D) the average number of individual hair strands per 1 square inch of scalp, based on samples taken from four locations on the head

54. What is the average hair density?

    A) approximately 2,200 hairs per square inch, totaling about 22,000 hairs on the scalp

    B) approximately 2,200 hairs per square centimeter, totaling about 22,000 hairs on the scalp

    C) approximately 2,200 hairs per 1 square inch, totaling about 100,000 hairs on the scalp

    D) approximately 2,200 hairs per 1 square centimeter, totaling about 100,000 hairs on the scalp

55. Natural blondes usually have the _____ hair density.

   A) lowest   C) lightest

   B) highest   D) most coarse

56. Natural redheads usually have the _____ hair density.

   A) lowest   C) lightest

   B) highest   D) most coarse

57. Which of the following correctly lists the natural hair colors in order from lowest to highest density?

   A) red, black, brown, blonde   C) blonde, black, brown, red

   B) red, blonde, black, brown   D) blonde, brown, red, black

SHORT ANSWER

58. What should you examine when you analyze a client's hair to determine its density? How do you determine whether the hair density is thin (low), medium, or thick (high)?

   _____

   _____

   _____

59. What steps should be taken to analyze the porosity of a client's hair? What characteristics of the hair will indicate low, normal, and high porosity?

   _____

   _____

   _____

60. Use the words from the word bank to complete the paragraphs below. Some words will be used more than once.

    Word bank: flat, low, high, processing, alkaline, moisture, raise, porosity, higher, average, overprocessed, porous, saturation, cuticle, process

    a. The hair's ability to absorb _____ is referred to as hair _____. Porosity is determined by the condition of the _____ layer and to what extent the "scales" of the _____ are raised.

    b. If the _____ is very healthy, the scales lie _____, which gives the hair _____ porosity. Chemical services performed on hair with _____ porosity require a solution that has _____ alkalinity to _____ the cuticle and allow _____ and _____ to occur evenly and thoroughly.

    c. If the _____ is raised in some places, the hair is considered to have _____ porosity, but the hair is still healthy. Chemical services performed usually _____ as expected.

    d. When hair has been _____ previously, it will appear damaged, dry, fragile, and brittle with a _____ porosity. Chemical services performed on overly _____ hair require less _____ solutions, with a lower pH, to prevent additional overprocessing and damage.

Indicate whether each statement is true or false. For any false statements, explain why they are false.

61. It's best to test the elasticity of hair when it is dry.

    T   F   _____

62. When testing for hair elasticity, you should check two areas of the head (front hairline and nape) because hair elasticity varies around the head.

    T   F   _____

63. Hair elasticity is an indicator of the hair's ability to stretch and return to its original length without breaking.

    T   F   _____

64. Dry hair with average elasticity will stretch up to 50 percent of its length and return to that same length without breaking. Wet hair stretches about 20 percent of its length.

    T   F   _____

65. The strength of the side bonds in the cortex is directly related to hair's elasticity.

    T   F   _____

66. Hair with low elasticity may require a solution with a lower pH to minimize further damage; additionally, it might not maintain a strong curl pattern when chemical services are performed.

    T   F   _____

67. If hair feels brittle and breaks easily, you should take precautions to accommodate its high elasticity.

    T   F   _____

SHORT ANSWER

68. How should you analyze the elasticity of a client's hair? How will you know whether a client's hair has low, average, or high elasticity?

    _____

    _____

    _____

69. When hair grows at a perpendicular or 90-degree angle to the head (or in an otherwise straight direction from the head), what are three possible hair patterns that might emerge?

    _____

    _____

    _____

70. What causes a natural part?

_____

_____

_____

71. What is the term for hair flowing in the same direction, and what causes it?

_____

_____

_____

72. While conducting your hair analysis on a client, you notice hair that has grown in a circular pattern. What is the term for that? What is causing it?

_____

_____

_____

73. If hair grows straight up or at a different angle than the other hair, it's called a cowlick. Where are cowlicks typically found on the head?

_____

_____

_____

MATCHING

74. Match each phrase with "dry hair and scalp" (D) or "oily hair and scalp" (O) based on which condition it relates to.

_____ Excessive shampooing and changes in climate can aggravate this hair.

_____ Overactive sebaceous glands are responsible for this condition.

_____ For this hair, cosmetologists should recommend a shampoo that returns the scalp to its natural pH.

_____ The lack of sebum can cause this kind of hair to look dull and lifeless.

_____ This kind of hair should avoid products with a high alcohol content.

_____ Make sure not to confuse this type of hair with overly porous hair.

_____ This kind of hair should avoid harsh products to avoid exacerbating its condition.

_____ This kind of hair should be rinsed hair thoroughly after shampooing.

_____ Products for this hair type should include emollients.

ROLE PLAY

75. Take some time to research and identify (1) four possible shampoos that you, as a cosmetologist, would recommend to a client who has dry hair and a dry scalp and (2) four shampoos that you would recommend to someone with oily hair and scalp from a range of products and prices. Follow the website link or use a separate sheet of paper to fill in the chart to keep this information organized. Note the benefits advertised for each one, as well as any specific ingredients that you think would help these conditions.

    Next, partner with a classmate and role play a cosmetologist and a client. The first client should describe their dry hair/scalp to the cosmetologist and include factors such as climate and hair care routines. The cosmetologist will then explain how each product they researched might benefit them. The client should ask questions and decide on the best product based on the discussion. Then switch roles—this time the person in the role of client has an oily scalp and needs recommendations to improve that condition.

    The point is to engage in a realistic discussion—one that is very likely to occur in any salon—discovering where you might need more information and learning about the current available products. It might feel awkward at first, but if you practice having this conversation with your classmate now, you will be more prepared for your real-life clients.

+ BONUS

Visit: bonus.milady.com/cos-wb/toc

SHAMPOO TYPE	DRY HAIR	DRY HAIR	DRY HAIR	DRY HAIR	OILY HAIR	OILY HAIR	OILY HAIR	OILY HAIR
Name								
Hair Texture								
Price								
Benefits								
Specific Ingredients								

Hair Growth

CROSSWORD

76. Complete the crossword puzzle using the clues provided.

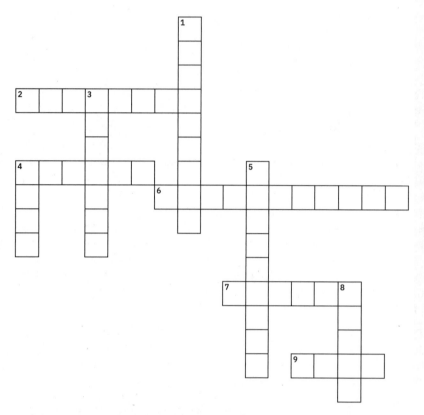

Across

2. Type of long pigmented hair on the scalp and body.
4. Short, fine hair that covers a fetus; generally sheds within a few weeks of birth.
6. One of two primary functions of vellus hair is to help regulate body _____.
7. Short, fine unpigmented body hair often referred to as peach fuzz.
9. Type of terminal hair that is not pigmented.

Down

1. All are capable of producing either vellus or terminal hair, depending on genetics, age, and hormones.
3. Terminal hair is coarser than vellus hair and may or may not have a _____.
4. Vellus hair can appear anywhere on the skin except on the palms, soles, and _____.
5. The type of gland missing from the follicles that produce vellus hair.
8. One of two primary functions of vellus hair is to help evaporate _____.

WORD SCRAMBLE AND MATCHING

77. Unscramble the names of the hair growth phases below. Then match them with their features and descriptions. Each phase will be used three times.

a. aengan   b. geltone   c. gnaecta

_____ Marked by hair shedding—a natural part of the hair's growth cycle—with 50 to 100 hairs lost each day

_____ Brief transition period between the other two phases

_____ Known as the growth phase

_____ The follicle canal shrinks and detaches from the dermal papilla, the hair bulb disappears, and the shrunken root end forms a rounded club

_____ Just under 10 percent of scalp hair is in this phase at any time, with the phase lasting three to six months

_____ The final hair cycle phase, also known as the resting phase

_____ 90 percent of hair is in this phase at any time, with the phase lasting from two to six years, and up to ten

_____ New cells are produced in the follicle faster than any other cell in the body, with an average monthly growth rate for healthy scalp hair of about 0.5 inch (1.25 centimeters)

_____ Less than 1 percent of scalp hair is in this one- to two-week phase at any time

TRUE OR FALSE

Indicate whether the statements below are true or false. For any false statements, explain why they are false.

78. Scalp massage can stimulate blood microcirculation, which provides nutrients to the hair follicle.

    T   F   _____

79. It has been scientifically proven that stimulation or scalp massage increases hair growth.

    T   F   _____

80. Minoxidil and finasteride are the only scientifically proven treatments to help stop hair loss and possibly regrow hair

    T   F   _____

81. Minoxidil and finasteride, both treatments for hair loss, are awaiting approval by the Food and Drug Administration (FDA).

    T   F   _____

82. Gray hair is less resistant than pigmented hair.

    T   F   _____

83. Genetics determines hair growth rate.

    T   F   _____

84. Once the hair grows 0.2 to 0.8 inch (a centimeter or two) away from the skin, it will be the same color it was before shaving.

    T   F   _____

85. Shaving and cutting hair causes it to grow back with a coarser texture.

T   F   _____

DISCOVERIES AND ACCOMPLISHMENTS

In the space below, write notes about key concepts discussed in this chapter. Share your discoveries with some of the other students in your class and ask them if your notes are helpful. You may want to revise your notes based on good ideas shared by your peers.

Discoveries:

_____

_____

_____

_____

_____

_____

_____

List at least three things you have accomplished since you decided to enroll in school.

Accomplishments:

_____

_____

_____

_____

_____

_____

_____

1. Cosmetologists should have a thorough understanding of the properties of the hair and scalp because _____.

   A) they are physicians specialized in a medical branch of science that involves the study of the hair and its structure

   B) understanding how the hair structure is formed, and how hairstyling and chemical services alter hair, will lead to safer, smarter services

   C) they are responsible for informing clients about the parts of the hair that will be affected by the hair services availed by them

   D) they are licensed to diagnose, treat, prescribe, or work on unhealthy hair and scalp

2. Which of the following refers to the study of the hair, including its diseases and care?

   A) hematology   C) trichology

   B) rheumatology   D) podiatry

3. Identify the part of the hair that is located below the surface of the epidermis.

   A) the hair root   C) the hair cuticle

   B) the cortex   D) the hair shaft

4. Which of the following statements is true of the hair bulb?

   A) It is the living portion of the hair found above the epidermis.

   B) It contains living cells that form the hair strand.

   C) It produces sebum that lubricates the hair and skin.

   D) It is the nonliving part of the hair attached to the hair shaft.

5. The _____ muscle is an involuntary muscle in the dermis that attaches to the hair follicle.

   A) adductor longus   C) arrector pili

   B) deltoid   D) soleus

continued

6. Identify a true statement about the hair cuticle.

   A) It protects the cortex.

   B) It is the fibrous protein layer of the hair.

   C) It contributes to about 90 percent of the hair's weight.

   D) It is part of the hair root.

7. Which of the following is a function of the cortex?

   A) It contributes to 50 percent of the hair's weight.

   B) It is responsible for the hair's strength, elasticity, and color.

   C) It contains living cells that form the hair strand.

   D) It produces sebum that lubricates the hair and skin.

8. The _____ is the innermost layer found in coarse hair and beard hair and is also known as the hair's pith or core.

   A) hair bulb   C) medulla

   B) hair cuticle   D) cortex

9. Which of the following statements best describes keratinization?

   A) It is the process by which sebaceous glands enhance the production of keratin by melanocytes.

   B) It is the process by which the amount of keratin in the skin helps determine skin color.

   C) It is the process by which newly formed cells in the hair bulb mature, fill with keratin, move upward, lose their nucleus, and die.

   D) It is the process by which sebum, lipids, keratin, sweat, and water form a hydrolipidic film to protect the skin from drying out.

10. Which of the following refers to tiny grains of pigment in the cortex that give natural color to the hair?

   A) collagen   C) keratin

   B) elastin   D) melanin

continued

11. The _____ of the hair refers to the amount of movement or shape of the hair strand.

    A) growth pattern   C) elasticity

    B) wave pattern   D) porosity

12. _____ is the diameter of an individual hair strand.

    A) Hair texture   C) Hair porosity

    B) Hair density   D) Hair elasticity

13. Identify a difference between fine hair and coarse hair.

    A) Fine hair requires strong chemicals, whereas coarse hair requires relatively weaker chemicals.

    B) Fine hair is typically dry and frizzy, whereas coarse hair is usually flat and limp.

    C) Fine hair has the smallest diameter, whereas coarse hair has the largest diameter.

    D) Fine hair requires higher heat during thermal services, whereas coarse hair requires lower heat during thermal services.

14. Which of the following hair colors generally has the highest density?

    A) blonde   C) black

    B) brown   D) red

15. Which of the following statements best describes hair porosity?

    A) It is the hair's ability to stretch and return to its original length without breaking.

    B) It is the diameter of an individual hair strand.

    C) It measures the number of individual hair strands on 1 square inch of scalp.

    D) It refers to the hair's ability to absorb moisture.

16. Hair with _____ porosity has a very healthy cuticle where the scales lie flat.

    A) low   C) average

    B) medium   D) high

continued

17. The hair's ability to stretch and return to its original length without breaking is referred to as hair _____.

   A) elasticity   C) porosity

   B) density   D) texture

18. People with dry hair and scalp should _____.

   A) shampoo their hair frequently

   B) use strong soaps and detergents

   C) avoid using products containing emollients

   D) avoid products with high alcohol content

19. People with oily hair and scalp should _____.

   A) use a shampoo that changes the pH value of the scalp to around 10

   B) thoroughly rinse hair after shampooing

   C) use products that activate sebaceous glands

   D) use excessively harsh products as they can curb oil production

20. In the context of the main types of body hair, which of the following is short, fine, unpigmented body hair often referred to as peach fuzz?

   A) lanugo hair   B) vellus hair

   C) terminal hair   D) fetus hair

21. In the context of the hair growth cycle, the _____ phase is the growth phase.

   A) transition   C) catagen

   B) telogen   D) anagen

continued

22. Which of the following occurs during the anagen phase of the hair growth cycle?

    A) The hair sheds.   C) New hair is produced.

    B) The follicle canal shrinks.   D) The hair bulb disappears.

23. Which of the following occurs during the catagen phase of the hair growth cycle?

    A) The hair sheds.

    B) The follicle canal shrinks and detaches from the dermal papilla.

    C) New hair is produced.

    D) The hair bulb appears, and the enlarged root end forms a rounded club.

24. Which of the following statements is true of the telogen phase of the hair growth cycle?

    A) It is the final hair cycle phase.

    B) Less than 1 percent of scalp hair is in the telogen phase at any time.

    C) About 90 percent of scalp hair is in the telogen phase at any time.

    D) It lasts two to six years.

25. Which of the following is a myth about hair?

    A) Shaving and cutting hair makes it grow back darker and coarser.

    B) Scalp massage can stimulate blood microcirculation.

    C) Gray hair is the same as pigmented hair in terms of texture.

    D) Genetics determines the growth rate of hair.

finished!

Ch. 08: Hair and Scalp Disorders and Diseases

Why Study Hair and Scalp Disorders and Diseases?

SHORT ANSWER

1. In your own words, explain why you think it's important for cosmetologists to have a thorough understanding and knowledge of hair and scalp disorders.

   _____

   _____

   _____

2. In addition to your text, identify two possible resources that you would consider consulting for information about hair and scalp disorders and explain why you chose them.

_____

_____

_____

Hair Loss

SHORT ANSWER

3. What are three specific internal and external factors that can affect hair health?

_____

_____

_____

4. Imagine one of your clients asks you if diet supplements or other changes to their nutrition plan can serve as a "quick fix" to improve the health of their hair. What will you tell them?

_____

_____

_____

5. What role do androgens and thyroid hormones play in the loss or thinning of hair?

_____

_____

_____

6. List three examples of styling techniques, processes, or tools that might hinder hair growth.

_____

_____

_____

7. Match the types of alopecia listed below with their description, characteristics, and/or image. The number in parentheses ( ) after each type indicates how many times the type is used.

   a. alopecia areata (4)   c. androgenic alopecia (6)   e. alopecia totalis (1)
   b. alopecia (1)   d. alopecia universalis (1)   f. postpartum alopecia (2)

Study tip: Once you've correctly completed this activity, you might find it helpful to use the information from the matches to create a set of flash cards. You can write the types of alopecia on the front of the card and their characteristics on the back. Use them to test yourself or pair up with a partner.

_____ The partial or complete loss of hair from where it typically grows; common types are androgenic, areata, and postpartum

_____ One type of this pattern hair loss that generally manifests in a horseshoe shape

_____ Temporary hair loss that occurs one to five months after delivery, with hair growth cycles regulating within six to twelve months

_____ Caused by an autoimmune disorder where the immune system attacks the hair follicle; specifically, white blood cells stop hair growth during the anagen phase, which causes hair to enter the telogen (resting) phase

_____ Occurs in people of all sexes, ages, races, and ethnic backgrounds, and most often begins in childhood

_____ Hair loss characterized by the miniaturization of terminal hair and a shortened anagen (growth) phase

_____ One type of this pattern hair loss typically appears as a diffuse thinning over the crown, top of head, and temple area

_____ More advanced form of alopecia areata that involves the loss of terminal hair on the body and scalp

_____ One example of this type of hair loss is commonly experienced by women after menopause

_____ Hair loss in round or irregularly shaped patches

_____ Can affect anyone and is caused by genetics, age, or hormonal changes

_____ When more hairs than usual enter the telogen (resting) stage after pregnancy, causing hair loss

_____ More advanced form of alopecia areata that involves the loss of terminal scalp hair

_____ The scalp where the hair occurs usually normal in appearance, showing no obvious signs of inflammation, skin disorder, or disease

_____ Common type of hair loss, with approximately 50 percent of people experiencing some degree of hair loss after puberty and as early as their teenage years

LABELING

8. Label each image of alopecia shown below with its type.

   Study tip: To get a more complete sense of what alopecia might look like on a client, use the Internet to search for various images of alopecia and take some time to study the different types and their distinct features.

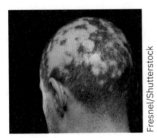
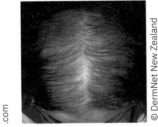
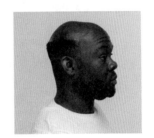

Fresnel/Shutterstock.com

© DermNet New Zealand

_____   _____   _____

ROLE PLAY

9. As a cosmetologist, you will likely encounter a variety of clients who are experiencing hair loss or thinning hair, so you will be in the unique position to guide them as a knowledgeable _and_ sensitive resource they can trust with an emotionally challenging condition. To prepare, you will need to develop a plan so that you can have an effective, supportive, and informative conversation with your clients about their hair loss. Read through each step and fill in the specifics, including any facts your clients might find useful, and answer the questions on a separate sheet of paper.

   1. Research and confirm your scope of practice regarding hair loss guidance in your state. Write the link to it and/or summarize what it says.

   2. Review hair loss types and possible causes. Jot down some notes from your text, or other research.

   3. Research current products and treatments available for hair loss/thinning hair, and identify those that are within your scope of practice (e.g., hair weave services, local wig companies, dietary supplements) and those that are not within your scope of practice (e.g., the latest medical and surgical options).

   4. Write out three or four initial fact-finding questions, as well as potential follow-up comments and questions that you would like to ask your client to obtain the information needed to provide them with appropriate guidance for their specific hair loss concerns. (e.g., diet, medications/medical conditions, hereditary patterns, stress, hair products and hair care routines). This step is your opportunity to refine your phrasing and focus on demonstrating care and sensitivity toward your clients.

5. Try out your script with a partner to further refine your approach and exchange tips and suggestions for having this conversation with your clients in the future.

Tip: Once you have outlined your plan for discussing hair loss with your clients here, you may want to type it up and keep it handy for future reference so that you can update it occasionally and make revisions based on how your conversations go.

MATCHING

10. Match the hair loss treatments and options with their descriptions. More than one treatment or option might match a description, so be sure to indicate all that apply.

    a. Minoxidil   c. Surgical options
    b. Finasteride   d. Nonmedical options

_____ Wigs and toupees, with guidance from a cosmetologist

_____ Hair transplant, which involves the removal of hair follicles from one or more areas of the head

_____ Rogaine© is the most well-known brand of this hair loss treatment

_____ Stimulates hair growth; slows the rate of hair loss

_____ More convenient and effective than minoxidil

_____ Permanent options

_____ Can cause birth defects in a male fetus, so can't be prescribed for people with childbearing potential

_____ Topical medication applied to the scalp

_____ Hair weavings and hair extensions completed by a cosmetologist

_____ Takes several months see results, and benefits end when an individual stops using the products

_____ Available in two different strengths: 2 percent (regular-strength solution) and 5 percent (extra-strength solution)

_____ Oral prescription medication

Hair Disorders

CROSSWORD

11. Complete the crossword puzzle using the clues provided.

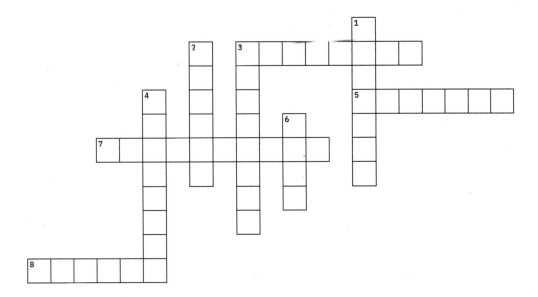

Across

3. A type of congenital canities present in people who are born without pigment in the skin, hair, and eyes.

5. The source of pigment in hair and skin.

7. One of two types of canities; present at birth.

8. If extreme, experiencing this or having an illness can contribute to graying hair.

Down

1. Canities results from the loss of the hair's natural _____.

2. A variety of canities where alternating bands of gray and pigmented hair appear throughout the length of the hair strand.

3. One of two types of canities; when the hair follicle produces less melanin as the result of aging and genetics.

4. Technical term for gray or white hair.

6. Except for the absence of pigment, gray hair is the _____ as pigmented hair.

12. Match each of the following hair disorders with their descriptions.

a. Monilethrix   c. Trichoptilosis   e. Hirsuties
b. Fragilitas criniumis   d. Hypertrichosis   f. Trichorrhexis nodosa

_____ Technical term for split ends

_____ Technical term for knotted hair

_____ Hair that grows longer and thicker than usual

_____ Technical term for beaded hair

_____ Growth of terminal body hair on face and chest; primarily affects women

_____ Technical term for brittle hair

Scalp Disorders

SHORT ANSWER

13. What is the name of the fungus that causes pityriasis, the technical term for dandruff? Briefly explain how it causes dandruff, and list three other factors that can affect dandruff.

_____

_____

_____

14. What type of agent (ingredient) is contained in antidandruff shampoos? How often should they be used to control dandruff?

_____

_____

_____

15. Is dandruff contagious?

_____

_____

_____

16. How are dandruff and dry scalp similar? What is the difference between them?

_____

_____

_____

17. What are the two main types of dandruff? Briefly describe each one.

_____

_____

_____

18. What should you do, as a cosmetologist, if you notice that your client has seborrheic dermatitis (dandruff accompanied by redness and inflammation, which is often also seen in the eyebrows or beard)?

_____

_____

_____

FILL IN THE BLANK

19. The table below lists fungal and parasitic infections and their causes, symptoms, method of spread, and other characteristics. In each row, three columns are missing information for that infection. Fill in the missing information based on the clues in the other columns.

NAME OF INFECTION	CAUSES	SYMPTOMS	METHOD OF SPREADING	OTHER NOTABLE CHARACTERISTICS
	Mites called *Sarcoptes scabiei* that lay eggs inside the skin			Mites cannot live longer than 24 to 48 hours without a host.
Tinea favosa				Scars may result; hair will not grow back in scarred areas.

NAME OF INFECTION	CAUSES	SYMPTOMS	METHOD OF SPREADING	OTHER NOTABLE CHARACTERISTICS
Tinea				This is the general technical term for ringworm.
		Using a magnifying glass, can see small nits attached to the hair; adult louse about the size of a sesame seed		They feed on human blood.
		Similar to tinea capitis in appearance; skin may be very inflamed		This primarily affects the beard and mustache areas of the face.
			Person-to-person; via infected skin and hair, as well as unclean bathtubs, swimming pools, and personal articles	This is also known as ringworm of the scalp.

WORD SCRAMBLE AND LABEL

20. Unscramble the words below and then use them to label the correct scalp disorder. One term will not be used.

   a. Cuslpdeisoi pscitias _____

   b. Ntiae vfsaoa _____

   c. Enait saciipt _____

   d. Aenit rbbaea _____

   e. Istpyaisir _____

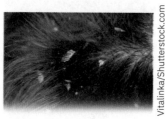
Vitalinka/Shutterstock.com

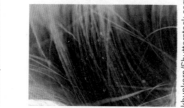
khunkorn/Shutterstock.com

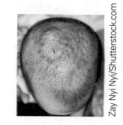
Zay Nyi Nyi/Shutterstock.com

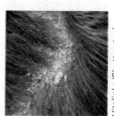
Vitalinka/Shutterstock.com

_____ _____ _____ _____

21. Which one of the following is *not* a type of bacterial infection of the scalp?

    A) folliculitis

    B) carbuncle

    C) psoriasis

    D) furuncle

22. Bacterial scalp infections are caused by either _____ or staphylococci bacteria.

    A) spirillum

    B) streptococci

    C) bacillus

    D) tinea barbae

23. What is the term for an inflammation caused by ingrown hairs where hair is plucked or shaved?

    A) folliculitis capitis

    B) tinea barbae

    C) tinea folliculitis

    D) folliculitis barbae

24. How do carbuncles present in a person?

    A) widespread across a large part of the body

    B) clusters of small red bumps or white-headed pimples

    C) as a cluster of boils

    D) as a single boil

25. What is another term for a boil?

    A) furuncle

    B) carbuncle

    C) blackhead

    D) vesicle

26. What is the best way to help prevent the spread of bacterial infections when performing services for clients?

    A) wear nitrile gloves and a face mask

    B) request a physician's note from a client confirming they are infection-free

    C) properly and consistently practice state board–approved cleaning and disinfection procedures

    D) sequester clients in a private room with high-grade ventilation

DISCOVERIES AND ACCOMPLISHMENTS

In the space below, write notes about key concepts discussed in this chapter. Share your discoveries with some of the other students in your class and ask them if your notes are helpful. You may want to revise your notes based on good ideas shared by your peers.

Discoveries:

_____

_____

_____

_____

_____

_____

_____

List at least three things you have accomplished since you decided to enroll in school.

Accomplishments:

_____

_____

_____

_____

_____

_____

_____

1. Cosmetologists should have a thorough understanding of hair and scalp disorders and diseases because _____.

   A) improving the appearance of certain scalp conditions that are medical disorders is the responsibility of cosmetologists

   B) identifying the differences between common and irregular hair loss helps them better recommend hair loss treatments to clients

   C) they are required to know that conditions that signal health problems seldom warrant a physician's attention

   D) they are licensed to diagnose, treat, prescribe, or work on unhealthy scalp

2. Why should cosmetologists have a thorough understanding of hair and scalp disorders and diseases?

   A) because cosmetologists are required to differentiate between common and irregular hair loss in order to treat hair and scalp disorders

   B) because cosmetologists are required to perform procedures that are listed under any medical license or podiatry license

   C) because cosmetologists' infection control duties include recognizing communicable scalp and hair conditions, as well as when a client should be turned away and referred to a physician

   D) because cosmetologists are required to tell a client that a specific disease or disorder is present

3. Which of the following statements is true of androgenic alopecia?

   A) It is hair loss characterized by a lengthened anagen phase.

   B) It is also known as alopecia areata.

   C) It is hair loss characterized by terminal hair miniaturization.

   D) It is a fungal infection.

4. Alopecia areata is _____.

   A) temporary hair loss after pregnancy

   B) also known as androgenetic alopecia

   C) an autoimmune disorder

   D) characterized by obvious signs of scalp inflammation

5. _____ include testosterone; they affect the dermal papilla and production of keratinocytes, resulting in hair follicle miniaturization and reduced hair growth.

   A) Estrogens   C) Thyroid hormones

   B) Androgens   D) Pancreatic hormones

continued

6. Which of the following statements related to hair loss treatments is true?

   A) Minoxidil is an oral prescription medication.

   B) Minoxidil comes in two different strengths: two percent and five percent minoxidil.

   C) Finasteride is less effective and convenient to take than minoxidil.

   D) Finasteride is prescribed for people with childbearing potential.

7. Which of the following statements related to the treatment of hair loss is accurate?

   A) A cosmetologist is licensed to perform surgical procedures as treatments for hair loss.

   B) A cosmetologist is allowed to help clients determine if their hair loss is typical or potentially concerning.

   C) Salon services, such as a hair spa, are the only proven treatment for hair loss.

   D) Advising clients facing hair loss problems on when to seek the help of a healthcare provider is out of a cosmetologist's scope of practice.

8. Identify a true statement about canities.

   A) It is the growth of terminal hair on a female's body in areas that typically do not have terminal hair.

   B) Acquired canities is present at birth.

   C) It is the technical term for gray or white hair and results from the loss of the hair's natural pigment.

   D) Congenital canities is a result of age and genetics.

9. As people age, the hair follicle produces less melanin, resulting in gray or white hair. This is termed _____.

   A) acquired canities   C) hypertrichosis

   B) congenital canities   D) trichoptilosis

10. Ringed hair is _____.

   A) a condition in which the hair grows longer or thicker than usual

   B) the technical term for split ends

   C) a variety of canities characterized by alternating bands of gray and pigmented hair throughout the hair strand's length

   D) typically characterized by brittleness and the formation of nodular swellings along the hair shaft

continued

11. Which of the following statements is true of hypertrichosis?

    A) It is a condition in which hair grows shorter or thinner than usual.

    B) It is hair loss characterized by terminal hair miniaturization and a shortened anagen phase.

    C) It is treated using methods such as photoepilation, electrolysis, and laser hair removal.

    D) It is characterized by brittleness and the formation of nodular swellings along the hair shaft.

12. What is the technical term for split ends?

    A) monilethrix

    B) canities

    C) hirsuties

    D) trichoptilosis

13. What is the only way to treat trichoptilosis?

    A) softening the hair with conditioners

    B) waxing

    C) sugaring

    D) cutting split ends

14. Which of the following is a true statement about trichorrhexis nodosa?

    A) Trichorrhexis nodosa is a condition in which the hair grows longer or thicker than usual.

    B) Trichorrhexis nodosa is caused by a gene mutation and has no recognized treatment.

    C) Trichorrhexis nodosa near the scalp often results from chemical straighteners or excessive thermal pressing.

    D) Trichorrhexis nodosa near the scalp is caused by a naturally occurring fungus called malassezia.

15. Which of the following is an accurate statement about monilethrix?

    A) People with monilethrix experience sparse hair growth.

    B) People with monilethrix should bleach their hair.

    C) Monilethrix has several recognized treatments.

    D) Monilethrix is the technical term for split ends.

continued

16. Fragilitas crinium is _____.

    A) characterized by brittleness and the formation of nodular swellings along the hair shaft

    B) typically treated using electrolysis, photoepilation, laser hair removal, shaving, tweezing, and depilatories

    C) caused by mechanical and chemical abuse, exposure to UV rays, and pulling the hair tightly into braids or ponytails

    D) hair loss characterized by terminal hair miniaturization and a shortened anagen phase

17. Pityriasis is characterized by _____.

    A) red spots at the openings of the hair follicles

    B) brittleness and the formation of nodular swellings along the hair shaft

    C) excessive production and shedding of skin cells

    D) dry yellow crusts on the scalp called scutula

18. Identify an accurate statement about dandruff.

    A) It is not contagious.

    B) Its technical term is fragilitas crinium.

    C) It is caused by dermatophyte fungus.

    D) It cannot be controlled by antidandruff shampoos.

19. The technical term for classic dandruff is _____, and it is characterized by scalp irritation, large flakes, and an itchy scalp.

    A) hypertrichosis   C) pityriasis steatoides

    B) pityriasis capitis simplex   D) trichoptilosis

20. Identify an accurate statement about pityriasis steatoides.

    A) When pityriasis steatoides is accompanied by redness and inflammation, it is called pediculosis capitis.

    B) Pityriasis steatoides is extremely contagious.

    C) Pityriasis steatoides is a less severe case of dandruff than pityriasis capitis simplex.

    D) Cosmetologists should not perform services on anyone who has pityriasis steatoides.

continued

21. Tinea is _____.

    A) caused by a parasite

    B) the technical term for ringworm

    C) a highly contagious condition caused by mites called *Sarcoptes scabiei*

    D) an infestation of the hair and scalp with head lice

22. Which of the following is most likely a scabies symptom?

    A) yellow crusts on the scalp called scutula, which have a distinctive odor

    B) scales and painful circular lesions

    C) greasy or waxy scales, mixed with sebum

    D) intense itching and a rash that may have blisters and bumps that resemble acne

23. Identify an accurate statement about head lice.

    A) They cause tinea barbae, which primarily affects the beard and mustache areas of the face.

    B) They cause scabies, which is a highly contagious condition.

    C) They usually live up to four days without a host.

    D) They are transmitted mainly from head-to-head contact with an infected person.

24. _____ is the technical term for a boil and is an infection of the tissue surrounding the hair follicle.

    A) A carbuncle   C) Canities

    B) A furuncle   D) Hirsuties

25. Folliculitis barbae, also known as pseudofolliculitis barbae, is _____.

    A) an infection of the hair follicles caused by head lice

    B) an inflammation of the hair follicles caused by ingrown hair

    C) a type of carbuncle caused by staphylococci

    D) an inflammation of the scalp caused by malassezia

finished!

ch. 09: Principles of Hair Design

Why Study Hair Design?

FILL IN THE BLANK

1. Complete the sentences below using the words from the word bank.

    Word bank: moves, resource, do-it-yourself, emphasize, educated, client, best, social media, product, expectations, moves, service, minimizing, skill, technical, judgment, reacts, styling

    As a cosmetologist, you should study and have a thorough understanding of hair design principles

    so that you'll know why a particular hairstyle will or will not be the _____ choice for a client.

    You will also be able to apply hair design principles to help you achieve your _____

Word bank: moves, resource, do-it-yourself, emphasize, educated, client, best, social media, product, expectations, moves, service, minimizing, skill, technical, judgment, reacts, styling

vision and meet the creative _____ of your clients. You'll have skills to create looks that

_____ the client's best attributes while _____ areas of concern.

In addition, honing your eye for design and combining that with your _____ expertise is

more important than ever with the prevalence of _____ influencers, _____ (DIY)

consumers, and clients who are becoming more _____ about their hair and preferred

_____ choices. Formal hair design education will help you understand how hair looks,

_____, and _____ to styling; it will also help you develop artistic _____ and

_____, which will set you apart as a quality _____ because you'll be providing a

premium _____ experience for the informed _____.

Design Philosophy

2. What are the five steps for forming your own design philosophy?

   _____

   _____

   _____

3. Before starting your design plan for a client, what should you do first?

   _____

   _____

   _____

4. Why is it important to take calculated risks—that is, leave your comfort zone—as you refine your design philosophy? What are three ways that you, as a cosmetologist, can continue to evolve your designs?

_____

_____

_____

MIND MAPPING

5. Mind mapping is a method used to create a visual representation of a group of connected ideas. In this activity, follow the link below or use a sheet of paper to create a mind map for your personal sources of inspiration and creativity. Start the map with a center circle that represents your sources for ideas, creativity, and inspiration. In the circle, write heading that refers to your sources of ideas (e.g. "My Design Philosophy"). From there, sketch out the categories where you typically find inspiration, such as celebrities/DIY influencers, colors, patterns, nature, art, music, or people on the street. Then brainstorm some specific examples of those categories of inspiration and add them to your mind map. (Note: For an example of a mind map, see Figure 1-10 in *Milady Standard Foundations*.)

Now, think about any patterns you notice and what that might tell you about your design philosophy or how that might help you refine it. When you feel that your mind map is complete, write two or three sentences summarizing what you discovered in this process and describe how you think that will help shape your design philosophy. Keep this with you and refine it as you grow through cosmetology school and beyond.

+ BONUS

Visit: bonus.milady.com/cos-wb/toc

Five Elements of Hair Design

SHORT ANSWER

6. What are the five basic elements of hair design?

_____

_____

_____

7. What is the relationship between form and space in terms of hair design? What are five items that might occupy the space in a hair design?

_____

_____

_____

8. What is the role of haircolor in a hair design?

_____

_____

_____

RESEARCH

9. Although design lines have existed through the years, the styles have changed. For this project, look up some images of the design lines in hairstyles from the late 1980s and early 1990s and paste them next to the corresponding term. Then look at the images of the design lines from your textbook in the third column. Could you tell they use the same lines, even if the hairstyles are different?

DESIGN LINE	1980S/1990S STYLE	CURRENT STYLE
a. Horizontal		
c. Diagonal		

DESIGN LINE	1980S/1990S STYLE	CURRENT STYLE
d. Curved		
b. Vertical		
e. Contrasting		
f. Transitional		 Oladimeji Odunsi/Unsplash

10. Describe the effect of the basic types of lines.

    a. Horizontal lines

    _____

    _____

    _____

    b. Vertical lines

    _____

    _____

    _____

    c. Diagonal lines

    _____

    _____

    _____

    d. Curved lines

    _____

    _____

    _____

FILL IN THE BLANK

11. Fill in the blanks below by explaining the elements of hair design.

    Color   _____

    Form   _____

    Design texture _____

    Line   _____

    Space   _____

12. Match each type of line with its effect or role in a hair design. Some lines will be used more than once.

    a. Single lines   c. Contrasting lines   e. Directional lines
    b. Parallel lines   d. Transitional lines

Type of Line   **The Effect or Role in Hair Design**

_____ Best for clients requiring the lowest maintenance when styling their hair

_____ Usually create distinct looks and work best for clients who can pull off a strong style

_____ Examples of this type of line seen in crimped hair or crinkle waves

_____ Lines with a definite forward or backward movement

_____ Most often used in one-length, blunt hairstyles, or simple one-dimensional designs using human or synthetic hair extensions

_____ Usually curved lines that blend and soften horizontal or vertical lines; used frequently when texturizing a haircut along with haircolor placement and color blending

_____ Horizontal and vertical lines that meet at a 90-degree angle, creating a hard edge

_____ Repeating lines in a hairstyle; can be straight or curved; the line repetition creates more interest in the design

SHORT ANSWER

13. Describe one specific technique for temporarily changing hair texture.

_____

_____

_____

14. How can chemicals be used to alter hair texture permanently?

_____

_____

_____

15. With so many product options available to temporarily redefine natural hair texture and create alternate designs, how do you plan to stay on top of the trends and available products?

_____

_____

_____

16. Explain why you think haircolor is important to the client psychologically in the overall look of a hair design.

_____

_____

_____

17. How can you use color to create a bold, dramatic accent?

_____

_____

_____

18. For the hair designs below, use colored pens or pencils to show how color can be used to create each of the following:

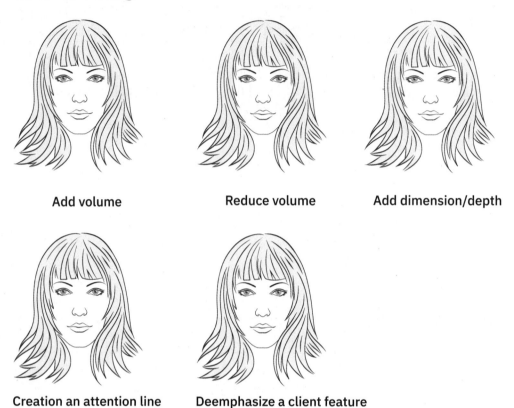

Add volume   Reduce volume   Add dimension/depth

Creation an attention line   Deemphasize a client feature

Five Principles of Hair Design

19. As a cosmetologist, it's important to train your artistic eye to notice and identify the principles of art and design in real-life everyday settings. For this activity, use the Internet, magazines, or your own photos to identify five examples of designs that demonstrate a pleasing use of proportion and five examples where the design seems to ignore or misuse the principles of proportion. Avoid looking at people. You instead may want to look at how proportions are used/misused in buildings, signage, landscapes, streets, plates of food, or anything else in the world around you.

Once you've gathered your examples, study them closely and write a short summary of what you like or dislike about the use of proportion in them, and mention any suggestions you might have for improving them.

20. Match each of the following principles of art and design with its description.

    a. proportion   c. rhythm   e. harmony
    b. balance   d. emphasis

    _____ Where the eye is drawn to first; also known as focus

    _____ Creation of unity in a design; the most important of the art principles

    _____ Establishing equal or appropriate proportions to create symmetry

    _____ Regular pulsation or recurrent pattern of movement in a design

    _____ Comparative relationship of one thing to another

FILL IN THE BLANK

21. Complete the sentences below using words from the word bank.

    Word bank: upswept, large, wave, taller, chin, shorter, volume, petite, proportions, above, longer, broad, proportion, smaller, head, body, curves

    The _____ measured from top to the _____ is classically used to establish the _____

    of the entire _____.

    Clients with _____, fuller proportions look best with medium or _____ styles with softer

    _____.

    Styles cropped _____ shoulder-length with gentle _____ patterns usually flatter

    _____, _____ frames.

    You would typically create a style with more _____ for a client with _____ hips or

    _____ shoulders.

    If a _____ person wore a tall constructed _____ style, it would likely appear out of

    _____.

22. How do you know if a hair design has symmetrical balance?

_____

_____

_____

23. Explain how balance is achieved in a hair design that might actually be considered asymmetrical.

_____

_____

_____

24. Which feature of a design does the principle of harmony refer to? What is the role of harmony in a design?

_____

_____

_____

25 What elements make a hairstyle harmonious?

_____

_____

_____

26. List the four physical characteristics of a client that an artistic and suitable (harmonious) hairstyle will address.

_____

_____

_____

27. What is your current favorite song? List it here: _____

   Next, play your song several times and, as you do so, sketch out a hair design that is inspired by the song. Consider rhythm, emphasis, balance, and harmony, and think about aspects such as color, texture, or ornamentation. When you're finished, share your sketch with a classmate (without telling them your song) and ask them to describe the principles of hair design they see in it. Does their description match your song? Does your style have harmony? Next, take a look at your classmate's sketch and try to identify the same aspects of their hairstyle. How accurate were your guesses?

Head Forms

SHORT ANSWER

28. List three ways in which knowing the reference points and head shapes can help you as a cosmetologist.

   _____

   _____

   _____

LABEL

29. Label each of the reference points of the head depicted below. Some reference points are shown twice, from different angles.

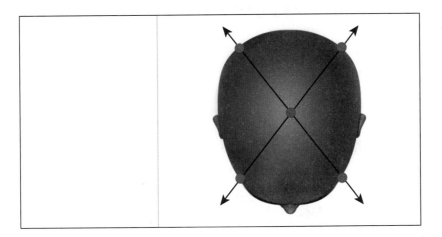

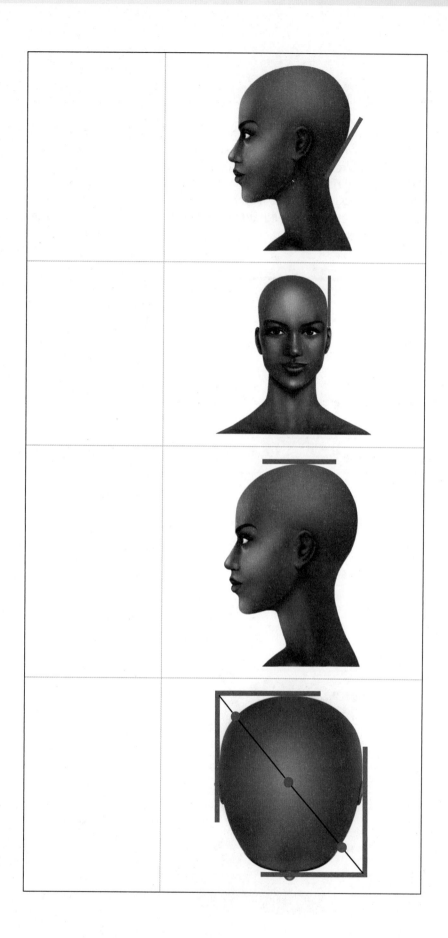

30. Match the reference point with the description of how to find it on the head. One reference point will be used twice.

   a. parietal ridge
   b. occipital bone

   c. apex
   d. four corners

   Reference Point   How to Locate the Reference Point

   _____ Feel the back of the skull or place a comb flat against the nape and see where the comb leaves the head

   _____ One of two ways to find this reference point: make two diagonal lines crossing the apex, which then point directly to the front and back

   _____ Find the area by placing a comb flat on the side of the head; this reference point is where the head starts to curve away from the comb

   _____ Locate the area by placing a comb flat on the top of the head; the comb will rest on the highest point

   _____ One of two ways to find this reference point: place two combs flat against the side and back, then locate the back at the point where the two combs meet

LABEL

31. Label the main areas of the head.

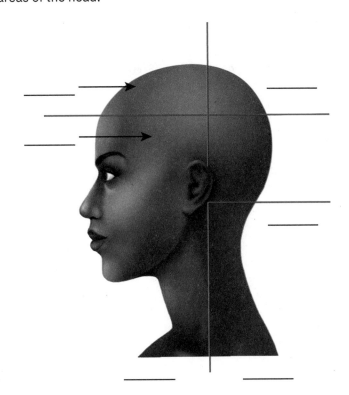

32. Match each area of the head with its description.

a. Top   c. Front   e. Nape   g. Bang area
b. Side   d. Crown   f. Back

Area of the Head   **How to Locate the Area/Type of Hair in the Area**

_____ Includes all hair from the back of the ear forward, below the parietal ridge

_____ Triangular section that begins at the apex and ends at the front corners; when combed into a natural falling position, this area falls no farther than the eyes' outer corners

_____ Make a parting from the apex to the back of the ear and let hair fall naturally; this hair is everything that falls in front of the ear

_____ This hair lies on the head shape

_____ Located by making a parting or drawing a line from the apex to the back of the ear; consists of all the hair that falls naturally behind the ear (*Hint:* When you identify the front, you also identify this area.)

_____ The area between the apex and the back of the parietal ridge; can feature cowlicks or whorls, making it extremely important to pay special attention to this area in styling and cutting

_____ Back part of the neck, consisting of the hair below the occipital bone

DRAW

33. Draw a diagram of the bang area as viewed from the top of the head, and label the back, bang area, and sides.

Hair Type and Texture

34. When selecting a hairstyle for your client, what are two major considerations? Give the names and identify their types.

_____

_____

_____

35. In general, how many universal curl patterns are recognized? Why is it important to familiarize yourself with these patterns?

_____

_____

_____

36. The relationship between which two factors is important to note when choosing a style for your client?

_____

_____

_____

37. How is hair density measured? How is it described?

_____

_____

_____

38. Match each of the following hair textures with its styling tips.

a. Wavy, medium hair   e. Curly, medium hair   i. Coily/Afro-texture
b. Straight, coarse hair   f. Very curly, medium hair   j. Curly, coarse hair
c. Curly, fine hair   g. Straight, fine hair   k. Wavy, coarse hair
d. Very curly, fine hair   h. Wavy, fine hair   l. Straight, medium hair

Type of Hair   **Styling Tip**

_____ Chemical services may take longer to process

_____ Remove some interior weight with texture shears

_____ Responds well to rollers and thermal styling

_____ May appear fuller when diffused with heat and the appropriate haircut and style

_____ Recommend styling aids or chemical services to achieve the most flattering style

_____ Responds well to blowdryer and flat iron

_____ Close cropping is great for styling ease and low maintenance

_____ Use products containing moisture; cut dry

_____ Responds well to keratin-based chemical treatments and smoothing

_____ Responds well to short, cropped layers along with braided, loc, and twisted styles

_____ When left natural, gives a soft, romantic look

_____ Offers the most versatility in styling

Hairstyle and Facial Shapes

39. What determines facial shape? Describe how you would identify your client's facial shape.

_____

_____

_____

40. What are the seven basic facial shapes?

_____

_____

_____

41. What is a good technique for explaining to a client how certain hairstyles are more suited for particular facial shapes?

_____

_____

_____

FILL IN THE BLANK

42. The chart below has a row for each facial type, and columns for a description of the facial contour, the objective for creating a hair design for that shape, and a recommended styling choice. Complete the chart by filing in the missing information for each row.

FACIAL SHAPE	DESCRIPTION OF FACIAL CONTOUR	OBJECTIVE FOR THE FACIAL SHAPE	STYLING CHOICE
Heart		To create the illusion of forehead width	
	Wide at the temples, narrow at the middle third of the face, and squared off at the jaw		Soften the hair around the temples and jaw by bringing the shape or silhouette close to the head form. Create volume in the area between the temples and jaw by adding width around the ear area.

FACIAL SHAPE	DESCRIPTION OF FACIAL CONTOUR	OBJECTIVE FOR THE FACIAL SHAPE	STYLING CHOICE
Oblong	Long, narrow face with hollow cheeks		
Oval		Can wear any hairstyle unless there are other considerations, such as eyeglasses, nose length and shape, or profile	
	Round hairline and round chin line; wide face	Slimmer face; the illusion of an elongated face	
Triangle		Create the illusion of forehead width	
	Narrow forehead, extreme width through the cheekbones, and narrow chin		Increase the fullness across the jaw line and forehead while keeping the hair close to the head at the cheekbone line. Avoid hairstyles that lift away from the cheeks or move back from the hairline on the sides near the ear area.

ROLE PLAY

43. Gather three or four examples of hairstyles that you like or find interesting from magazines, the Internet, or photos you've taken with your phone. Partner with a classmate. Take turns being the client and the cosmetologist.

In the role of client, show your partner, the cosmetologist, the hairstyle examples you found. For each one, ask the cosmetologist their opinion of how it might look with your facial shape and whether they would recommend it. As the client, practice passion for a particular hairstyle and object to the cosmetologist's recommendation (you can even pretend to have a different head shape!). The cosmetologist should respond to you, the client, with a description of facial shapes and explain the results that the various hairstyle examples might have, while also exhibiting sensitivity, knowledge, confidence, and calm persuasion. While these conversations can be difficult, they are good practice for working with clients in a salon.

Profiles and Proportions

44. Complete the sentences below using the word bank.

Word bank: unique, angles, proportion, complement, big, flatter, profiles, small

In terms of _____ and proportions, a hair design should look great from all _____.

Every part should _____ the client's _____ physicality. The style should never be

too _____ or too _____ compared to the client's total body _____. Mainly, it

should _____ the client's overall features.

45. What does the term *profile* refer to in terms of hair design?

_____

_____

_____

46. Why is it important to take care with hair partings?

_____

_____

_____

47. Match each of the following parts of the face with their importance for the cosmetologist.

a. Bottom third   b. Top third   c. Middle third

Profile	Description
_____	Balance the eyes and nose with the hair design
_____	Consider the shape of the jaw and chin
_____	Flatter the shape and size of the forehead

48. Label each image with the type of profile that's depicted below. Then fill in a brief description of styling recommendations for that profile.

TYPE OF PROFILE	IMAGE	STYLING RECOMMENDATIONS

CREATE

49. Imagine that you've just completed a facial analysis for a client who is ready for a new hairstyle. Choose one facial feature from each third of the face (e.g., narrow forehead, close-set eyes, and large chin) to represent the features you identified in your client. Next, design a hairstyle that you think would enhance, flatter, or minimize the various features of your client based on the information in your text and the above crossword. Sketch it out on a separate sheet of paper and write a few sentences to explain your design choices.

SHORT ANSWER

50. What are the three different ways that you can part the bang area? Describe the effect of each type of part.

_____

_____

_____

51. When recommending a hairstyle for your client, which specific components of your client's glasses should you consider?

_____

_____

_____

52. Complete the crossword on appropriate styling tips for client facial features.

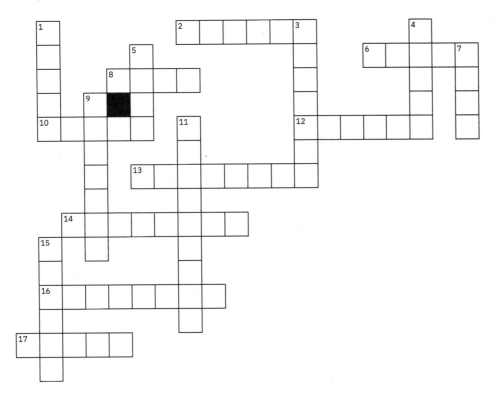

Across

2. Direct hair away from the face at this kind of forehead. Lighter highlights may be used at the temples to create the illusion of width.
6. Move the hair up and away from the face along the type of chin line.
8. Draw the hair away from the face and use a center part to help elongate and narrow this kind of nose.
10. If the client desires, use bangs with little or no volume to cover this forehead.
12. Use curved lines at this jaw line.
13. Slight hair lightening at the corners of these eyes will give the illusion of width (hyphenated word).
14. If the client desires, direct bangs over this kind of forehead with an outwardly directed volume.
16. Direct hair forward in the chin area for this type of chin.
17. Use straight lines at the jaw line for this kind of jaw.

Down

1. For clients with this nose, move the top hair off the forehead to give the illusion of length.
3. To add length to the face and make these eyes appear proportional, you can use a higher half-bang (hyphenated word).
4. Hair should be either longer or shorter than this type of chin line to avoid drawing attention to it.
5. Direct hair forward over the sides of this kind of forehead.
7. Hair should be full and fall below this kind of jaw to direct attention away.
9. Asymmetrical, off-center styles are flattering for this kind of nose
11. Bring hair forward at the forehead with softness around the face with this kind of nose
15. Select a style where the hair moves away from the face, creating the illusion of wider facial features with this nose

Complete each sentence by filling in the blanks.

Word bank: voluminous, dramatic, thickness, width, oval, height, wide, round, crown, Side, center, eye, back

53. Zigzag partings are known to create a _____ effect.

54. Center partings are used for _____ faces, but they also give an _____ illusion to _____ and _____ faces.

55. _____ partings start right above the _____ of either the left or right _____, back to just in front of the _____ area.

56. Diagonal _____ partings create the illusion of _____ or _____ in a hairstyle, making them an excellent choice for _____ hairstyles. They also create a more even _____ on either side of the part.

Sideburns

57. List the four components that should be considered when determining the most suitable length and shape for the client's sideburns.

_____

_____

_____

58. Describe how ear size and placement determine whether the sideburns are considered short, medium, or long relative to these features.

_____

_____

_____

59. How will a client's facial features and structure affect the appearance of a sideburn's length? Provide an example.

_____

_____

_____

60. Use the Internet, magazines, or your own photos to locate two or three examples of interesting sideburn designs and styles. Assess them based on the design principles that you have been studying, and determine whether they complement the person in the picture. Explain how they follow or ignore the guidelines for designing sideburns. (*Hint:* "Porkchop" and "mutton chops" might be useful search terms.)

_____

_____

_____

DISCOVERIES AND ACCOMPLISHMENTS

In the space below, write notes about key concepts discussed in this chapter. Share your discoveries with some of the other students in your class and ask them if your notes are helpful. You may want to revise your notes based on good ideas shared by your peers.

Discoveries:

_____

_____

_____

_____

_____

_____

_____

List at least three things you have accomplished since you decided to enroll in school.

Accomplishments:

_____

_____

_____

_____

_____

_____

_____

1. Cosmetologists should study and have a thorough understanding of hair design principles because _____.

   A) improving the appearance of certain hair and scalp conditions that are medical disorders is the responsibility of cosmetologists

   B) hair design principles will assist them in achieving their styling vision

   C) they are required to inform clients about hair design principles before performing any services on them

   D) they are licensed to diagnose, treat, prescribe, or work on unhealthy hair and scalp

2. A _____ includes objectives, goals, and step-by-step planning developed by artists to mold their unique vision into a piece of art.

   A) design line   C) design philosophy

   B) profile   D) reference point

3. Which of the following guidelines is most likely to help you in bringing a design to life and becoming a great stylist?

   A) Never envision the result before beginning the design.

   B) First practice your techniques and your planned design on a staff member or a person other than the client.

   C) Limit positive risks and keep yourself in your comfort zone.

   D) Decide which tools are needed to achieve your design and ensure that they are available and ready for use.

4. Which of the following is one of the five basic elements of three-dimensional hair design?

   A) balance   C) rhythm

   B) elasticity   D) color

continued

5. In the context of the types of design lines, _____ lines help build height and length in a hair design.

    A) vertical   C) horizontal

    B) diagonal   D) curved

6. In the context of the basic elements of hair design, identify a true statement about form.

    A) It refers to the directional wave patterns or illusion of motion in the hair.

    B) It is two-dimensional, meaning it has length and width but no depth.

    C) It is also referred to as space.

    D) It is a hairstyle's mass or general outline.

7. In the context of the basic elements of hair design, _____ is the area surrounding the form or the area a hairstyle occupies.

    A) space   C) volume

    B) mass   D) design texture

8. Which of the following terms refers to the directional wave patterns or illusion of motion in the hair?

    A) form   C) volume

    B) design texture   D) design line

9. In the context of the principles of hair design, _____ is the comparative relationship of one thing to another.

    A) proportion   C) balance

    B) rhythm   D) harmony

continued

10. In the context of the principles of hair design, which of the following statements best describes emphasis?

    A) It relates to establishing equal or appropriate proportions to create symmetry.

    B) It is where the eye is drawn first before traveling to the rest of the design.

    C) It is a regular pulsation or recurrent pattern of movement in a design.

    D) It refers to a design's unity and is the most important art principle.

11. Which of the following principles of hair design refers to a design's unity and is the most important art principle?

    A) balance   C) harmony

    B) proportion   D) rhythm

12. _____ on the head mark where the head's surface changes, such as the ears, jawline, occipital bone, and apex.

    A) Side bonds   C) Reference points

    B) Design lines   D) Hair follicles

13. In the context of standard reference points, the _____ is the head's widest area, starting at the temples and ending at the bottom of the crown.

    A) parietal ridge   C) occipital bone

    B) fringe area   D) apex

14. In the context of the areas of the head, which of the following statements best describes the crown?

    A) It is a triangular section that begins at the apex and ends at the front corners.

    B) It is the area between the apex and the back of the parietal ridge.

    C) It is the highest point on the top of the head.

    D) It is the back part of the neck and consists of the hair below the occipital bone.

continued

15. Hair type is categorized by two defining characteristics. Identify them.

   A) growth patterns and hair porosity

   C) directional pattern and hair texture

   B) hair porosity and side bonds

   D) hair elasticity and hair pigment

16. In the context of hair type and texture, a _____ is defined as a very tight curl.

   A) plait

   C) cornrow

   B) loc

   D) coil

17. In the context of hair types, which of the following is a quality of straight fine hair?

   A) It lacks body or volume.

   C) It offers the most styling versatility.

   B) It has an extremely wide silhouette.

   D) It has the highest elasticity.

18. Identify the hair type that offers the most styling versatility.

   A) straight medium hair

   C) very curly fine hair

   B) wavy medium hair

   D) curly coarse hair

19. A good way to determine a client's facial shape is to _____.

   A) understand the structure and type of skin on the client's face

   B) divide the face into three zones: forehead to eyebrows, eyebrows to end of nose, and end of nose to bottom of chin

   C) identify the parietal ridge, which is the highest point on the top of the head

   D) leave all of their hair hanging around the face to better observe the face

20. Identify the face shape that is around 1.5 times longer than its width across the brow, has a forehead that is marginally broader than the chin, and has no areas that visibly dominate the others.

   A) the oval face shape

   C) the square face shape

   B) the round face shape

   D) the triangular face shape

continued

21. Which of the following hairstyles is the most flattering for oblong facial shapes?

   A) medium-length styles

   B) shoulder-length styles

   C) waist-length styles

   D) chin-length styles

22. To help balance the heart face shape, you should _____.

   A) style the hair close to the head with no volume

   B) avoid bangs or fringes

   C) gradually decrease the silhouette's width while styling the middle third of the shape in the cheekbone area

   D) keep the silhouette at its narrowest at the jaw and neck area

23. Identify a true statement about a concave profile.

   A) It can be complemented by softly styling the hair at the apex with a downward movement.

   B) It has a prominent forehead and chin, with other features receding inward.

   C) It can be complemented with an arrangement of curls or bangs over the forehead.

   D) It has a receding forehead and chin.

24. In the context of hair partings, a _____ is the basic parting for bang sections and gives a symmetrical balance to facial features.

   A) center parting

   B) diagonal parting

   C) triangular parting

   D) curved parting

25. Which of the following factors should be considered for determining the most suitable length and shape for a client's sideburns?

   A) the type of melanin in their hair

   B) wave patterns

   C) hair porosity and hair elasticity

   D) face shape, natural hair growth, and ear size and placement

finished!

Ch. 10: Hair Service Preparation

Why Study Hair Service Preparation?

FILL IN THE BLANK

Complete the sentences below using the words from the word bank.

> **Word bank:** scalp massage, loyalty, canvas, sebum, reputation, buildup, rinsing, massage, hygiene, debris, business, conditioning, scalp, vitality, cleanse, relief

1. Proper hair cleansing, _____, and _____ provide a clear _____ for styling and finishing.

2. To maintain good health and _____, it's essential to _____ and condition the hair

    and _____.

3. In addition to removing excess _____, dirt, environmental _____, and product

    _____, a gentle massage builds _____ and provides _____ to the scalp area.

4. You should offer _____ during the shampoo or conditioning process, or both.

5. Performing a _____ makes it a pleasurable and memorable experience that can build

    client _____, repeat _____, and your _____ as a stylist.

SHORT ANSWER

6. Why is it recommended to perform scalp treatments at prescribed intervals—even for normal scalps?

    _____

    _____

    _____

7. List three reasons that cosmetologists should study and have a thorough understanding of scalp
    care, shampooing, and conditioning.

    _____

    _____

    _____

Three-Part Client Service Process

SHORT ANSWER

8. In your own words, describe how having a three-part, step-by-step process for your services can
    benefit both you, as the cosmetologist, and the client.

    _____

    _____

    _____

9. Match each part of the client service process with its purpose. Some parts might be used more than once.

   a. Pre-service   b. Service   c. Post-service

**Part of the
Service**   **Purpose**

_____ Help your client through the scheduling and payment process and close the service by offering rebooking dates

_____ Accomplish the actual service the client has requested, such as a shampoo, haircut, hair coloring, and/or chemical service

_____ Assemble materials and organize your station

_____ Meet with your client and perform an effective consultation to gain information about service expectations

_____ Care for your client after the procedure has been completed

_____ Clean and disinfect your implements

_____ Opportunity to share product recommendations with your client based on your initial consultation

_____ Opportunity to retail home care purchases

SEQUENCE

10. Number the following pre-service steps in the order they should occur. The first and last steps have been provided for you.

   _____ Review schedule.

   ___1___ Wear gloves.

   _____ Greet client.

   _____ Clean tools.

   ___19___ Perform consultation.

   _____ Rinse and dry tools.

   _____ Eliminate distractions.

_____ Immerse implements in EPA-registered disinfectant.

_____ Clean and disinfect station.

_____ Remove implements.

_____ Escort client to workstation.

_____ Store implements.

_____ Remove gloves and wash hands.

_____ Fill disinfectant container.

_____ Collect implements to bring to your station.

_____ Review intake form and service record card (for returning clients). Have an intake form ready for new clients.

_____ Prepare self by taking care of personal needs before client arrives.

_____ Wash hands.

_____ Clear head.

SHORT ANSWER

11. When you greet the client during the pre-service part, what are three gestures you can make to help build your relationship with them?

_____

_____

_____

12. Before your client arrives, what should you remind yourself of as you take a few breaths to relax?

_____

_____

_____

13. Why is it important to take care of your own personal needs before you meet with your client?

_____

_____

_____

14. Just before your client leaves, what are three things you should say to them?

_____

_____

_____

SEQUENCE

15. Number the following post-service steps in the order they should occur.

_____ Record information on the intake form and service card.

_____ Prepare station for the next customer.

_____ Thank client.

_____ Advise client on at-home maintenance.

_____ Clean and disinfect tools and implements.

_____ Schedule the next appointment.

_____ Determine if client is satisfied.

_____ Put on gloves.

_____ Escort client to reception desk, write up service ticket, and recommend products.

Client Consultation

Indicate whether the following statements are true or false. For any false statements, explain why they are false.

16. It is appropriate to ask your client whether they find shampooing and conditioning services to be pleasurable.

    T   F   _____

17. It is prohibited to ask your client whether they are taking any medications that contraindicate a wet shampoo service or scalp massage.

    T   F   _____

18. The answer your client gives when you ask about the last time they shampooed (or how often they shampoo their hair) will allow you the option to decline service.

    T   F   _____

19. When removing extensions or protective styles, it's important to first detangle the hair properly before the shampoo service. Once the hair is detangled, you can then use a clarifying shampoo to remove buildup.

    T   F   _____

20. You should ask whether your client has been using any natural nonprofessional treatments, such as coconut oil, olive oil, or shea butter, so that you can determine if a shampoo/treatment is actually needed.

    T   F   _____

21. Occasionally, you may have a client whose physician requests that they use a dry shampoo for a medical reason.

    T   F   _____

22. Because you are an experienced professional, you are better qualified than the client to determine the ideal water temperature for shampooing and conditioning services.

    T   F   _____

23. As uncomfortable as it might be, you should ask your client whether they have had any negative or concerning experiences with prior shampoo and conditioning services.

   T   F   _____

24. You have an obligation to ask whether a client has neck problems or other health issues that might be aggravated during the shampooing, conditioning, or massage services.

   T   F   _____

SHORT ANSWER

25. What are two ways that you can get a good view of the scalp?

   _____

   _____

   _____

26. What is the purpose of a scalp analysis?

   _____

   _____

   _____

27. What are five conditions of the scalp that require you to decline the service and recommend that the client seek medical attention?

   _____

   _____

   _____

Professional Draping

28. Complete the sentences below.

    Before draping a client, make sure you do the following:

    • Use a protective neck _____—absorbent tissue paper or _____ that stretches to fit

    comfortably around the client's neck—and/or a _____ between the client's neck and the

    cape's band to ensure _____ for the client.

    • Ensure each cape has been _____ before use.

    • Ask the client to _____ their _____ and glasses and _____ all personal items as

    desired.

    • To _____ you as a professional, even if the client chooses not to remove _____,

    _____ them of the _____ of their _____ getting damaged or lost during the service.

29. What are two possible outcomes of improper draping? What should you do if your client
    experiences these outcomes?

    _____

    _____

    _____

30. Why is professional draping an important aspect of every service?

    _____

    _____

    _____

31. What is another term for shampoo draping?

_____

_____

_____

32. List the three types of draping used in a salon.

_____

_____

_____

33. What type of material is used for a shampoo cape?

_____

_____

_____

34. Describe a cutting and styling cape.

_____

_____

_____

35. What are three examples of the services that require a chemical draping? At what point in the service is the chemical cape removed from the client?

_____

_____

_____

36. Number the following steps for a shampoo draping from 1 to 10, beginning to end.

_____ Place a towel, folded lengthwise and diagonally, across client's shoulders and cross the ends under their chin.

_____ Place shampoo cape over the towel and fasten securely in the back.

_____ Remove shampoo cape and towels and place them in a designated laundering place.

_____ Proceed with the scheduled service.

_____ Proceed with shampoo service.

_____ Invite client to sit comfortably in the chair. If needed, turn their collar to the inside of their shirt.

_____ Escort them back to your workstation.

_____ Place another towel over the cape and secure in the front by crossing the ends under.

_____ Make sure they are comfortably seated in the styling chair. Then use second towel of the original draping to completely towel dry the hair. Pin long hair up and out of the way.

_____ Secure neck strip around client's neck. Place and fasten a cutting or styling cape over the neck strip. Fold the neck strip down over the cape so no part of the cape touches their skin.

Hair Brushing

37. List three benefits of correct hair brushing.

_____

_____

_____

38. How do the recommendations for brushing straight to wavy hair textures before shampooing differ from those for tighter curl patterns?

_____

_____

_____

39. What is at risk for your client if you skip detangling and brushing curly or textured hair before shampooing?

_____

_____

_____

40. List the four circumstances under which brushing, massage, or scalp treatment should be avoided.

_____

_____

_____

41. What type of bristle is recommended for brushing straight to wavy hair textures? Why?

_____

_____

_____

42. List the four types of brushes that can be used to detangle hair.

_____

_____

_____

43. What are two alternatives to using brushes to detangle hair?

_____

_____

_____

44. Identify each brushing/detangling implement shown below.

NAME	IMPLEMENT
	KonstantinDmitriev /Shutterstock.com

45. Number the following steps for hair brushing from 1 to 12, beginning to end.

_____ For straight or wavy hair, use the front of the comb to part their hair using a half-head parting. For coily hair, finger detangle, then perform a shampoo and conditioning.

_____ Drape your client for the shampoo.

_____ Hold the hair in your nondominant hand between the thumbs and fingers.

_____ Ask the client to remove all jewelry, glasses, and hair ornaments and put them in a safe place.

_____ Rotate the brush by turning your wrist slightly and sweeping the bristles the full length of the hair shaft.

_____ Lay the brush (held in the dominant hand) with bristles down on the hair and close to the scalp.

_____ Invite your client to the salon chair and assist them into a comfortable position.

_____ Repeat brushing three times on each section of hair.

_____ Further subsection the hair 1 inch (2.5 centimeters) from the front hairline to the crown. For 4a to 4c textures, you may need to twist and braid the detangled sections as you complete them.

_____ Continue brushing until the entire head has been brushed.

_____ For very curly or coily hair, now use the front of the comb to part the hair using a half-head parting.

_____ To confirm you can proceed with the service, examine the condition of the scalp to be sure there are no abrasions or contraindications. If there are scalp contraindications, you must decline the service.

Scalp Massage

Indicate whether each statement is true or false. For any false statements, explain why they are false.

46. Massage is a method of manipulating the scalp by rubbing, kneading, or stroking it with the hands. Tapping is also part of a scalp massage.

    T   F   _____

47. Benefits of scalp massage include slowing down scalp microcirculation and calming tenseness.

    T   F   _____

48. The basic requirement for a healthy scalp is cleanliness.

    T   F   _____

49. Scalp massages are recommended for relaxation but, in certain situations, they can also address scalp conditions such as dryness, minimal flaking, excess oiliness, and tight scalp.

    T   F   _____

50. Depending on the client's needs, you should consider using your fingernails to touch, lightly scrape, or gently scratch the scalp during the massage.

    T   F   _____

51. When massaging during the conditioning phase, the conditioner is distributed throughout the hair, followed by massage manipulations, which allows the conditioning product to penetrate more evenly, improves the scalp's microcirculation, relaxes the scalp and neck, and restores hair to a more balanced state.

    T   F   _____

52. As you develop your massage technique, you should begin to incorporate stiff, mechanical movements throughout the service to show your client that you have skills and confidence.

    T   F   _____

53. To prevent tangling throughout the service, you should make sure that you are manipulating the scalp, not the hair.

    T   F   _____

MATCHING

54. Indicate whether each description is related to effleurage (E) or petrissage (P).

Effleurage (E) or Petrissage (P)?	Description
_____	Usually done with the balls of the fingers in forward-to-backward movements
_____	Most often used for scalp massage
_____	Intended to help soothe muscles

_____ Uses stroking and circular hand movements

_____ Gentle pushing and kneading of the scalp with the palms, fingers, and thumbs

_____ Gentle and rhythmic to relax your client, stimulate the microcirculation, and bring nutrients to the scalp

_____ Often used in a therapeutic massage to loosen up dead skin cells from the scalp

SHORT ANSWER

55. What should you encourage your client to do while you are performing the scalp massage? How long should a scalp massage last?

_____

_____

_____

56. Why might you ask a client to sit up at the shampoo bowl during a conditioning massage?

_____

_____

_____

SEQUENCE

57. Number the steps of the scalp massage from 1 to 8, beginning to end. Steps 2 and 3 have been provided.

_____ Resume Procedure 10-5, Shampooing and Conditioning, step 21 if deep conditioning or step 22 if ready to rinse the hair.

_____ Hold back of client's head with your left hand. Place the stretched thumb and fingers of your right hand on client's forehead. Move your hand slowly and firmly upward to 1 inch (2.5 centimeters) past the hairline. Repeat four times.

_____ Cup client's chin in your left hand. Place your right hand at base of the skull and rotate the head gently. Reverse the position of your hands and repeat.

_____ Place your fingertips again on each side of the client's head, this time 1 inch (2.5 centimeters) back from where you placed your fingertips in the preceding step. Slide your hands firmly upward, spreading the fingertips until they meet at the top of the head; rotate and move the client's scalp. Repeat four times.

_____ Place the palms of your hands firmly against client's scalp. Lift the scalp in a rotary movement, first with your hands placed above client's ears and then with your hands placed at front and back of client's head.

_____ Place your fingertips on each side of client's head. Slide your hands firmly upward, spreading the fingertips until they meet at the top of the head. Repeat four times.

_____ Repeat the preceding movement over entire head, moving back toward nape.

_____ Place fingers of both hands at client's forehead. Massage around hairline by lifting and rotating. For textured hair, avoid circular movements to avoid introducing tangles. Use smooth, gliding movements.

ROLE PLAY

58. Partner with a classmate to practice the effleurage and petrissage massage techniques on each other's scalps—however, do not tell each other which technique you are using. When you've each completed the massages, each partner should guess which technique was used on them. If they guess correctly, ask them how they knew which type it was. If they were wrong, discuss what led them to that answer.

Scalp Treatments

SHORT ANSWER

59. What are the two keys to creating an ideal environment for healthy hair and scalp?

_____

_____

_____

60. Describe the role of scalp exfoliators and give two examples of their typical ingredients.

_____

_____

_____

61. List at least three precautions to take when exfoliating a scalp.

_____

_____

_____

MATCHING

62. Match the type of scalp treatment with its description. Each type will be used four times.

   a. Normal scalp   c. Oily hair and scalp
   b. Dry hair and scalp   d. Antidandruff

**Type of Scalp
Treatment**   **Description**

_____ Purpose is to maintain a clean and healthy scalp

_____ May be the result of over exfoliation of the scalp

_____ Products used in these treatments also dry the hair, so should be paired with a deep hair conditioning to restore moisture

_____ Should be used when there is a natural oil deficiency on the scalp and hair

_____ Manipulate the scalp using a kneading technique to reduce any hardened sebum that has collected in the scalp's pores

_____ Can be affected by weather changes, so these clients will benefit from having a scalp treatment performed with every season change

_____ Recommended shampoos, conditioners, and topical lotions used in this treatment contain antifungal agents

_____ Scalp steamer, which resembles a hooded dryer, can be used to help restore the hair's moisture balance; is also an effective tool to soften hair with tighter textures and aid in detangling

_____ Generally includes a gentle brushing at the root area on straight to wavy textures

_____ Pre-brushing not recommended with this treatment because you risk overstimulating delicate scalp issues

_____ Treatment for excessive oiliness caused by overactive sebaceous glands

_____ Environmental elements, chemicals, and hair texture can contribute to this condition

_____ Used for a condition caused by a fungus called malassezia that sits on the scalp and creates dryness, itchiness, and discomfort

_____ Treatment generally includes a scalp massage lasting up to 10 minutes for relaxation and to improve scalp vitality

_____ Using a deep cleansing shampoo during the shampoo and conditioning phase recommended

_____ Select scalp preparations containing moisturizing and emollient ingredients

CREATE

63. If you can, think about a scalp massage or treatment that you or someone you know experienced. What was it like? Did you enjoy it? Now, write one or two brief paragraphs describing the *ideal* scalp massage and treatment that you would like to receive. Be specific regarding what conditions you would like treated, any special considerations for your needs, the treatment products that you prefer, the duration, the atmosphere, and so on. If you wish, use the Internet to find more information about the variety of equipment, products, and types of scalp treatments and massages available, and mention any that appeal to you as you design your ideal scalp treatment.

Shampoo Types

TRUE OR FALSE

Indicate whether the statements below are true or false. For any false statements, explain why they are false.

64. Hair should be shampooed as often as necessary to keep the hair and scalp in good condition.

   T   F   _____

65. Although the shampoo service provides a good opportunity to ensure the hair and scalp are properly cleansed and nourished, it is not the best time to educate your client about the importance of home hair care or suggest hair-care products for home use.

   T   F   _____

66. Excessive shampooing promotes the fatty or oily secretion (sebum) that lubricates the skin and preserves the hair's softness.

    T   F   _____

67. As a general rule, oily hair needs to be shampooed more often than normal or dry hair.

    T   F   _____

FILL IN THE BLANK

Complete the sentences below using the word bank. Some words will be used more than once.

> **Word bank:** surfactant(s), calcium, hair, lipophilic, fragrance, oil, moisturizers, water, hydrophilic, impurities

68. Deionized _____ has had _____ that would make a product unstable—such as

    _____ and magnesium and other metal ions—removed.

69. A _____ is a cleansing or surface-active agent. Each _____ molecule has two ends: a

    hydrophilic, or _____-attracting, head and a lipophilic, or _____-attracting, tail.

70. A push–pull process is created during the shampooing process when the _____ head

    attracts water, and the _____ tail attracts oil and causes the oils, dirt, and deposits to roll up

    into little balls that are lifted off by the _____ and rinsed from the _____.

71. Shampoo formulas contain _____, _____, and other ingredients such as _____,

    oils, proteins, foam enhancers, and _____.

SHORT ANSWER

72. What does a pH scale measure?

    _____

    _____

    _____

73. Label the following pH scale with the correct numbers at the far ends and center. Then add a line where the pH most closely matches the pH of hair.

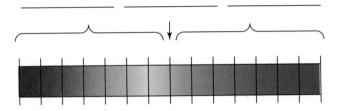

74. What does a higher pH rating indicate about a shampoo?

_____

_____

_____

75. Which type of shampoo—slightly more alkaline or slightly more acidic—most closely matches the ideal pH of hair?

_____

_____

_____

76. What are two possible effects of using a high pH shampoo?

_____

_____

_____

77. Match each type of water (hard or soft) with its description. The types will be used more than once.

Type of Water   **Description**

_____ Contains minerals that reduce the ability of soap or shampoo to lather

_____ Allows soap and shampoo to lather freely; preferred for shampooing

_____ Rainwater or chemically treated

_____ Can change the results of hair-coloring service

_____ Contains small amounts of minerals

_____ Well water

SHORT ANSWER

78. What is water's role in the cosmetology industry? Why do you need to know about the type of water in your salon?

_____

_____

_____

79. How can you find out what type of water is in your salon?

_____

_____

_____

CASE STUDY

80. For this activity, arrange to have both hard and soft water available. Using different water types and a professional shampoo product, compare the product's lathering ability, its cleansing ability, and the appearance of hair afterward for different swatches of hair (such as natural hair, color-treated, relaxed, and permed). Record your results in the space provided.

_____

_____

_____

81. Match each type of shampoo with its purpose.

	SHAMPOO	PURPOSE
_____	pH-balanced shampoos	a. Contain special ingredients that are very effective in reducing dandruff or relieving other scalp conditions
_____	Conditioning shampoos	b. Wash away excess oiliness, while preventing the hair from drying out
_____	Medicated shampoos	c. Designed to make the hair appear smooth and shiny
_____	Clarifying shampoos	d. Used to brighten, to add a slight hint of color, or to eliminate unwanted color tones
_____	Balancing shampoos	e. Special solutions available for hair enhancements
_____	Dry or powder shampoos	f. Balanced to the pH of skin and hair
_____	Color-enhancing shampoos	g. Cleanse the hair without the use of soap and water
_____	Shampoos for hairpieces and wigs	h. Used when product buildup is evident, after swimming, and prior to all chemical services
_____	Vegan shampoos	i. Ideal for clients who live in dryer climates and have curly or brittle hair
_____	Shampoos for thinning hair	j. Help temporarily strengthen the hair as they cleanse, using artificial protein molecules to cling to the hair's natural protein
_____	Strengthening shampoos	k. Contain volume-boosting ingredients to give illusion of additional volume and density, while encouraging a clean environment for healthy hair growth
_____	Shampoos with keratin protein added	l. Add strength to weak, damaged, or brittle hair
_____	Oil shampoos	m. manufactured as wetting agents for compatibility with hair and soft water sources; gentle on artificial hair color and beneficial for maintaining the hair's natural oils; favorable for all hair types
_____	Sulfate-free shampoos	n. typically for clients interested in making specific environmental, ethical, dietary, or lifestyle choices

82. Complete the sentences below using the word bank. Not all words in the word bank will be used.

    Word bank: open, softness, before, warmer, dullness, rinsing, pressure, hardness, after, close, vibrancy, temperature, shine, chemical, during, cooler

    Always remember to monitor the _____ and _____ of the water _____ and

    _____ the professional service. _____ tepid water is adequate for _____

    shampoo and _____ product, and _____ water works well to _____ the

    cuticle post-service, helping to add _____ and _____ to the hair.

SHORT ANSWER

83. What is the most widely purchased hair-care product?

    _____

    _____

    _____

84. With the large variety of shampoo types and hair types, what is the key to selecting an appropriate shampoo for your client?

    _____

    _____

    _____

85. What determines the efficacy of the more recent true color-depositing shampoos (and conditioners) that are designed to add rich pigments to the hair and refresh hair color between services?

    _____

    _____

    _____

86. List two reasons that a dry shampoo might be used.

_____

_____

_____

87. What is the ideal pH level for shampoos, to prevent dryness and hair damage during cleansing?

_____

_____

_____

88. What is a risk when using a shampoo with keratin protein added to it?

_____

_____

_____

89. What is unique about the ingredients used in vegan shampoos?

_____

_____

_____

RESEARCH

90. Use the internet or go to a store to identify three or four vegan shampoos. Review their ingredients and familiarize yourself with what sets them apart from other shampoos. List the most common vegan ingredients on a sheet of paper. In a few sentences, answer these questions:

Would you use a vegan shampoo? If so, which one would you select, and why?

If you already use a vegan shampoo, explain why you do.

If you do not (or would not) use a vegan shampoo, why would you choose another type of shampoo?

91. Complete the following crossword based on shampoo types. (*Hint:* The word *shampoo* will not be used in any answers.)

Across

4. Also known as soap-free shampoos, these _____-free shampoos are formulated with little to no alkaline base.
5. This type of shampoo is often dispensed with aerosol.
6. This shampoo is also called neutralizing shampoo and can cause dry hair to be drier.
8. This shampoo is formulated with a pH of 7 or higher and is good to use after swimming.
9. This shampoo helps relieve scalp conditions, including dandruff.
10. This shampoo adds strength to weak, damaged, brittle hair.
11. This shampoo is best for curly and brittle hair.

Down

1. This shampoo can help neutralize unwanted yellows in the hair. (2 words)
2. Shampoos with _____ protein added help to temporarily strengthen hair as it cleanses.
3. This shampoo is best for people who want to avoid all animal products and is usually plant-based.
7. This shampoo makes the hair smooth and shiny, and often contains biotin.

92. How should you shampoo a client who has a disability or is in a wheelchair?

_____

_____

_____

93. What is the best way to service a client who has a communication disability?

_____

_____

_____

94. What are three best practices for educating your client about the products you are using in their service?

_____

_____

_____

Conditioner Types

FILL IN THE BLANK

95. _____ deposit protein or moisturizer to help restore the hair's strength, to infuse moisture, to give it body, or to protect it against possible breakage.

96. _____ are designed to penetrate the cortex and reinforce the hair shaft from within to temporarily reconstruct the hair.

97. _____ treatments are chemical mixtures of concentrated protein and intensive moisturizer.

SHORT ANSWER

98. What are the four basic types of conditioners?

_____

_____

_____

99. What are humectants?

_____

_____

_____

100. Why is silicone often added to conditioners?

_____

_____

_____

101. Explain what conditioners do.

_____

_____

_____

102. List and describe four additional conditioning agents to be familiar with.

_____

_____

_____

103. A client who has coarse and extremely curly hair would benefit most from which of the following products?

    A) volumizing shampoo   C) spray-on thermal protection

    B) protein and moisturizing treatments   D) pH/acid-balanced shampoo

104. A client who has straight, fine hair would benefit most from which of the following products?

    A) leave-in conditioner   C) moisturizing treatments

    B) finishing rinse   D) volumizing shampoo

Indicate whether the following statements are true or false. For any false statements, explain why they are false.

105. The fatty acids in oils can replace the lack of natural lipids in the hair to help avoid dullness.

    T   F   _____

106. Oil treatments are ideal for dry scalp and hair.

    T   F   _____

107. Oils such as olive oil, coconut oil, and ucuuba butter can be used naturally or found in professional products.

    T   F   _____

108. It is not advisable to add essential oils to an oil treatment because it results in excessive oiliness and negates the treatment.

    T   F   _____

109. One risk of using oil treatments is that too much oil can lead to blocked hair follicles and excess buildup on the scalp, which could actually promote dry hair.

    T   F   _____

SHORT ANSWER

110. What does the term *co-wash* refer to?

    _____

    _____

    _____

111. What type of hair are co-washes best suited for?

    _____

    _____

    _____

112. What is often the foundation for weekly cleansing in the natural hair community and curly hair market?

_____

_____

_____

113. Explain why it is not recommended to use co-washing exclusively as a way to cleanse the hair.

_____

_____

_____

114. What are two possible disadvantages of using the co-wash method too much?

_____

_____

_____

115. What are two other terms for a deep-conditioning treatment?

_____

_____

_____

116. Why would you choose to use a hair mask for a client?

_____

_____

_____

DISCOVERIES AND ACCOMPLISHMENTS

In the space below, write notes about key concepts discussed in this chapter. Share your discoveries with some of the other students in your class and ask them if your notes are helpful. You may want to revise your notes based on good ideas shared by your peers.

Discoveries:

_____

_____

_____

_____

_____

_____

_____

List at least three things you have accomplished since you decided to enroll in school.

Accomplishments:

_____

_____

_____

_____

_____

_____

_____

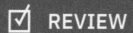

1. A cosmetologist should study and have a thorough understanding of scalp care, shampooing, and conditioning for all hair types because _____.

    A) the shampoo service is the last opportunity to establish the cosmetologist's position as a professional who attends to the clients' specific needs

    B) product category knowledge allows the cosmetologist to recommend the best preparations and services to the clients

    C) improving the appearance of certain scalp conditions that are medical disorders is the responsibility of the cosmetologist

    D) the cosmetologist needs to be licensed to diagnose, treat, prescribe, or work on unhealthy scalp

2. Identify a true statement about the pre-service hair-care procedure.

    A) It is an organized, step-by-step plan for accomplishing the client's requested service.

    B) It is an organized, step-by-step plan for caring for your client after the procedure has been completed.

    C) It is the time to perform an effective client consultation to gain information about service expectations.

    D) It allows you to close the service by offering rebooking dates and retail home care purchases.

3. Identify an accurate statement about the service hair-care procedure.

    A) It is an organized, step-by-step plan for caring for your client after a requested service has been completed.

    B) It is an organized, step-by-step plan for accomplishing the client's requested service.

    C) It is the time for assembling materials, organizing your station, and meeting your client.

    D) It is the time to perform an effective client consultation to gain information about service expectations.

4. Which of the following statements is true of the post-service hair-care procedure?

    A) It is an organized, step-by-step plan for accomplishing the client's requested service.

    B) It details helping your client through the scheduling and payment process.

    C) It involves an organized, step-by-step plan for cleaning and disinfecting your implements.

    D) It is the time to perform an effective client consultation to gain information about service expectations.

continued

5. What is the first step in removing extensions or protective styles?

    A) using a clarifying shampoo to remove build up

    B) detangling the hair properly prior to the shampoo service

    C) using a shampoo or conditioner to maintain hair health

    D) giving a scalp massage using coconut oil, olive oil, or shea butter

6. Identify the second step in removing extensions or protective styles.

    A) using a conditioner to maintain hair health

    B) massaging the scalp

    C) using a clarifying shampoo to remove build up

    D) detangling the hair properly

7. Which of the following questions most likely helps determine if a clarifying shampoo or treatment is needed for a client?

    A) Are you taking any medications that contraindicate a wet shampoo service or scalp massage?

    B) When was the last time you shampooed, and how often do you shampoo?

    C) Have you been using any natural nonprofessional treatments, such as coconut oil, olive oil, or shea butter?

    D) Have you recently removed hair additions such as braids, tape-ins, fusion extensions, or full head sew-in extensions from your hair?

8. A shampoo draping is _____.

    A) used for chemical services or treatments

    B) used for hair coloring and a permanent wave

    C) sometimes called a wet draping

    D) sometimes called a styling draping

9. Identify a true statement about a cutting or styling draping.

    A) It is sometimes called a wet draping.

    B) It is used for chemical services or treatments, such as hair coloring and a permanent wave.

    C) It involves the use of a cape that has a smaller neck strip, which allows a natural fall to the hair.

    D) It is done with a plastic shampoo cape.

continued

10. A chemical draping is _____.

   A) also known as a cutting draping

   B) done with a plastic shampoo cape

   C) used for treatments such as hair coloring and a permanent wave

   D) used when a client is in the salon for a shampoo and styling service

11. Hair brushing should be _____.

   A) done before bleach lightening services

   B) done after a semipermanent or permanent hair-color service to remove dust, dirt, and hair-spray buildup

   C) avoided before a chemical service even if the manufacturer recommends shampooing before the service

   D) avoided if the scalp is irritated

12. Which of the following statements associated with hair brushing is true?

   A) Brushes with natural bristles should be avoided for wavy hair textures before a scalp massage.

   B) Paddle brushes with rubberlike bristles are widely used to detangle wet hair.

   C) Correct hair brushing diminishes microcirculation to the scalp.

   D) When performing a scalp treatment, brushing should overstimulate the scalp.

13. Which of the following statements is true about scalp massage?

   A) It reduces scalp microcirculation.

   B) It increases scalp tenseness.

   C) It is a method of manipulating the scalp by tapping, kneading, rubbing, or stroking it with the hands.

   D) It is typically done by both manipulating the scalp and the hair simultaneously throughout the service.

14. In the context of a scalp massage, effleurage _____.

   A) is often used in a therapeutic massage to loosen up dead skin cells from the scalp

   B) involves gentle pushing and kneading of the scalp with the palms and fingers

   C) uses stroking and circular hand movements

   D) is usually done using the fingertips in backward-to-forward movements

continued

15. A petrissage scalp massage _____.

    A) uses stroking and circular hand movements

    B) involves gentle pushing and kneading of the scalp with the palms, fingers, and thumbs of the hand

    C) is seldom used in a therapeutic massage

    D) is usually done with the balls of the fingers in forward-to-backward movements

16. When using the techniques of effleurage or petrissage to give a scalp massage, _____.

    A) touch and scratch the scalp with your fingernails

    B) apply strong pressure using your fingertips

    C) begin the gentle stroking movements at the hairline

    D) discourage the client from taking deep breaths

17. The purpose of a normal scalp treatment is to _____.

    A) decrease microcirculation to the scalp

    B) replenish hardened sebum in the scalp's pores

    C) control dandruff by facilitating malassezia growth

    D) maintain a clean and healthy scalp

18. A dry hair and scalp treatment should be used when there is _____.

    A) excessive oiliness caused by overactive sebaceous glands

    B) a deficiency of the scalp and hair's natural oils

    C) dandruff on the scalp

    D) hardened sebum collected in the scalp's pores

19. An oily hair and scalp treatment should be used when there is _____.

    A) dandruff on the scalp

    B) a deficiency of the scalp and hair's natural oils

    C) excessive oiliness caused by overactive sebaceous glands

    D) a lack of moisture in the hair, especially dry, brittle hair

continued

20. Identify a guideline associated with antidandruff treatments.

   A) Avoid recommending additional salon treatments.

   B) Avoid hair brushing before an antidandruff treatment.

   C) Avoid recommending regular use of antidandruff home care products.

   D) Avoid using antidandruff shampoos containing mint as part of an antidandruff treatment.

21. In most shampoos, _____ is usually the first ingredient listed, which indicates that it is the main ingredient.

   A) surfactant

   B) water

   C) moisturizer

   D) foam enhancer

22. Which of the following statements associated with shampoos is true?

   A) The less alkaline a shampoo, the stronger and harsher it is.

   B) Hard water contains minerals that increase the ability of a shampoo to lather.

   C) A slightly acidic shampoo closely matches the ideal pH of hair.

   D) Cooler, rather than warmer and tepid, water is adequate for rinsing shampoo.

23. Identify an accurate statement about moisturizing shampoos.

   A) They are created by combining the surfactant base with direct-dye color pigments.

   B) They do not improve the hair's manageability.

   C) They do not remove as much artificial color from the hair.

   D) They cleanse the hair without soap and water.

24. Which of the following statements is true of leave-in conditioners?

   A) They need to be rinsed thoroughly.

   B) They restore protein and moisture and require a longer processing time or the application of heat.

   C) They are sometimes called daily conditioners.

   D) They are created with a low molecular weight to avoid weighing down the hair.

25. _____, usually found in a cream base, softens and improves the scalp's health and contains moisturizing and emollient ingredients.

   A) A spray-on thermal protector

   B) A scalp conditioner

   C) A medicated scalp lotion

   D) A scalp astringent lotion

finished!

Practical Skills
Self-Evaluation Checklist

Regular self-assessment helps you to improve your technical skills and achieve success. After performing each procedure, review the procedure steps in the textbook and rate yourself as "Competent" or "Needs Work," and write in comments on how you were successful or where you can improve. Rating yourself helps you identify your strengths and weaknesses and develop your own plan for improvement.

CRITERIA	COMPETENT	NEEDS WORK	COMMENTS
PROCEDURE 10-1 PRE-SERVICE PROCEDURE			
Cleaning and Disinfecting			
Basic Station Setup			
Stylist Preparation			
Greet Client			
Timing			
PROCEDURE 10-2 POST-SERVICE PROCEDURE			
Advised Client and Recommended Products			
Scheduled Next Appointment and Thanked Client			
Prepared Work Area and Implements for Next Client			
Timing			
PROCEDURE 10-3 DRAPING			
Preparation			
Procedure			
Timing			
PROCEDURE 10-4 HAIR BRUSHING AND DETANGLING			
Preparation			
Procedure			
Timing			
PROCEDURE 10-5 SHAMPOOING AND CONDITIONING			
Preparation			
Procedure			
Timing			
PROCEDURE 10-6 SCALP MASSAGE			
Preparation			
Procedure			
Timing			

Ch. 11: Haircutting

⚑ TRACK MY PROGRESS!

Use this simple tracker to record your progress as you work through the activities in each learning objective.

COMPLETED	# OF CORRECT ANSWERS	OBJECTIVE
☐	_____/2	**LO 1** - Explain why cosmetologists need a thorough understanding of haircutting.
☐	_____/28	**LO 2** - Define haircutting in terms of lines, sections, angles, elevation, finger angle, guidelines, and overdirection.
☐	_____/14	**LO 3** - Describe the role of growth pattern, density, texture, and wave pattern to determine the behavior of hair.
☐	_____/28	**LO 4** - Demonstrate and explain the uses of various haircutting shears.
☐	_____/6	**LO 5** - Demonstrate how to effectively hold haircutting shears.
☐	_____/19	**LO 6** - Demonstrate and explain the uses of the various haircutting tools.
☐	_____/6	**LO 7** - Demonstrate three body positions to ensure healthier posture while creating a haircut.
☐	_____/7	**LO 8** - List four strategies for proper safety in haircutting.
☐	_____/3	**LO 9** - Explain general haircutting techniques for any haircut.
☐	_____/36	**LO 10** - Perform the four basic haircuts.
☐	_____/19	**LO 11** - Outline cutting techniques for curly hair, bangs, razor cutting, slide cutting, and shear-over-comb.
☐	_____/10	**LO 12** - Explain three different texturizing techniques performed with shears.
☐	_____/12	**LO 13** - Explain clipper cut styles and techniques.

Why Study Haircutting?

SHORT ANSWER

1. In addition to using professional skills and artistry to perform a precise haircut for a client, what are three ways that applying a systematic plan can help you succeed?

_____

_____

_____

2. What are the four reasons that cosmetologists should study and have a thorough understanding of haircutting?

_____

_____

_____

Haircutting Lines, Sections, and Angles

FILL IN THE BLANK

Complete the sentences below by filling in the blanks.

3. The two basic lines used in haircutting are _____ and _____.

4. An _____ is what gives the hair _____ and _____.

5. All haircuts are made up of _____, _____, and _____.

6. A _____ is a thin, continuous mark used as a guide.

7. A _____ is the working area that the hair is separated into before cutting.

SHORT ANSWER

8. What are the two haircutting techniques that use diagonal lines to create angles? Briefly describe them.

_____

_____

_____

9. Describe how diagonal forward and diagonal back lines create movement.

_____

_____

_____

10. Match each type of straight line with its description.

    a. Horizontal   b. Vertical   c. Diagonal

**Type of Straight
Line**   **Description**

_____ Direct the eye from one side to the other

_____ Have a slanting or sloping direction

_____ Parallel to the floor and relative to the horizon

_____ Two types of these lines: forward and back

_____ Remove weight to create graduated or layered haircuts; used with higher elevations

_____ Between horizontal and vertical

_____ Build weight; create one-length and low-elevation haircuts

_____ Described in terms of up and down

11. Label the three types of straight lines in the accompanying figure.

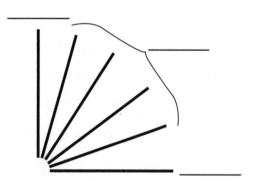

12. On each image below, draw the type of line that it demonstrates. Then label the line.

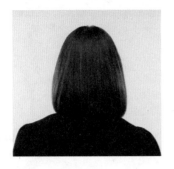 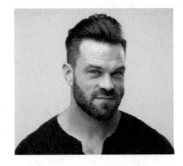 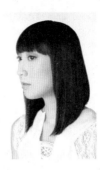

_____   _____   _____

SHORT ANSWER

13. Describe what a part (or a parting) is, and explain how it is used when performing a haircut.

_____

_____

_____

14. List the four types of sections used in haircutting.

_____

_____

_____

FILL IN THE BLANK

15. Complete the chart below, filling in the blanks and drawing the sections directly on the images.

TYPE OF SECTION	DESCRIPTION	DRAW
Horseshoe	Separates the head at the _____ to below the _____	

TYPE OF SECTION	DESCRIPTION	DRAW
Profile	Center _____ to center _____; facilitates sub_____	
_____	Also referred to as a pie-shaped section; rotates from a central point; used in layering and graduation	
_____	Taken from ear to ear and divides the head from front to back, starting behind the apex in the crown	

SHORT ANSWER

16. What are two other terms for *elevation*?

_____

_____

_____

17. Define graduation as it relates to haircutting.

_____

_____

_____

18. Which haircuts require elevation?

_____

_____

_____

19. Why should you usually cut hair, especially curly hair, a bit longer?

_____

_____

_____

DRAW

20. Sketch the elevations using lines to indicate the degrees for each type of elevation.

0-Degree Elevation   45-Degree Elevation   90-Degree Elevation   180-Degree Elevation

SHORT ANSWER

21. What is a finger angle?

_____

_____

_____

22. List four other names for the term *finger angle*.

_____

_____

_____

23. Label each type of finger angle depicted below.

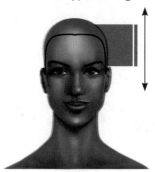 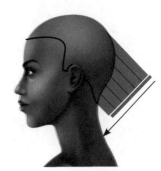 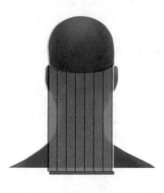

_____   _____   _____

MATCHING

24. Match the guideline terms with their descriptions. Some terms will be used more than once.

a. Guideline   c. Interior   e. Traveling
b. Perimeter   d. Stationary

Term	Description
_____	The hairstyle's outer line
_____	One of two types of guideline
_____	Also known as a movable guideline
_____	Does not move
_____	Also known as a guide
_____	One of two types of guideline
_____	The cut's inner or internal line
_____	Used in blunt (one-length) haircuts and in haircuts that use overdirection to create a length or weight increase
_____	Moves with you as you progress through the haircut
_____	Hair subsection that determines the length the hair will be cut
_____	Created by taking a small slice of the previous subsection and moving it to the next position, or subsection, where it becomes a new guideline

_____ All other sections are combed to this guideline and cut at the same angle and length

_____ Used when creating layered or graduated haircuts

_____ Usually the first section cut when creating a shape

LABELING

25. Describe the elevation, cutting line, and guidelines that are shown in each image below. Then, for each image, use the Internet or magazines to locate an example of an actual finished haircut that incorporates the haircutting techniques illustrated below, and paste those images onto the third row.

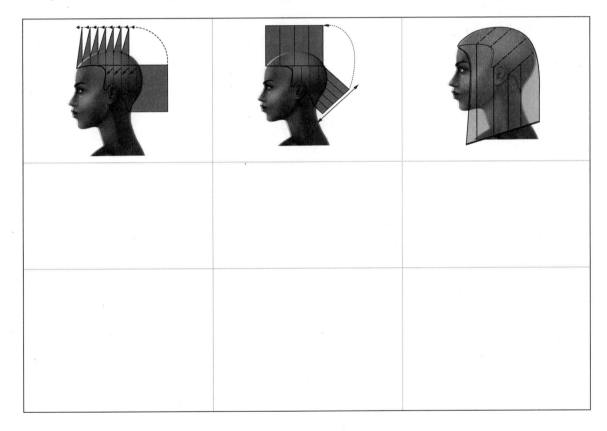

SHORT ANSWER

26. What is overdirection, and why is it used?

_____

_____

_____

27. Imagine you are working on a layered haircut and you want the hair to be longer toward the front. How would you use overdirection? What if you were creating shorter layers around the face and longer layers in the back?

_____

_____

_____

DRAW

28. On the outline of a head below, illustrate how you would overdirect hair for a long-layered look.

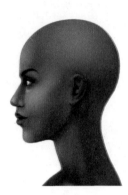

CASE STUDY

29. As a professional stylist, you will have numerous clients who bring in photographs of hairstyles as references. Therefore, learning how to evaluate a style and determine how it was achieved will be of great benefit to you. With that in mind, look through various magazines and select three particular cuts that appeal to you. Paste them on the chart below in the left column. In the right column, diagram and/or explain the techniques, angles, and elevations you would use to create the haircut and style.

PASTE PICTURE HERE	Procedure:
PASTE PICTURE HERE	Procedure:
PASTE PICTURE HERE	Procedure:

30. Find five photos of various haircuts. For each photo, write a description of the techniques you think were used to create the look. In your descriptions, be sure to use the terminology you studied in this chapter—for example, types of guidelines (traveling/stationary), degree of elevation, overdirection, and sectioning. If necessary, draw lines or add shading to the photo to further illustrate the areas you are describing.

When you're finished evaluating the haircuts in your photos, partner with a classmate to show each other your photos and descriptions. Discuss with each other whether your evaluation of each haircut is accurate. If you do not agree, explain why and feel free to demonstrate the techniques (overdirection, sectioning, finger angles, etc.) on each other—without cutting your hair!

Hair Analysis

SHORT ANSWER

31. What are the four characteristics of hair that determine its behavior?

_____

_____

_____

FILL IN THE BLANK

Complete the sentences below.

Word bank: perimeter, natural, neck, crown, dry, fringe, much, shorter

32. The hairline, _____, and _____ areas are where we often find strong growth patterns.

33. The hairline is the hair that grows along the _____ of the face, around the ears, and on the

_____.

34. Using too _____ tension when cutting areas that have strong or obvious growth patterns may

result in _____ areas when the hair is _____, because it will fall in its _____ position.

Indicate whether each statement below is true or false. For any false statements, explain why they are false.

35. Hair density is usually described as thin, medium, or coarse.

    T   F   _____

36. Wave and curl patterns can be categorized into letters and numbers from 1A to 4C, where the tightness of the curl goes from A to C.

    T   F   _____

37. Curly and coiled hair with thin/low density may appear to have less hair.

    T   F   _____

38. The amount of hair in a subsection should have no effect on your ability to see your guideline and control the hair.

    T   F   _____

39. Curl pattern and texture refer to the same thing.

    T   F   _____

FILL IN THE BLANK

40. As a cosmetologist, it is important to recommend haircuts to your clients that work well with their hair texture and density. Based on the combination of hair texture and density in the chart below, would you recommend the haircut to the client?

HAIR TEXTURE + DENSITY	TYPE OF HAIRCUT	RECOMMEND? (Y/N)
Medium + Thin	Graduated shape	
Fine + Thick	Blunt ends with texturizing	
Coarse + Thin	Razor cut to remove weight	
Medium + Thick	Any shape, as long as there is no texturizing	
Coarse + Medium	Kept long, cut without a razor	
Fine + Thin	Long layers with increased texturizing	
Medium + Medium	Long layers with some texturizing	
Coarse + Thick	Very short, razor cut	
Fine + Medium	Blunt cut with low elevation	

41. When healthy, hair with which texture is the most resilient? What is one recommendation for protecting it?

_____

_____

_____

42. What are three precautions to take when handling fine hair? What physical characteristics of fine hair require careful treatment of that texture?

_____

_____

_____

43. Label each type of hair curl/wave pattern shown below with its number/letter category and the description of it from the word bank. (*Hint:* There is little difference between 3A and 3B, so look closely.) Then go around the room and try to find a classmate with each type of curl pattern.

Word bank: straight, waves, spiral curls, very coily

Image									
Number/Letter									
Description									

44. Match each hair curl/wave patterns from the chart above with its special considerations for haircutting.

**Curl/Wave
Pattern Category**   **Special Considerations**

_____ Should be blown dry before cutting to account for shrinkage

_____ Typically will not shrink or recoil when combing for wet haircutting

_____ May require understanding how the client wears their hair most often when choosing a style, especially if worn curly

_____ Can usually be cut with ease either wet or dry

_____ May need to be stretched or thermal styled for cutting due to the tightness of the curl pattern

_____ May need to be cut dry to visualize the true shape

Haircutting Shears

SHORT ANSWER

45. What are three differences between cast and forged shears?

_____

_____

_____

46. Why is it important to know the Rockwell hardness gauge of your haircutting shears?

_____

_____

_____

47. In your own words, briefly describe the difference between the terms *shears* and *scissors* in relation to haircutting.

_____

_____

_____

48. Label the parts of the shear in the illustration below. Then in the chart below describe what each piece does.

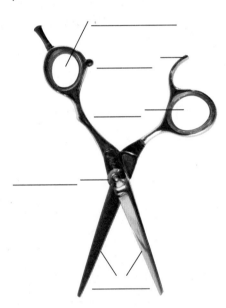

Part of the Shear	Description
Adjustment knob	_____
Pivot and adjustment area	_____
Finger tang	_____
Adjustment knob	_____
Ring-finger hole	_____
Cutting edge	_____
Thumb hole	_____
Finger tang	_____

49. Match each blade length with its features and functions. Lengths will be used more than once.

Word bank: short, mid-length, long

Blade Length   **Features and Functions**

_____ Best for a variety of cutting techniques, including cutting long lines in blunt styles, cutting on skin, slide cutting or slithering, and cutting around the face

_____ Ideal for refining a haircut, especially short haircuts

_____ Standard universal blade length

_____ Good for general cutting techniques, and ideal for precision cutting between your fingers

_____ Recommended for over comb techniques and free-form cutting on curlier hair

_____ Best for cutting shorter small sections, detail work around the ears and hairline, and point cutting

SHORT ANSWER

50. List the maintenance tasks that should be performed daily on your haircutting shears.

_____

_____

_____

51. Describe the cleaning and lubrication process for (1) the daily and (2) the weekly version of this maintenance task.

_____

_____

_____

52. What happens if the tension is too loose or too tight in your shears?

_____

_____

_____

53. How can you test whether the tension needs adjusting?

_____

_____

_____

54. Why should you be careful using cutting blades that extend past your middle finger?

_____

_____

_____

55. What are the lengths of long, short, and mid-length shears? Write them below in both inches and centimeters. (*Hint:* One inch is about 2.5 centimeters.)

_____

_____

_____

56. What is the purpose of texturizing shears?

_____

_____

_____

57. What are three aspects to consider when purchasing shears?

_____

_____

_____

58. What are the differences between right- and left-handed shears? How would you make right-handed shears into left-handed ones?

_____

_____

_____

59. What does the number of teeth in a texturizing shear indicate?

_____

_____

_____

60. What effects do texturizing techniques have on hair with wavy or curly patterns?

_____

_____

_____

MATCHING

61. Match the different texturizing shears shown below. Then identify what each shear is used for.

    a. Thinning shear   c. Chunking shear
    b. Texturizing shear   d. Blending shear

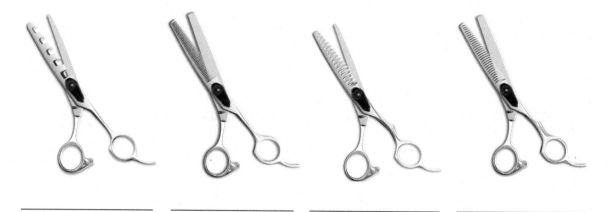

_____   _____   _____   _____

62. When purchasing shears, what is the role of a set of ring guards (or a finger-fitting system)?

_____

_____

_____

63. Which handle design is the most ergonomic?

_____

_____

_____

64. What are five guidelines to consider when you are choosing your professional haircutting shears?

_____

_____

_____

RESEARCH

65. Now it's time for you to conduct some research for your own haircutting shears! Use the Internet or beauty supply catalogues—or even consult with a haircutting professional—to identify three different types of shears that you think would work best for you: including where to purchase it, the cost, blade length and style, handle design, type of steel, and recommendations for usage. Be sure to check if it has a custom finger-fitting system, a maintenance kit or shear oil. or a warranty plan, and include any other features you find notable. Follow the website below to record your findings in the table or use a separate sheet of paper, and then write a few sentences about which shear you would buy and why.

+ BONUS
Visit: bonus.milady.com/cos-wb/toc

66. Match each blade edge with its description. Blade edges will be used more than once.

    a. Semiconvex   b. Convex   c. Beveled

**Type of Blade
Edge**   **Description**

_____ Very sharp edge; extremely quiet and smooth; glides through the hair easily

_____ Sharper than beveled edge but narrower

_____ Not smooth; can be noisy; has a stronger grip on hair

_____ Hair does not slip down the blades

_____ Best overall edge for the professional stylist

_____ Durable; great for beginning stylists

_____ Great for shear-over-comb; good for dry haircutting (not for slide cutting)

_____ Great for all kinds of cutting techniques, including slide cutting

_____ Excellent for dry cutting and taper cutting

SHORT ANSWER

67. List the four components of correctly fitting shears to your hand.

_____

_____

_____

68. Why should you avoid sharing shears with a colleague?

_____

_____

_____

69. What type of handle design will guarantee correct finger placement on the shear?

_____

_____

_____

70. What is being demonstrated in the image below?

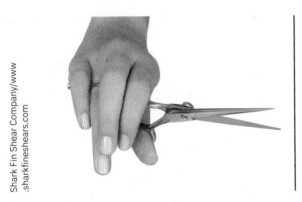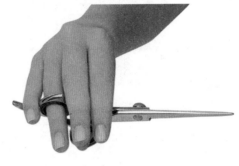

Shark Fin Shear Company/www .sharkfineshears.com

_____

_____

_____

71. Which of the following is *not* part of a properly fitted shear?

A) The ring-finger hole rests between the first and second knuckle.

B) The thumb hole will rest up to or over your knuckle.

C) Your cuticle will be centered underneath the center of the thumb ring guard.

D) There can be a little extra space around you finger and the finger hole.

72. On properly fitted shears, where should your pinky rest?

A) on the finger tang

B) on the ring finger hole

C) over the cuticle area

D) wrapped around the thumb ring guard

Holding the Shears and Comb

73. Why is it important to properly hold your shears?

_____

_____

_____

74. When holding the shears and comb, what is the role of the cutting hand? What is another term for the cutting hand?

_____

_____

_____

75. When holding the shears and comb, what is the role of the holding hand?

_____

_____

_____

76. What is the purpose of holding the comb and shears at the same time during the haircutting process?

_____

_____

_____

SEQUENCING

77. Number the steps for palming the shears from 1 to 3, beginning to end.

_____ Curl your fingers in to palm the shears, which keeps them closed while you comb or part the hair.

_____ Hold the comb between the thumb, index, and middle fingers, while holding the shears at the same time.

_____ Remove your thumb from the thumb grip, leaving your ring and little fingers in the grip and finger rest.

78. Number the steps for transferring the comb from 1 to 4, beginning to end.

_____ Place the comb between the thumb and index finger of your nondominant hand (the hand holding the subsection).

_____ Confirm that your fingers are in place at the correct cutting position.

_____ Cut the subsection.

_____ Comb a subsection into position.

Haircutting Tools

SHORT ANSWER

79. List three differences between cutting with shears and razor cutting.

_____

_____

_____

80. Where do you set the guide for razor cutting, compared to cutting with shears?

_____

_____

_____

81. What will happen if you use a razor on dry hair?

_____

_____

_____

82. List the five safety tips for cutting hair with a razor.

_____

_____

_____

MATCHING

83. Match the haircutting tools with their descriptions. Tools will be used at least once.

a. Haircutting razors
b. Clippers
c. Trimmers

d. Sectioning clips
e. Wide-tooth combs
f. Tail combs

g. Barber combs
h. Styling or cutting combs

Haircutting Tool   **Description**

_____ Smaller version of clippers

_____ Its narrow end allows the shears, clippers, or trimmers to get very close to the head

_____ Mainly used to detangle and are ideal for textured and relaxed hair

_____ Mainly used for a softer effect on the hair ends

_____ Also referred to as all-purpose combs and are used for most haircutting procedures

_____ May be used without a guard to shave hair right to the scalp (called balding) or with cutting guards of various lengths

_____ Used mainly to section and subsection the hair

_____ Two types are used: jaw or butterfly and duckbill

_____ Mainly used when creating short haircuts, short tapers, fades, and flat tops

_____ 6 to 8 inches (15 to 20 centimeters) long; have fine teeth at one end and wider teeth at the other

_____ Used mainly for close tapers on the nape and sides when using the shear-over-comb technique

_____ Mainly used to remove excess or unwanted hair at the neckline and around the ears and create crisp outlines; generally used on very short haircuts

84. Describe how to hold the razor for each method that's shown below.

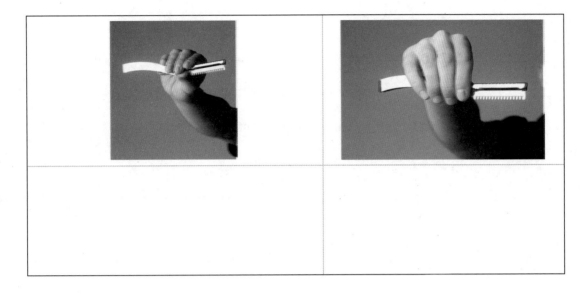

85. Wider teeth provide more tension when combing hair.

    T   F   _____

86. A wide-tooth comb may be ideal for textured hair.

    T   F   _____

87. The fine teeth of a comb are used for combing and parting the hair.

    T   F   _____

88. The finer teeth in a comb are useful when cutting around the ears, when dealing with challenging hairlines due to growth direction, and when cutting dense straight-wavy hair.

    T   F   _____

89. Match the type of tension—minimum or maximum—with its description.

Type of Tension   **Description**

_____ Used around the ears and on hairlines with strong growth patterns

_____ Achieved by combing the section straight and slightly pulling the hair

_____ Used for straight hair when you want a precise line

_____ Used when cutting dry hair to shape

_____ Involves combing the hair and holding the section straight without pulling the hair

TRUE OR FALSE

Indicate whether the statements below are true or false. For any false statements, explain why they are false.

90. You can use clippers with length guards to remove hair completely (great for cleaning up necklines and around the ears).

    T   F   _____

91. Clippers can be used without length guards, to taper hairlines from extremely short lengths into longer lengths, using the clipper-over-comb technique.

    T   F   _____

92. The clipper-over-comb technique is completely different from the shear-over-comb because the clippers move from bottom to top.

    T   F   _____

SHORT ANSWER

93. Which type of motor is preferred by most barbers? Why?

    _____

    _____

    _____

94. Which type of clipper motor is best for stylists who only use clippers a few times a week? Why?

_____

_____

_____

95. Match each tool used in clipper cutting with its description or function. Each tool will be used at least once.

    a. Clipper blades
    b. Clipper guard attachments

    c. Haircutting shears
    d. Thinning shears

    **Tool for Clipper
    Cutting**   **Description**

    _____ Can be attached to the clipper with a simple snap-on design

    _____ Allow you to cut all the hair evenly to an exact length from 1/16 inch (1.6 millimeters) to 1.25 inch (31.7 millimeters); the lower the number, the shorter the hair

    _____ Great for removing excess bulk and for blending one area with another

    _____ Used mainly for removing length and detailing the haircut

    _____ Detachable versions used in lieu of clipper guards

    _____ Interchangeable; available in a variety of styles, sizes, and lengths

96. Where on the head is the classic barbering comb typically used? Why?

_____

_____

_____

97. What are the finer- and wider-spaced teeth used for in a regular cutting comb?

_____

_____

_____

Trimmers

98. For each image below, describe how the trimmer is being used.

_____   _____   _____   _____   _____

99. In addition to haircutting, what are other uses for clippers and trimmers?

_____

_____

_____

100. What is a tattoo trimmer? What is it best used for?

_____

_____

_____

101. What is an alternative to using a comb with trimmers when trimming a beard?

_____

_____

_____

102. Describe how to maintain clippers and trimmers.

_____

_____

_____

103. For each image below, name the technique being used for trimming the facial hair.

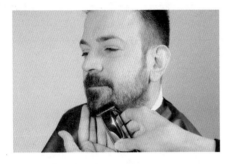

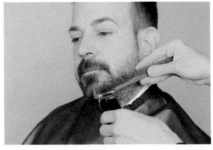

_____   _____

Demonstrate Proper Posture and Body Positions

SHORT ANSWER

104. What are three benefits of maintaining good body position during a haircut?

_____

_____

_____

105. What does good posture help you avoid?

_____

_____

_____

106. In addition to maintaining good posture and body position, what are two other precautions you can take while cutting hair to prevent problems in your body?

_____

_____

_____

107. What are three ways to ensure that you maintain good body position when cutting hair?

_____

_____

_____

108. Briefly describe how to center your weight when (1) working, (2) standing, and (3) sitting.

_____

_____

_____

109. How can positioning your hands properly and ergonomically help you during a haircut?

_____

_____

_____

110. What is a haircut where you would cut below the fingers?

_____

_____

_____

Safety in Haircutting

111. Briefly list the four general safety strategies for haircutting. What are two other ways you can prevent accidents?

    _____

    _____

    _____

112. What is one way to ease knee and leg fatigue when standing to perform haircuts?

    _____

    _____

    _____

RESEARCH

113. According to your text, cosmetologists are required by law in some states to wear closed-toe shoes in the salon. Does your state require you to wear closed-toe shoes? Use the Internet or go to the library to learn more about the safety requirements in your state as they relate to haircutting. Make a note of the sources you used for your answers so that you can stay up to date on the safety laws in your state.

Haircutting Techniques

SHORT ANSWER

114. List the four basic haircuts.

    _____

    _____

    _____

115. Define weight line.

_____

_____

_____

116. How many haircuts can you create with the four basic types?

_____

_____

_____

117. Match each basic type of haircut with its description. Each type will be used at least once.

a. Blunt
b. Graduated

c. Layered
d. Long-layered

Basic Type of Haircut | **Description**

_____ Has no elevation or overdirection

_____ Compared to a graduated haircut, this cut has less weight and the ends appear farther apart

_____ Most common elevation is 45 degrees

_____ Cut at a 90-degree elevation and then overdirected to maintain length and weight at the perimeter, which results in elevating length and weight from 0 degrees (in natural fall) to 180 degrees when overdirected

_____ Slow or immediate buildup of weight caused by cutting the hair with tension

_____ When creating this cut for fine hair, use a stationary guide at the center profile and overdirect into the center section with a high elevation

_____ Hair cut at higher elevations, usually 90 degrees

_____ Resulting shape will have shorter layers at the top and increasingly longer layers toward the perimeter

_____ Has a visual buildup of weight, and the hair ends appear to be stacked

_____ Cut with a stationary guide; all hair comes to single hanging level, forming a weight line

118. Identify the basic haircut type shown in each photo below.

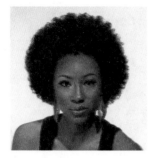 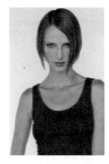 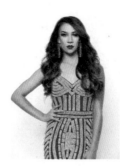 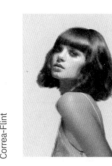

Hair: Sherri Jesse Photo: Kristen Correa-Flint

Hair: Gareth Palmer Photo: Kristen Correa-Flint

_____ _____ _____ _____

TRUE OR FALSE

Indicate whether the statements below are true or false. For any false statements, explain why they are false.

119. It is important to understand how curly hair behaves and shrinks after it is cut and dried.

    T   F   _____

120. It is not necessary to consider density and texture when making cutting decisions about hair that has a curl pattern—you only need to focus on the client's face shape and the desired result.

    T   F   _____

COLLAGE

121. Using the Internet, your text, and magazines, find depictions of the four basic haircuts (blunt, graduated, layered, and long-layered) done on straight, wavy, curly, and coily hair. How do they look different? Keep these images with you to remind yourself that even a basic haircut can look very different depending on a client's curl pattern.

122. For each statement, indicate whether it's a do or a don't when performing haircuts on clients who have curly hair patterns.

Do or Don't?	When Performing Haircuts for Clients Who Have Curly Hair
_____	Leave lengths longer
_____	Stretch the hair as you cut it
_____	Use minimal tension and/or the wide teeth of your comb when cutting
_____	Use a razor on curly hair that is fine or damaged
_____	Elevate less than when working with straight hair to achieve strong angles
_____	Cut textured hair when dry
_____	Maintain consistent hair dampness while cutting wet
_____	Cut curly hair shorter than desired

SHORT ANSWER

123. Why is it important to familiarize yourself with products that are appropriate for curly hair?

_____

_____

_____

124. What are two techniques you can use instead of a razor to remove bulk and weight from curly hair?

_____

_____

_____

125. What is the "big chop"? What are three questions you can ask a client who is considering this move?

_____

_____

_____

126. This exercise requires samples of straight, wavy, curly, and coily hair. Take each sample of hair and, without adding any tension, measure the length of the sample from top to tip. Then wet each sample of hair as you would if you were performing a shampoo service, and measure them again. What is the difference? Fill out the table below and see if your results match the shrinkage guide in your textbook.

You can find the shrinkage percentage by:

1. Dividing the length when dry by the length when wet.
2. Subtracting that number from 1.
3. Multiplying the result by 100.

For example, if the length when dry is 6 inches and when wet it's 10 inches, then you would divide 6/10 = 0.6. Next, subtract 1 − 0.6 = 0.4. Finally, multiply 0.4 × 100 = 40, and that's 40 percent shrinkage!

HAIR TYPE	LENGTH WHEN DRY	LENGTH WHEN WET	SHRINKAGE %	SHRINKAGE % IN TEXTBOOK
Straight				0%
Wavy				1–20%
Curly				20–50%
Coily				50–90%

127. Indicate whether each statement below is something that should (Do) or should not (Don't) be done when performing a haircut.

Do or Don't?   **When Performing Haircuts**

_____ Charge based on haircut style, not gender

_____ Use the mirror to see your elevation

_____ Work with your guideline

_____ Use a large subsection

_____ Cross-check the haircut

_____ Reduce the size of your subsection before cutting if you cannot see the guide

_____ Replace the blade during the cut with coarse hair textures

_____ Turn the client sideways so that you can see one side in the mirror while working on the opposite side

_____ Say "women's cut" or "men's cut"

_____ Ensure your lines and sections are clean and balanced

_____ Place an even amount of hair in each subsection

_____ Check that both sides are even by standing in front of your client

FILL IN THE BLANK

Complete the sentences below.

128. _____ is parting the same haircut in the opposite way that you _____ it, to

check for _____ and _____ precision.

129. Maintain _____ tension by using the _____ teeth of the _____ and not

_____ the subsection too _____.

130. When selecting a style for the client, consider existing _____ because it can give the

illusion of _____, _____, or brightness.

LABELING

131. Identify the specific type of blunt cut shown in each image below.

_____   _____   _____   _____

132. Number the main steps of the procedure for performing a blunt cut, using the numbers 1 through 12. One step has been numbered for you.

_____9_____ Once the haircut is complete, start in the center back, and comb from scalp to ends. Make sure the hair is at zero degrees with no elevation.

_____ Section from front hairline down to the nape.

_____ Part hair in center, using the nose as a reference point.

_____ Place the comb on top of the ear and section straight across to the opposite ear. There should now be four quadrants with the back two sections from the top of the ear down to the nape.

_____ Create your guideline.

_____ Continue adding ½- to ¼-inch subsections until you complete the entire two back quadrants.

_____ a. Dry the hair for final styling: If the hair will be styled curly, add styling product, work it throughout the hair with your hands, and dry with a diffuser.
b. Dry the hair for final styling: If the hair will be styled straight, blowdry the hair straight and smooth.

_____ Starting in the left back quadrant, create a horizontal or horseshoe ½- to ¼-inch section from left to right.

_____ Moving to the front right quadrant, continue dropping down ½- to ¼-inch subsections, cutting horizontally using the previous guide from the back right quadrant.

_____ Once the hair is dry, visually check for a horizontal line all around the head and clean up the perimeter line as needed.

_____ Move to the front left quadrant and repeat the steps, using horizontal or horseshoe sections throughout the entire cut.

_____ Stand in front of your client and, starting at the scalp area, slowly measure the right and left sides of the haircut.

SHORT ANSWER

133. List three questions or prompts for use in a client consultation when a blunt haircut is being considered.

_____

_____

_____

134. Until you become more familiar and comfortable with performing blunt cuts, what are some other questions you would want to ask a client who is considering this type of cut?

_____

_____

_____

FILL IN THE BLANK

135. For each topic listed below, provide a tip specifically related to performing blunt cuts.

Topic	Tip for Blunt Cuts
Combing the sections	_____
Curl patterns	_____
Tension	_____
Natural growth patterns	_____
Ears	_____
Hair moisture – cutting wet	_____
Crown and hairline	_____

LABELING

136. Identify the specific type of graduated haircut shown in each image below.

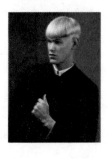 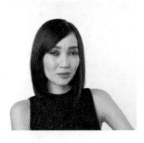 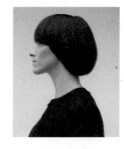 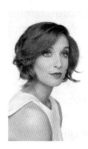

_____   _____   _____   _____

137. Number the general steps of the procedure for performing a graduated haircut, using the numbers 1 through 14. One step has been numbered for you.

_____ Section the hair from front hairline to the apex.

_____ Part the hair in the center, using the nose as a reference point.

_____ Move to the back quadrant and comb the entire back section in its natural fall from the crown to the nape.

___8___ Repeat, dropping the ¼- to ½-inch guide using horizontal or horseshoe subsections followed by a vertical cutting line.

_____ Complete the crown, occipital, and nape areas. Continue cutting using vertical ¼- to ½-inch subsections until the entire back nape, occipital, and crown have been cut at 45 degrees. Once these sections are complete, move to the front two sections.

_____ Section from the apex to behind the right and left ears and secure the right and left quadrants with clips.

_____ Cut at 45-degree angle using vertical line. Once the traveling guide is established, the remaining hair will be cut at a 45-degree angle using a vertical line.

_____ Check the hair vertically or horizontally at a 45-degree elevation.

_____ Dry the hair to check the line for accuracy in the mirror to ensure a graduation of length.

    a. If the hair will be styled straight, blowdry the hair straight and smooth and recheck the lines and angles using a horizontal or vertical angle.

    b. When drying curly hair, use a diffuser and visually check the line for balance using your mirror.

_____ Section horizontally from left to right and cut with no elevation; use the first ¼- to ½-inch horizontal or horseshoe subsection to create a guide.

_____ Move to the right side of the head and begin with the horseshoe or horizontal subsections. Comb the hair from scalp to end using the previous guide from the back. Continue cutting hair using vertical subsections.

_____ Cut your desired length with no elevation using a horizontal cutting line. The cutting tool and comb should be horizontal when cutting the guide.

_____ Check the right and left sides and adjust accordingly. Stand in front of your client and starting at the scalp area, slowly measure the right and left sides of the haircut and adjust accordingly.

_____ Continue to cut each section at a 45-degree angle. Once the guide is matched from the back/previously cut section, use the guide from the bottom to continue the 45-degree haircut. Repeat on the left side of the head.

138. List three questions or prompts for use in a client consultation when a graduated haircut is being considered.

_____

_____

_____

139. Until you become more familiar and comfortable with performing graduated cuts, what are some other questions you would want to ask a client who is considering this type of cut?

_____

_____

_____

FILL IN THE BLANK

140. For each topic listed below, provide a tip specifically related to performing graduated haircuts.

Topic	Tip for Graduated Haircuts
Fine and thin hair	_____
Neckline	_____
Coarse textures and curly hair	_____
Tension	_____
Hair with medium density	_____

LABELING

141. Identify the type of uniform-layered haircut shown in each photo below.

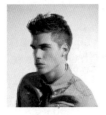   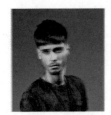   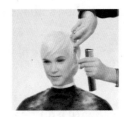

_____   _____   _____

142. Number the general steps of the procedure for performing a uniform-layered haircut, using the numbers 1 through 12. One step has been numbered for you.

_____5_____ Begin dropping down 1½-inch subsections from the first quadrant. Cut the hair using your razor at 90 degrees, working from the center of the first quadrant toward the side, then back to the center toward the opposite side.

_____ Pick up your shears and begin cutting the second quadrant in the center back using a palm-to-palm or overcutting technique.

_____ Move to quadrant 4 and continue the cut by slicking vertical ½-inch or less vertical subsections. Repeat with quadrant 5

_____ Begin creating a zero-degree guideline. The razor can then be placed on top of the middle and index fingers. Continue to create your guideline.

_____ Once the hair is dry, check the mirror. Measure each quadrant on the head at a 90- degree angle. If the nap is 6 inches, then the entire haircut should be 6 inches when held out at 90 degrees.

_____ Once you get to the top of the ear, quadrant 1 is complete. The remaining quadrants will be cut using your shears.

_____ Starting in the back-nape area, establish your guide by using a razor with guard. Create a horizontal or horseshoe-shaped ¼- to ½-inch section from left to right.

_____ Once the guide is established, hold the guide out at a 90-degree angle and measure the hair's length

_____ With the interior layers complete, use the nose as a guide and section the hair down the center using a zero-degree elevation to make sure the entire exterior is even.

_____ Use your index and middle fingers to guide the hair and continue cutting the hair with vertical subsections at a 90-degree angle.

_____ Move to quadrant 3 and continue cutting as you move into the center of the front section, holding the hair at a 90-degree angle to complete this section.

_____ Continue getting the guide using zero elevation and a horizontal cutting line, working from the center to the left ear and then from the center to the right ear.

143. List three questions or prompts for use in a client consultation when a uniform-layered haircut is being considered.

_____

_____

_____

144. Until you become more familiar and comfortable with performing uniform-layered cuts, what are some other questions you would want to ask a client who is considering this type of cut?

_____

_____

_____

145. How would you create a shag haircut?

_____

_____

_____

DRAW

146. Using the head images and profile outlines provided below, sketch your version of a finished long-layered haircut design for a client with wavy hair and for a client who has curly hair. (If you prefer to sketch a shag haircut for wavy/curly hair, indicate that on your drawings.) Make your drawings as detailed and specific as possible to highlight the layers, and include any labeling, heavier lines, or arrows that you think will help emphasize the features of your long-layered haircuts.

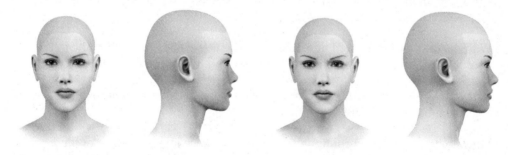

Long-Layered Haircut for Wavy Hair   **Long-Layered Haircut for Curly Hair**

SHORT ANSWER

147. List three questions or prompts for use in a client consultation when a long-layered haircut is being considered.

_____

_____

_____

148. Until you become more familiar and comfortable with performing long-layered cuts, what are some other questions you would want to ask a client who is considering this type of cut?

_____

_____

_____

149. For each topic listed below, provide a tip specifically related to performing long-layered haircuts.

Topic	Tip for Long-Layered Haircuts
Coarse hair texture	_____
Thin hair density	_____
Long hair that falls below shoulder blades	_____
Medium/thicker hair density	_____
Long-layered shapes with thickness at the bottom	_____

Beyond Basic Haircutting Techniques

SHORT ANSWER

150. Why is it important to evaluate your client's curl or wave pattern before performing the techniques that go beyond the basic haircuts?

_____

_____

_____

151. What are three possible outcomes if you do not evaluate your client's curl or wave pattern?

_____

_____

_____

TRUE OR FALSE

Indicate whether the statements below are true or false. For any false statements, explain why they are false.

152. The term *bangs* means the same thing as *fringe*.

   T   F   _____

153. When cutting the bangs, the hair should be either damp or completely dry.

   T   F   _____

154. To determine where the bang area begins, you should place a comb on the top of the head so that the middle of the comb is balanced on the apex—it begins where the comb leaves the head in front of the apex.

   T   F   _____

155. You should use medium to maximum tension when combing and preparing to cut bangs.

   T   F   _____

156. The amount of hair and sectioning for the bangs is solely based on the width of your client's head.

   T   F   _____

157. You will get better results and your client will be more comfortable if you ensure the client's eyes are closed and the brow area is relaxed and in its natural resting position.

   T   F   _____

158. What is a possible outcome if you work with hair that is outside of the natural distribution when creating or shaping bangs?

_____

_____

_____

159. What are the recommendations for cutting bangs on clients who have strong cowlicks or low facial hairlines?

_____

_____

_____

MATCHING

160. Match the bangs with the corresponding description or image. Some descriptions will fit two types of bangs; all types will be used at least once.

a. Asymmetric
b. Side-swept

c. Versatile
d. Curly

e. Square

Type of Bangs	Description or Image
_____	Used mostly on mid-length to long hair; works great for clients with natural side parts
_____	To create, take a triangle section at the top of the head; create two or three horizontal subsections and create your desired length in the center, adding slight length on both corners
_____	Designed for all hair lengths; makes a statement and can vary from subtle to bold

_____

_____ To create, use shears or a razor (like asymmetric bangs but only longer) to work off the natural side part and take vertical 90-degree sections to create a stationary guide and overdirect to the guide

_____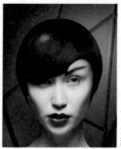

Eli Mancha

_____ Twisting strands and point cutting can add texture and volume for this type of hair; can also be cut dry

_____ Designed for all hair lengths; can be worn on either side

_____ Created using shears and can be worn heavy or soft

_____ Created with shears by sectioning an offset triangular section and overdirecting each section to the stationary guide

_____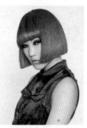

Hair: Courtney Von Burge
Photo: Kristen Correa-Flint

_____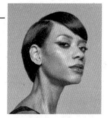

_____ To create, use a standard triangle, section the bang area, then create horizontal subsections and create your guide using zero tension; when complete, blowdry and then check the line to ensure it is balanced

_____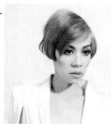

Hair: Teddy Button Photo:
Kristen Correa-Flint

161. Explain what slide cutting is.

_____

_____

_____

162. List four reasons to use slide cutting.

_____

_____

_____

163. How much moisture should hair have when you are slide cutting?

_____

_____

_____

164. What is the goal of cutting on the curve?

_____

_____

_____

SEQUENCE

165. Number the main steps of the shear-over-comb technique, from 1 to 4.

_____ Place the comb, teeth first, into the hairline and turn the comb so the teeth are angled away from the head.

_____ Stand or sit directly in front of the section you are working on. The area you are cutting should be at eye level.

_____ Angle the comb farther away from the head as you reach the area you are blending to avoid cutting into the length (weight).

_____ With the still blade of the shears parallel to the spine of the comb, move the comb up the head, continually opening and closing the thumb blade smoothly and quickly.

166. Briefly describe the shear-over-comb technique for cutting hair.

_____

_____

_____

167. Should you use the shear-over-comb technique on wet or dry hair? Why?

_____

_____

_____

168. Why is it recommended to cut with an even rhythm when using the shear-over-comb technique?

_____

_____

_____

Texturizing

TRUE OR FALSE

Indicate whether each statement below is true or false. For any false statements, explain why they are false.

169. Texturizing is the process of removing excess bulk while shortening the length; it is also used to cut for effect within the hair length, causing wispy or spiky results.

    T   F   _____

170. Texturizing techniques can add or remove volume, make hair move, and blend one area into another.

    T   F   _____

171. There is no need to check your client's curl pattern before performing texturizing techniques.

T   F   _____

SHORT ANSWER

172. Describe how to remove weight and taper the ends using a razor.

_____

_____

_____

173. When free-hand slicing with a razor, how do vertical and horizontal movements, respectively, affect how much hair you remove?

_____

_____

_____

174. Describe the basic method for using thinning shears to remove bulk or weight. What should you do for longer lengths?

_____

_____

_____

175. What are precautions or tips for using thinning shears to remove bulk/weight on coarse hair textures? Blunt haircuts? Curly hair?

_____

_____

_____

176. Match the types of texturizing techniques for shears with their descriptions and images. Each type will be used three times.

a. Point cutting   c. Free-hand notching   e. Slicing

b. Notching   d. Effilating   f. Carving

Type of Texturizing Technique for Shears   **Descriptions and Images**

_____

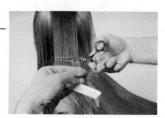

_____ This can be done on wet hair to remove length by holding the hair and turning your wrist so that the tips of the shears point to the ends of the hair on dry hair. This technique is performed to soften the line, remove weight, and create a seamless effect.

_____

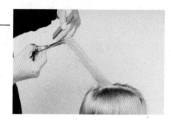

_____ This technique is generally used on the section's interior rather than at the ends.

_____ A version of slicing that creates a visual separation in the hair; works best on short hair (1.5 to 3 inches [4 to 7.5 centimeters] in length).

_____ A technique that removes weight and adds movement through the hair length.

_____ Another version of point cutting, performed with straight or notching shears, but more aggressive and creates a chunkier effect.

_____

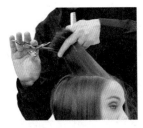

_____ Also known as slithering, this is the process of thinning the hair to graduated lengths with shears.

_____

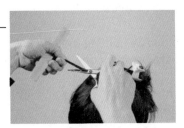

_____ Uses the tips of the shears on hair ends to create a broken edge.

_____

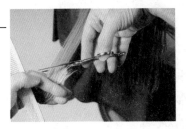

_____ Snip out hair pieces at random intervals. This works well on curly hair, where you want to remove some density.

_____ To perform this technique, place the still blade into the hair and rest it on the scalp. Move the shears through the hair, gently opening and partially closing them as you move.

_____

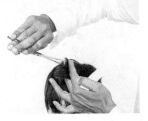

_____ The hair strand is cut by a sliding movement of the shears with the blades kept partially opened. It is used to reduce volume and create movement.

_____ This technique involves placing the tips of your shears about 2 inches (5 centimeters) from the ends. Close your shears as you quickly move them out toward the ends.

_____ In this technique, you fan out the hair section to be cut and never completely close the shears.

177. Match the types of razor texturizing techniques with their descriptions and images. Each type will be used three times.

a. Free-hand slicing with razor on the ends

b. Razor-over-comb

c. Razor rotation

Type of Texturizing Technique for Razors   **Descriptions and Images**

_____ Use this technique by holding the ends of a small piece of hair with your fingertips and slicing down one side toward your fingers.

_____ This is mainly for shorter haircuts and great for tapering the nape area or softening weight lines.

_____

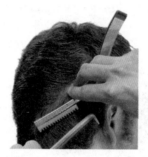

_____ To perform this technique, make small, gentle strokes on the hair's surface with the razor, and move the comb down as you move the razor down.

_____ This is used on the ends of the hair to produce a softer perimeter or create separation throughout the shape.

_____

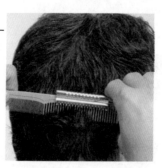

_____ This is very similar to razor-over-comb technique, except you make small circular motions, which helps soften the texture of the area and gives the haircut direction.

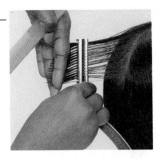

_____ Place the razor on the hair's surface and allow the comb to follow the razor through the area that was just cut.

LABELING

178. Three basic haircuts and their texturizing enhancements are shown below. Label each one.

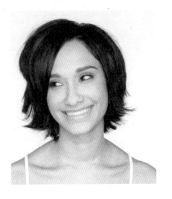

_____

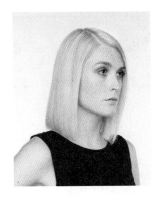

_____

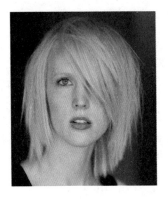

_____

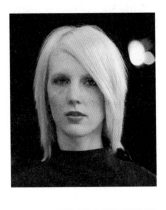

_____

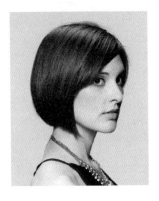

_____

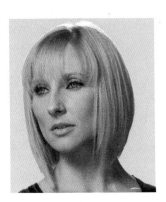

_____

Basic Clipper Techniques

179. What does the clipper-over-comb technique allow you to do with the hair, and what type of haircut can you create with it?

_____

_____

_____

180. Compare the clipper-over-comb technique with the shear-over-comb technique.

_____

_____

_____

SEQUENCE

181. Number the main steps for using the clipper-over-comb technique from 1 to 4.

_____ Hold the comb stationary and cut the length against the comb, moving the clippers from right to left. (If you are left-handed, move the clippers left to right.)

_____ Although your movements should be fluid, remember to stop momentarily to cut the section. Remove the comb from the hair and begin the motion again, using the previously cut section underneath as your guideline. Continue working up the head toward the weight or length.

_____ Place the comb, teeth first, into the hairline, and turn the comb so that the teeth are angled slightly away from the head. Always work against the hair's growth patterns to ensure that you are lifting the hair away from the head and cutting evenly.

_____ Stand directly in front of the section on which you are working. The area you are cutting should be at eye level.

182. List five questions for use in a client consultation when you're preparing to perform a clipper cut.

_____

_____

_____

183. What are two questions you would ask during a client consultation when you're preparing to perform a fade? What are some other questions to ask while you're familiarizing yourself with this type of cut?

_____

_____

_____

TRUE OR FALSE

Indicate whether each statement below is true or false. For any false statements, explain why they are false.

184. When using clippers, the distance between the comb and the scalp determines the amount of hair to be cut.

   T   F   _____

185. The fade technique combines artistry with tool knowledge to achieve the best results.

   T   F   _____

186. A fade is a tapered haircut where the hair transitions from one length to the next, creating a faded look with all soft lines.

   T   F   _____

187. A bald fade is when you clip the hair down to the bare skin.

   T   F   _____

188. There is no need to examine the hair's curl pattern and growth direction when preparing to perform a clipper cut because clippers are powerful enough to compensate for those variations.

   T   F   _____

189. A line up is when straight lines or sharp angles are shaped in the natural hairline, using clippers or trimmers, to change the look of an existing hairline.

   T   F   _____

190. Partner with a classmate to engage in a style consultation for some type of clipper cut, and take turns playing the role of stylist and client.

   - In the role of the stylist, use the questions from the text and any others that you think would be helpful while learning these techniques.

   - As the client, try to provide challenging or unexpected answers to your classmate's questions.

   - Each scenario should end with the stylist making a professional recommendation and describing in detail how they will perform the clipper haircut based on their consultation with the client.

DISCOVERIES AND ACCOMPLISHMENTS

In the space below, write notes about key concepts discussed in this chapter. Share your discoveries with some of the other students in your class and ask them if your notes are helpful. You may want to revise your notes based on good ideas shared by your peers.

Discoveries:

_____

_____

_____

_____

_____

_____

_____

List at least three things you have accomplished since you decided to enroll in school.

Accomplishments:

_____

_____

_____

_____

_____

_____

_____

1. Identify a reason why cosmetologists should study and have a comprehensive understanding of haircutting.

    A) because haircutting is the basic foundational skill upon which all hair designs are built

    B) because they are licensed to diagnose, treat, prescribe, or work on unhealthy hair and perform any service required in the process

    C) because haircutting services are listed under a podiatry license, and performing procedures that are listed under any podiatry license is a primary responsibility of cosmetologists

    D) because they are required to inform clients about the parts of the hair that will be affected by haircutting

2. Which of the following refers to the working area that the hair is separated into before cutting?

    A) a layer   C) a section

    B) an angle   D) a perimeter

3. The degree at which a subsection of hair is lifted from the head when cutting is known as _____.

    A) the cutting position   C) the finger angle

    B) overdirection   D) elevation

4. Which of the following occurs when a hairstylist combs the hair away from its natural falling position, rather than straight out from the head, to increase the design's length?

    A) lifting   C) projection

    B) overdirection   D) graduation

5. In the context of haircutting, the density of the hair determines _____.

    A) the direction the hair grows from the scalp

    B) whether the hair is fine, medium, or coarse

    C) the size and number of subsections needed to complete a haircut

    D) the amount of movement in the hair

continued

6. Identify a guideline that you should follow to maintain your sheers and keep them in excellent shape.

   A) Sharpen your shears on a three- to six-month cycle or every time the sharpening technician comes to the salon.

   B) Thoroughly wipe the inside of the blades after every client using a soft cloth saturated with scissor oil.

   C) After disinfecting your shears with soap and water, take the shears apart by loosening the screw to dry the area.

   D) Put shear oil directly under the adjustment knob once every week.

7. Identify a true statement about texturizing shears.

   A) They are used mainly for creating smoother edges.

   B) They are also known as swivel shears or curved shears.

   C) They are used primarily to remove bulk from the hair.

   D) They are only appropriate for a left-handed cutter.

8. Which of the following is an advantage of palming the shears?

   A) It enables a hairstylist to hold the comb and the shears at the same time.

   B) It keeps the points of the shears open.

   C) It decreases strain on the little finger while combing the hair.

   D) It allows hairstylists to rest their cutting hand.

9. When working with a razor, _____.

   A) the ends are cut at an angle and the line is not blunt

   B) the ends of the hair are cut blunt

   C) the guide is usually below your fingers

   D) you can only cut horizontal or vertical lines, not diagonal lines

10. _____ is the pressure applied when combing and holding a subsection of hair and is created by stretching or pulling the subsection.

   A) tension   C) graduation

   B) lifting   D) overdirection

continued

11. Which of the following is a function of trimmers?

    A) They are primarily used for a softer effect on the hair ends.

    B) They are mainly used to create a taper.

    C) They are used to clean up the hair on the neck that grows below the design line.

    D) They are primarily used to section and subsection the hair.

12. Identify a guideline that you should follow to maintain proper body posture and position when working.

    A) When standing, keep your knees locked rather than slightly bent.

    B) When sitting, keep both feet hanging rather than on the floor.

    C) Keep your body weight centered and firm.

    D) Bend at the waist if you need to lean slightly one way or the other.

13. When cutting with a vertical or diagonal cutting line, which of the following is the best way to maintain control of a subsection, especially regarding elevation and overdirection?

    A) cutting palm-to-palm   C) cutting on the insides of knuckles

    B) cutting below the fingers   D) cutting over the fingers

14. Which of the following is a safety measure you should take to avoid injuring your client during a haircutting service?

    A) Take special care not to accidentally cut the client's skin when cutting around the ears.

    B) Never palm the razor when combing or parting the hair.

    C) Do not cut past the first knuckle when cutting palm-to-palm.

    D) Keep the points of the shears open at all times.

15. Identify a strategy for proper safety in haircutting.

    A) When working with a razor, learn without a guard.

    B) Do not cut past the first knuckle when cutting below your fingers.

    C) Never palm the shears when combing or parting the hair.

    D) Discard used blades in a puncture-proof container.

continued

16. Identify a true statement about a blunt haircut.

    A) It is cut with a traveling guide.

    B) The hair is cut with elevation and overdirection.

    C) It is best for coarse and thick hair types.

    D) All the hair comes to one hanging level, forming a weight line.

17. For basic haircutting techniques, a _____ haircut is an immediate or slow buildup of weight caused by cutting the hair with tension, low to medium elevation, or overdirection.

    A) graduated   C) blunt

    B) pageboy   D) layered

18. A _____ haircut is achieved by cutting the hair with elevation or overdirection; the hair is cut at higher elevations, usually 90 degrees.

    A) layered   C) one-length

    B) blunt   D) graduated

19. In a _____ haircut, the hair is cut at a 90-degree elevation and then overdirected to maintain length and weight at the perimeter.

    A) pageboy   C) long-layered

    B) blunt   D) graduated

20. Which of the following guidelines should you follow when cutting bangs?

    A) Avoid cutting bangs on clients with cowlicks or high facial hairlines.

    B) When cutting bangs, ensure the hair is either damp or completely dry.

    C) Never cut beyond the bang area if you are blending into the sides.

    D) When combing and preparing to cut bangs, use tension instead of the hair's natural lift.

21. The term _____ refers to where and how hair is moved over the head.

    A) projection   C) distribution

    B) tension   D) elevation

continued

22. Which of the following is a method of layering the hair in which the fingers and shears glide along the edge of the hair to remove length?

   A) slicing

   C) texturizing

   B) slide cutting

   D) point cutting

23. Which of the following terms refers to the process of removing excess bulk without shortening the length of the hair?

   A) beveling

   C) graduation

   B) lifting

   D) texturizing

24. _____ is a texturizing technique performed on hair ends using the tips of the shears to create a broken edge.

   A) Point cutting

   C) Effilating

   B) Carving

   D) Free-hand slicing

25. In the context of basic clipper techniques, a _____ is a tapered haircut where the hair transitions from one length to the next, creating a faded look with no hard lines.

   A) zero-elevation haircut

   C) layer

   B) fade

   D) line up

finished!

Practical Skills
Self-Evaluation Checklist

Regular self-assessment helps you to improve your technical skills and achieve success. After performing each procedure, review the procedure steps in the textbook and rate yourself as "Competent" or "Needs Work," and write in comments on how you were successful or where you can improve. Rating yourself helps you identify your strengths and weaknesses and develop your own plan for improvement.

CRITERIA	COMPETENT	NEEDS WORK	COMMENTS
PROCEDURE 11-1 BLUNT HAIRCUT			
Preparation			
Procedure			
Post-Service			
Timing			
PROCEDURE 11-2 GRADUATED HAIRCUT			
Preparation			
Procedure			
Post-Service			
Timing			
PROCEDURE 11-3 UNIFORM-LAYERED HAIRCUT			
Preparation			
Procedure			
Post-Service			
Timing			
PROCEDURE 11-4 LONG-LAYERED HAIRCUT			
Preparation			
Procedure			
Post-Service			
Timing			
PROCEDURE 11-5 BASIC CLIPPER CUT			
Preparation			
Procedure			
Post-Service			
Timing			
PROCEDURE 11-6 TAPER FADE ON STRAIGHT HAIR			
Preparation			
Procedure			
Post-Service			
Timing			
PROCEDURE 11-7 CLASSIC FADE ON CURLY HAIR			
Preparation			
Procedure			
Post-Service			
Timing			

Ch. 12: Hairstyling

🏳 TRACK MY PROGRESS!

Use this simple tracker to record your progress as you work through the activities in each learning objective.

COMPLETED	# OF CORRECT ANSWERS	OBJECTIVE
☐	_____ /4	**LO 1** - Explain professional hairstyling and how it can enhance your beauty career.
☐	_____ /7	**LO 2** - Detail the steps for an effective hairstyling consultation.
☐	_____ /10	**LO 3** - Describe professional hairbrushes, combs, and implements, and their specific uses.
☐	_____ /24	**LO 4** - Identify the different types of styling aids and their many uses.
☐	_____ /25	**LO 5** - Explain the features and benefits of professional blowdryers and the safety precautions to take when using them.
☐	_____ /36	**LO 6** - Describe the different types of thermal irons used by salon professionals, including safety precautions to take when using them, and demonstrate curling iron and smoothing techniques.
☐	_____ /24	**LO 7** - Discuss thermal pressing in terms of type of pressing, tools, products, and procedures.
☐	_____ /20	**LO 8** - Describe and demonstrate natural textured styles.
☐	_____ /17	**LO 9** - Describe and demonstrate curl formation and teasing techniques.
☐	_____ /34	**LO 10** - Explain the different types of wet sets and demonstrate how to perform them.
☐	_____ /10	**LO 11** - Describe the importance of updo preparation, sectioning, pinning, and balance, and create two foundational updos for styling long hair.

Why Study Hairstyling?

SHORT ANSWER

1. Why is it important for you, as a hairstylist, to understand the natural hair movement?

_____

_____

_____

2. Describe what is meant by the term *natural hairstyling*.

_____

_____

_____

3. What is your responsibility to your clients, as a cosmetologist, related to being aware of current hair trends or modern looks?

_____

_____

_____

4. Listed below are the eight reasons that cosmetologists should have a thorough understanding of hairstyling. As you review them, consider them to be mini-goals that will inspire your learning. Rewrite each reason to study hairstyling as a personal goal. Then, after reflecting or doing some research, include one or two specific ways that you plan to achieve that goal. An example is provided for the first reason. Finally, for further inspiration, partner with a classmate to review each other's mini-goals and briefly discuss your plans to achieve them.

ORIGINAL REASON TO STUDY HAIRSTYLING	MINI-GOAL VERSION OF THE REASON	WHAT I CAN DO TO ACHIEVE THE MINI-GOAL
1. Hairstyling is an important, foundational skill that allows you to display your creativity and deliver a client's desired specific outcome.	Example: I want to master the basics of hairstyling so that I can be creative and meet or exceed my clients' expectations and hairstyle requests.	Example: (1) I am going to identify five friends or relatives who are willing to let me practice hairstyles on them during this chapter. (2) I will focus on my listening skills so that I can *really* hear my clients' requests and translate them.
2. Clients rely on you to teach them about their hair and how to style it so that they can have a variety of options based on their lifestyle and fashion needs.		
3. Professional cosmetologists should be prepared to work with and style every hair type.		

ORIGINAL REASON TO STUDY HAIRSTYLING	MINI-GOAL VERSION OF THE REASON	WHAT I CAN DO TO ACHIEVE THE MINI-GOAL
4. Styling techniques and product recommendations should always target the specific hair texture.		
5. Clients look to you for special-occasion hairstyles.		
6. Hairstyling skills enable you to help clients be as modern as they want to be.		
7. Proficient hairstyling skills make you a true hairdresser.		
8. Learning basic hairstyling techniques is the first step in becoming a wedding specialist or participating in photo shoots and editorial work.		

Hairstyling Consultation

SHORT ANSWER

5. What is the difference between co-washing and co-styling?

_____

_____

_____

6. During the consultation, what would you specifically ask a client with coily hair textures, damaged hair, or color-treated hair?

_____

_____

_____

7. During the consultation, what would you specifically ask a client with curly/coily hair about their care regimen?

_____

_____

_____

8. Match the qualities that you should examine during the hair and scalp analysis with the description of what you're looking for.

a. Diameter   d. Density   g. Porosity/elasticity
b. Feel   e. Condition   h. Scalp health
c. Pattern   f. Length

HAIR OR SCALP QUALITY	WHAT YOU ARE LOOKING FOR
_____	Is the hair long enough to execute the desired hairstyle?
_____	Does the hair feel oily, dry, hard, soft, rough, or smooth?
_____	Is the hair straight, wavy, curly, or coily?
_____	Is the scalp's condition healthy and properly cared for? Are there scalp conditions present such as alopecia, seborrhea, eczema, or psoriasis?
_____	How well does the hair absorb and retain moisture? How well does the hair appear to retain a hairstyle?
_____	Is the hair coarse, medium, or fine?
_____	Is the hair damaged? Does it exhibit breakage? For clients with previously braided styles, check the hairline for traction alopecia caused by excessive pulling, tight extension braids, locs, or tightly sewn and braided-in weaves.
_____	Are there any areas where the hair is thin?

9. Complete the sentences below using words from the word bank. Each word will be used once.

   Word bank: wash 'n' go, curly, maintenance, weekly, sets, natural, locs, maintained, standard, styling, protective

   When you have a client seeking a _____ hairstyle, you need to ask not only the

   _____ consultation questions but also questions about their daily/ _____

   hair-care _____ routine, _____ /coily _____ regimen, and haircut and

   style determinations. This will help you determine which looks are best suited and _____

   , such as curly or coily (_____) styles, braids, _____ styles, _____ , or

   natural textured _____ or styles.

10. Partner with a classmate to practice your client consultation technique for a client who has a natural hairstyle. The tone of your conversation should be confident, authentic, and knowledgeable. You will take turns playing the role of stylist and client, and then discuss suggestions to improve when finished. Before you meet for this activity, independently prepare for each role by familiarizing yourself with the 10 questions about a natural hair home care regimen from your textbook and preparing possible answers to the questions from both a stylist's and a client's perspective. Then locate a photo of a natural hairstyle you would like the stylist to create for you, including reasons you want it, and use that to start the consultation.

11. Imagine that a client tells you they are going to the prom in a month, and they would like you to create a hairstyle for them—one that will flatter them, make them feel beautiful, last throughout a night of dancing, and impress their friends. You're excited to contribute to their special evening and know that it might earn you some referral business for other special-occasion services. How would you go about making a plan to give the client the perfect hairstyle? Write a short paragraph about it below.

   _____

   _____

   _____

Brushes, Combs, and Implements

12. Match each type of brush with its description and/or function. Each brush will be used at least once.

a. Vent
b. Edging
c. Wet and dry

d. Styling
e. Paddle
f. Oval grooming

g. Round
h. Detangling
i. Teasing

Type of Brush	Description/Function
_____	Small brushes with nylon bristles or boar hair used to create "baby hair" after applying edge control
_____	Has a half-round head with a rubber pad for cushion and grip; typically has nine rows of round-tipped nylon pins
_____	Has a mix of boar bristles and nylon pins; the boar bristles help distribute the scalp oils and groom the cuticle, and the nylon pins help the bristles gently penetrate the hair
_____	Slender nylon and natural bristles with a tail for sectioning and a narrow row of bristles, pins, or both
_____	Has a pneumatic (air-cushioned) pad and glides through wet hair to detangle and refresh styles between shampoos
_____	Cylindrical base can be wood, metal or ceramic; bristles can be nylon, boar, or a combination of both
_____	Top-of-the-line versions are heat resistant, antistatic, and ideal for styling precision haircuts, providing any type of controlled styling, and smoothing the hair; provides a beveled blow-out look, adding smoothness with a bend on the ends of the hair
_____	Speeds up drying times due to their special brush heads and wide-spaced pins; creates more natural styles because it does not force the hair into a specific shape
_____	Well suited for mid-length or longer hair; the go-to brush for smooth flat blow-outs; can be used on all wave patterns to smooth highly textured hair's cuticle layer
_____	Helps reduce pressure on the hair and scalp, minimizing damage and split ends
_____	Designed for backbrushing hair; the brush tips' sides are ideal for smoothing the hair's surface into the finished style

_____ Has a large, flat base with a pneumatic (air-cushioned) pad; some have ball-tipped nylon bristles and staggered pin patterns to enhance the grip on the hair and keep the hair from snagging

_____ Particularly suited for fine-to-medium hair; achieves smooth, flat styles with highly textured hair

_____ Comes in various diameters; smaller versions can curl the hair; large versions generally smooth, add volume, and bevel the hair's ends

SHORT ANSWER

13. What are three things to look for in damaged brushes?

_____

_____

_____

14. What are the three qualities that a professional comb should have?

_____

_____

_____

15. What is the function of combs and picks?

_____

_____

_____

16. Why is it important to use only high-quality professional combs and picks?

_____

_____

_____

17. Complete the chart below by filling in the missing information—either the type of comb/pick or its description.

TYPE OF COMB OR PICK	DESCRIPTION/FUNCTION	IMAGE
	A tool used in finishing a style and producing different looks; available in different lengths, sizes, materials, and teeth variations. Those with shorter teeth and teeth spaced farther apart will remove less curl than a longer-toothed feather comb.	
Tail		
Hair pick		
	Also known as all-purpose combs, they finely comb each cutting section and style the hair. Ideal for finger waves, detangling, parting and sectioning the hair, wet sets, and thermal styling.	
Teasing		
	These have fine combing and styling abilities—the pick portion can lift and separate the curls, while the teeth are ideal for creating smooth finishes.	
Wide-tooth		

18. Partner with two or three other classmates who have different lengths and types of hair and practice sectioning each other's hair with various clips and clamps. If possible, you may want to try this on both wet *and* dry hair.

    Do some work better than others to hold the hair? Which ones? How do your "clients" like the feel of the clips/clamps? Practice until (1) you feel comfortable knowing which clamp or clip to use on which types of hair and (2) your "clients" confirm that the clips feel secure without hurting them.

19. What are lightweight clips used for?

_____

_____

_____

20. What kind of hair requires heavy-duty clamps?

_____

_____

_____

21. Describe sectioning clamps and what they are used for.

_____

_____

_____

Styling Aids

SHORT ANSWER

22. List the three general factors that a stylist should consider when choosing a styling product to apply to a client's hair.

_____

_____

_____

23. What is the range of hold that a styling product might have on hair?

_____

_____

_____

24. What is the main difference between pomade and edge control?

_____

_____

_____

25. Briefly describe the chemistry involved in the use of hair spray.

_____

_____

_____

26. List three examples of natural oils that are used as styling aids.

_____

_____

_____

MATCHING

27. Match each type of styling aid with its description. Each type will be used at least once.

a. Hair spray
b. Sheen
c. Natural oil/styling oil
d. Styling lotion
e. Styling cream

f. Gel
g. Foam
h. Setting lotion
i. Setting foam
j. Volumizer

k. Serum
l. Edge control
m. Pomade

Type of Styling Aid	Description
_____	Oil that gives hair a luminous appearance during and after styling; can be used on all hair types and is offered in many varieties, ranging from aerosol cans to spray bottles

_____ Smooths and controls the fine hair around the face's perimeter (also known as baby hair); offers hold and produces a sleek finish

_____ Typically offers low to medium hold with a natural-looking shine and minimal frizz

_____ A light whipped version of setting lotion used to perform wet sets, including roller sets, finger waves, rod sets, two-strand twist, braid sets, coils, wraps, and molds; creates smooth, sleek finishes on textured hair to define curls and add soft control, with shine

_____ Light, airy whipped styling product that resembles shaving foam and builds moderate body and volume into the hair

_____ Also referred to as shine spray or gloss

_____ Lubricant that adds shine and gloss to hair; derived from organic materials

_____ Adds volume, especially at the base, when wet hair is blown dry

_____ Used on highly textured or chemically relaxed hair

_____ Creamy consistency and alcohol-free, allowing for a light hold with a natural effect

_____ Also known as spritz; comes in various formulas and holds to aid in all stages of styling

_____ Greasy, waxy, or oily styling aid that gives hair a shiny and slick appearance, or a matte finish; keeps the hair in place with either a light or strong hold

_____ Quick-drying liquid delivered to the hair via spray bottle

_____ Also known as silicone; adds gloss and sheen to the hair while creating textural definition

_____ Thickened styling preparation that comes in a tube, bottle, or large container and creates a strong hold

_____ Also known as mousse

_____ Concentrated liquid solution that sets hair; can be diluted with water to create a softer hold

28. What are three examples of tools that heat protectants protect the hair from?

_____

_____

_____

29. At what point in the hairstyling service are heat protectants typically applied to the hair? Are they applied to dry, damp, or wet hair?

_____

_____

_____

30. Are heat protectants usually found in other styling aids?

_____

_____

_____

31. What are three examples of the various forms (compositions) of blowdry styling aids?

_____

_____

_____

32. List at least five ways that properly using blowdry styling aids can help you and your client achieve their style goals.

_____

_____

_____

33. Your text recommends that stylists keep at least three different kinds of blowdry styling aids on hand for different hair textures and style goals. For this exercise, use the Internet or beauty supply catalogues to identify three blowdry styling aids that would be appropriate for a range of hair types and hairstyles. Use your workbook, a separate sheet of paper, or follow the link for a table to record your findings. When you've completed your research, write one or two sentences explaining why you identified these three products to add to your stylist toolkit.

+ BONUS

Visit: bonus.milady.com/cos-wb/toc

	BLOWDRY STYLING AID #1	BLOWDRY STYLING AID #2	BLOWDRY STYLING AID #3
Name/Brand of Product			
Size			
Cost			
Source (Store or Website)			
Appropriate for What Type of Hair/Hair Texture?			
Advertised Benefits			
Directions for Use			
Method of Dispensing/Composition (e.g., spray bottle/liquid)			

SEQUENCE

34. Number the steps for applying dry shampoo from 1 to 5.

    _____ Brush the hair to remove excess product.

    _____ Massage the roots to encourage further absorption.

    _____ Apply dry shampoo to the root area on dry hair and then down to where the natural oil line ends.

    _____ Blowdry the roots.

    _____ Wait up to 10 minutes to give the powder time to absorb the oil.

Indicate whether each statement below is true or false. For any false statements, explain why they are false.

35. Dry shampoos can be used as a style enhancer to add texture and volume to hair.

T   F   _____

36. Working hair sprays allow you to spray and then move the hair during the dry-down phase.

T   F   _____

37. Working hair sprays are usually packaged in aerosol form.

T   F   _____

38. After blowdrying and before or after ironing the hair, you can improve the style by using your fingers to lift the hair, add noticeable texture, augment movement, or create more defined results.

T   F   _____

39. Finishing hair sprays are only used to hold the completed style by applying your choice of product in light layers until you reach the desired amount of hold.

T   F   _____

SHORT ANSWER

40. Describe the physical characteristics of pomade.

_____

_____

_____

41. At what point in the hairstyling service are pomades applied? How long will pomade generally last in a hairstyle?

_____

_____

_____

42. Describe how pomades can be used to build texture. What other types of styles can they be used to create?

_____

_____

_____

43. Match each type of pomade to its description.

    a. Hair wax pomade   c. Hybrid pomade   e. Hair paste pomade
    b. Water-based pomade   d. Clay pomade

Type of Pomade   **Description**

_____ Water soluble

_____ Excels at creating all structured styles

_____ Good choice for creating mussed styles or less structured, textured details

_____ Has a low-to-moderate shine factor; usually has a medium hold factor

_____ Popularized by the "greasers"—a rebellious cultural movement in the 1950s—and was used to comb quiff, pompadour, and jellyroll hairstyles

_____ Excels at molding rockabilly-type quiffs and pompadours, as well as styles with strong side parts

_____ Fairly stiff consistency that softens in your hands; easily applied to the hair

_____ Formulated with both water and oil

_____ Easy to shampoo out; available in soft-, medium-, and hard-hold formulas

SHORT ANSWER

44. As you style your client's hair, is it acceptable to talk about the products you're using and explain why you chose them? Why or why not?

_____

_____

_____

45. Why should you make home care recommendations to your clients—both styling tips and professional products?

_____

_____

_____

Blowdryers

SHORT ANSWER

46. What are the two main ways a blowdryer might be used?

_____

_____

_____

47. List three hairstyles that are often dried under hooded dryers.

_____

_____

_____

48. In addition to drying certain hairstyles, what are two other possible uses for hooded dryers?

_____

_____

_____

49. What can a blowdryer do that a hooded dryer cannot? Why not?

_____

_____

_____

50. Why is it important to conduct careful and thorough research when selecting a blowdryer or other thermal tools such as styling irons? Provide an example of a claim that is often made about features of these tools.

_____

_____

_____

TRUE OR FALSE

Indicate whether the statements below are true or false. For any false statements, explain why they are false.

51. The power of a blowdryer's air velocity and heat is likely to have very little influence on your ability to work faster or more easily without damaging the hair, so this is a minor consideration when making your purchasing decision.

    T   F   _____

52. Even though it might seem costly, the purchase of a professional tool such as a blowdryer should be viewed as an investment in your work, not as an expense.

    T   F   _____

53. When choosing a blowdryer, barrel length is an important consideration, especially if you frequently hold the barrel when blowdrying.

    T   F   _____

54. Extremely loud blowdryers can actually cause physical and mental fatigue; long-term use can even cause varying degrees of hearing loss.

    T   F   _____

55. Blowdryers manufactured for consumers to use at home are cheaper and therefore a good alternative to professional-grade versions—they last just as long, perform equally well, are safe for heavy-duty use, and dry and style with the same speed and effect.

    T   F   _____

56. Easy maintenance of a blowdryer is an important consideration when choosing a blowdryer because clogged filters are known to reduce airflow, slow drying time, and shorten the motor's life span.

    T   F   _____

57. Complete the sentences below using the words from the word bank. Each word will be used once.

    Word bank: balanced, study, pressure, hand, hold, wrist, use, trade, heavy, blowdrying, stores

    One of several tips to keep in mind when shopping around for a blowdryer recommends that you

    _____ it, _____ it, and _____ its features and benefits. Two places to test

    blowdryers are at professional _____ and at _____ shows. To test the blowdryer,

    hold the blowdryer in your _____, as if you are _____ hair. Ask yourself: Does it feel

    _____? Is it applying _____ on my _____? Does it feel too _____?

SHORT ANSWER

58. When shopping for a specific blowdryer, what should you determine in terms of what a manufacturer might make for one?

    _____

    _____

    _____

59. Describe what a diffuser can do.

    _____

    _____

    _____

60. Why would you use picks and straightening combs/picks with a blowdryer?

    _____

    _____

    _____

61. Complete the chart by filling in the descriptions (which might be a comparison, in some cases) for the features of each type of blowdryer motor. One example has been provided for you.

MOTOR FEATURE	AC MOTORS	DC MOTORS	EC MOTORS
Noise Level			
Cost			
ACLI Safety Plug			
Cord			
Life Span	Working life span of up to 1,200 hours	Working life span typically up to 700 hours	Significantly longer life span than AC or DC motors
Weight			
Air Velocity/Heat Output			

TRUE OR FALSE

Indicate whether the statements below are true or false. For any false statements, explain why they are false.

62. You should partially towel dry the hair before blowdrying to speed up the drying time.

    T   F   _____

63. Always direct the hot air away from the client's scalp to avoid scalp burns.

    T   F   _____

64. Hold the blowdryer still when drying a section, except when using the cool shot button.

    T   F   _____

65. When blowdrying, direct the hot air from the scalp toward the ends of the hair to smooth the cuticle; avoid ruffling the cuticle; and create a sleek, shiny hair surface.

    T   F   _____

66. What kind of tension is recommended to straighten the hair with blowdrying?

_____

_____

_____

67. On which three types of hair should you avoid using tension? What should you do instead?

_____

_____

_____

68. While blowdrying, where do you place the nozzle of the blowdryer? What are two reasons for this placement?

_____

_____

_____

69. How can you use blowdrying to achieve more volume at the root? Less volume?

_____

_____

_____

SEQUENCE

70. Number the steps of the procedure for blowdrying straight or wavy hair to achieve maximum volume from 1 to 8.

   _____ Build desired shape from the bottom up, working from the nape up toward the crown. Secure hair with clips above the area you are working on.

   _____ While moving in the desired direction, direct airflow toward the top of the brush and ends of the hair. Dry using a 45- to 90-degree angle to create fullness.

_____ Place clean neck strip on client and drape with cutting or styling cape.

_____ Repeat over entire head, directing the hair at the sides either away or forward. The bang area can be dried either onto the forehead or away from the face.

_____ Apply mousse, volumizing spray, or flexible gel.

_____ Work in sections, lifting and drying then brushing them in the desired direction when they are completely dry.

_____ While turning the brush downward and away from the scalp, allow the brush to pick up and lift a section of hair and begin drying.

_____ Using a paddle brush or classic styling brush, distribute hair into the desired shape.

Thermal Irons

SHORT ANSWER

71. What are two names for the process of using thermal irons?

    _____

    _____

    _____

72. How is the shell handle maneuvered?

    _____

    _____

    _____

73. List the four ways that thermal irons are used.

    _____

    _____

    _____

74. List the four basic types of thermal irons.

_____

_____

_____

75. Label the basic parts of a typical curling iron.

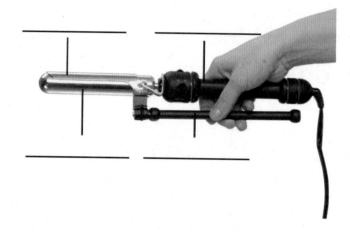

76. What are the two types of clamp irons?

_____

_____

_____

77. What is the heating source for each type of clamp iron?

_____

_____

_____

78. What are some of the types of curls you can create with clamp irons?

_____

_____

_____

Indicate whether each statement below is true or false. For any false statements, explain why they are false.

79. The Marcel iron is the most common type of iron used by consumers.

    T   F   _____

80. A large percentage of salon stylists who used spring irons before attending beauty school typically use them for various styling purposes in the salon setting.

    T   F   _____

81. Spring irons feature a spring-loaded clamp controlled by the index finger and palm.

    T   F   _____

82. When using a spring iron on short hair, you must insert a heat-resistant styling comb right at the scalp to protect it from burning; then clamp the iron at the base of the curl placement and rotate in place.

    T   F   _____

83. For what type of hair do some stylists prefer to use conventional Marcel irons?

_____

_____

_____

84. What is another term for Marcel irons?

_____

_____

_____

85. Describe the handles of a Marcel iron.

_____

_____

_____

86. Describe how to begin the procedure for creating Hollywood wave curls, including where on the head, the direction of the iron, and the recommended size of the subsection.

_____

_____

_____

87. What is the "twist and hold" technique? How do you use it when creating Hollywood wave curls?

_____

_____

_____

88. What kind of brush or comb should you use to finish a Hollywood wave style? What pattern do you comb or brush the hair into when finishing this style?

_____

_____

_____

89. What type of iron is best for messy, beachy curls? Why?

_____

_____

_____

LABELING

90. For each method of using a heated Marcel iron, indicate whether it's a Do or Don't.

DO OR DON'T?	WHEN USING A HEATED MARCEL IRON
	Discard the tested strip or wrap in the trash
	Use your hand or place the iron near your mouth or face to test the temperature
	Insert a heat-resistant comb into the hair between the scalp and the barrel of the iron when nearing the base of the section
	Ask your client to hold their ear down if you are curling at the hairline
	Press the hair against the shell
	Create subsections that are the same diameter or smaller than the barrel of the curling iron
	Pat or touch the hair or the iron once the hair is fed into the rod and shell
	Comb the hair from scalp to ends, opening and closing the Marcel iron as you feed the hair into it

SEQUENCE

91. Number the steps for ensuring a smooth styling session with a flat iron, from 1 to 5.

_____ If the hair is longer than 12 inches (30 centimeters), or is super curly or rough, divide the hair into two separate sections (e.g., root down to 6 inches (15 centimeters) in length; 6 inches (15 centimeters) down to 12 inches (30 centimeters).

_____ Take sections that are small enough to control the hair and be evenly heated throughout.

_____ Once all the sections are smooth, glide the flat iron from root to end until uniformly smooth.

_____ Brush the hair, lightly clamp the iron around the section, and smoothly move down the hair shaft to the ends.

_____ Comb or brush thoroughly and take two passes with the iron from root to end to warm up the hair.

Indicate whether each statement below is true or false. For any false statements, explain why they are false.

92. Professional flat iron plates are coated with ceramic, tourmaline, or titanium to ensure a smooth, snag-free glide.

   T   F   _____

93. Chasing is when you move the flat iron quickly through multiple sections of hair.

   T   F   _____

94. For best results, apply the crimping iron to wide, thick sections of hair.

   T   F   _____

95. The main difference between crimping irons and flat irons is that the crimping iron's plates create a zigzag or sawtooth pattern in the hair.

   T   F   _____

96. Avoid applying a styling spray before crimping the hair—it will interfere with the crimping iron's effectiveness.

   T   F   _____

SHORT ANSWER

97. Where should you leave hot irons to cool? Why?

   _____

   _____

   _____

98. How can you safely determine whether a thermal styling iron is too hot to use?

   _____

   _____

   _____

99. What materials should combs be made of if they are being used in thermal styling?

_____

_____

_____

100. Why should flat irons coated with titanium be avoided for fine, damaged, or fragile hair?

_____

_____

_____

FILL IN THE BLANK

101. Search your favorite magazine or online for pictures that depict various design textures created from the use of styling tools. Paste them in the spaces provided below or on a separate piece of paper. Then, write a brief explanation of what styling tools can be used to recreate the look.

HAIR STYLE	EXPLANATION

102. Identify each type of thermal styling tool or accessory shown below.

THERMAL STYLING TOOL OR ACCESSORY	IMAGE

103. On the thermometer below, indicate the recommended temperature and the type of hair texture (listed in the word bank) that can be styled with an iron at that temperature.

Word bank: coarse and coily, fine, fragile, medium, coarse

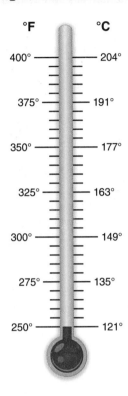

°F	°C
400°	204°
375°	191°
350°	177°
325°	163°
300°	149°
275°	135°
250°	121°

SEQUENCE

104. Number the steps for cleaning a thermal iron, from 1 to 5.

_____ If heated, allow it to cool to room temperature.

_____ Dry the barrel or plates using a dry, absorbent cloth.

_____ Rub the damp cloth on the iron's barrel or plates several times until the coating has been removed.

_____ Unplug your iron.

_____ Using a spray bottle, slightly dampen a cloth with water or rubbing alcohol.

105. Match the type of thermal iron—electric (E) or nonelectric (NE)—to the description of its disinfecting process. Some descriptions will apply to both types of thermal iron.

**Type of Thermal
Iron**   **Description of the Disinfecting Process**

_____ Clean with soap or detergent and water

_____ Disinfect with an EPA-registered disinfectant spray or wipe with a proven bactericidal, fungicidal, and virucidal solution, according to the manufacturer's instructions

_____ Must be disinfected.

_____ Completely dry with a new (clean) paper towel

_____ Remove all visible debris

_____ Totally immerse in an EPA-registered disinfectant with proven bactericidal, fungicidal, and virucidal activity, according to the manufacturer's instructions

REFLECTION

106. Now that you've practiced thermal iron styling procedures, think about what you knew about using those tools before you began this section compared to what you've studied. Write a few sentences in which you reflect on what you excel at and struggle with when it comes to thermal iron—Marcel, flat, spring, wand, and crimping—techniques. How can you make your demonstration flawless for your examination?

When you're finished, meet with a classmate and discuss your responses. Look for opportunities to fill in each other's gaps and help each other master the thermal iron techniques.

Thermal Pressing

TRUE OR FALSE

Indicate whether the statements below are true or false. For any false statements, explain why they are false.

107. Pressing combs are often used on highly textured hair for finishing or to reach edges around the hairline where a flat iron cannot reach.

    T   F   _____

108. For people with curly or coily hair, a permanent form of hair straightening, known as thermal pressing, may be the ideal way to switch to straight hair.

T   F   _____

109. In order to add pressing services to your menu, you will need education, training, practice, and experience to successfully use a pressing comb.

T   F   _____

MATCHING

110. Match each type of thermal press—soft, medium, or hard—with its description. Each type will be used at least once.

Type of Thermal Press	Description
_____	Removes about 60 to 75 percent of the curl
_____	Involves applying the thermal pressing comb once on each side of the hair
_____	Removes 100 percent of the curl
_____	Involves applying the thermal pressing comb once on each side of the hair, using slightly more pressure
_____	Also called a double press, which is one of two techniques used to achieve this type of press, and is accomplished by first passing a hot thermal iron through the hair
_____	Removes about 50 to 60 percent of the curl
_____	One of two techniques used to achieve this type of press, which involves applying the thermal pressing comb twice on each side of the hair

SHORT ANSWER

111. How long does a hair pressing generally last?

_____

_____

_____

112. Why might a base touch-up to a hair pressing style be required between full services?

_____

_____

_____

113. When performing a soft press, what size subsections should you use for medium-textured hair of average density? For coarse hair with greater density? For thin or fine hair with sparse density?

_____

_____

_____

FILL IN THE BLANK

Complete the sentences below using the words from the word bank. Some words will be used more than once.

> **Word bank:** brush, steel, electric, teeth, comb, grease, stove, paper, high/low, carbon, gas, cool, oil, thermostat, soot, on/off

114. _____ pressing combs are available in two forms: with a(n) _____ switch or with a(n) _____ that indicates _____ degrees of heat.

115. Regular pressing combs may be designed as electrical appliances or be heated on _____ or _____ stoves. When heating on a _____ stove, point the _____ up and keep the handle away from the _____.

116. After heating the _____ to the proper temperature, test it on a piece of _____. If it becomes scorched, allow the _____ to _____ slightly before applying it to the hair.

117. The teeth of the _____ can be cleaned using a small wire _____ to remove _____ or _____ buildup. Remove _____ or _____, which appears as black dust, from _____ -heated irons using _____ wool.

118. What should you apply to prepare a client's hair for a pressing treatment?

_____

_____

_____

119. What are three reasons burns caused by a thermal tool are dangerous? What should you apply immediately in case of a scalp burn?

_____

_____

_____

CASE STUDY

120. To familiarize yourself with the variety of thermal pressing oils and creams available, conduct some research using either the Internet or a beauty supply catalogue, or visit a beauty supply store. Identify two pressing creams and two pressing oils that interest you. Use the workbook, a separate sheet of paper, or follow the link to a table to record your findings so that you will have a quick reference guide when it comes time to assemble your products for thermal pressing services.

When you're finished with your research, write one or two sentences explaining why you chose these products over others that you rejected.

+ BONUS

Visit: bonus.milady.com/cos-wb/toc

FEATURES OF THERMAL PRESSING OILS AND CREAMS	PRESSING OIL #1	PRESSING OIL #2	PRESSING CREAM #1	PRESSING CREAM #2
Name/Brand				
Source (Store/Website)				
Method of Dispensing				
Size Options				
Cost				
Advertised Features				
Directions for Use				
Precautions				

121. What are six tips or precautions specifically related to temperature when performing thermal pressing services?

_____

_____

_____

122. What is an alternative to using thermal pressing tools to straighten hair that has a fine texture?

_____

_____

_____

123. What are two ways to prevent the release of vapor from hair during thermal pressing treatments?

_____

_____

_____

124. What kind of comb can you use instead of pressing short hair on the temples and the back of the neck?

_____

_____

_____

125. What is the key to ensuring the overall safety of your client and the health of their hair during thermal hair pressing services?

_____

_____

_____

MATCHING

126. Match each hair type with the safeguards and precautions applicable to pressing that kind of hair.

   a. Fine hair
   b. Short, fine hair
   c. Coarse hair
   d. Coily or curly hair
   e. Lightened hair
   f. Tinted hair
   g. Gray hair

Special Hair Type   **Safeguards and Precautions for Thermal Pressing**

_____ Because of the compact construction of its cuticle cells, this hair type requires more heat and pressure than others.

_____ Might require pre- and post-conditioning treatments, depending on the extent of the damage.

_____ May be harder to straighten. For good results, use a moderately heated pressing comb applied with light pressure. Avoid excessive heat, as discoloration or breakage can occur.

_____ Never recommended.

_____ Take extra care at the hairline. Pressing comb should not be too hot because the hair will burn easily.

_____ Apply enough pressure so that the hair remains straightened.

_____ Avoid using a high-heat pressing comb or too much pressure; consider flat ironing on high heat if the curl form is not highly textured. To avoid hair breakage, apply less pressure to the hair near the ends.

SHORT ANSWER

127. How can you protect yourself when first learning to use a heated comb?

_____

_____

_____

128. How do you straighten the hair using the back of the comb?

_____

_____

_____

129. How many times should you pass the comb through a section for fine to medium hair? Coarse or highly textured hair?

_____

_____

_____

SEQUENCE

130. Number the main steps for thermal pressing, from 1 to 7.

_____ Use the teeth of the pressing comb to separate and control the hair; use the back of the comb to straighten the hair.

_____ Separate the hair into small sections. Each section should take up only about half of the pressing comb's width.

_____ Move the pressing comb through the hair and the perimeter (edges) with the recommended tension, as outlined in this chapter. Finish by styling the hair with thermal tool of choice.

_____ Wash and dry the hair. Apply a heat protectant product. Then lightly apply a pressing oil or cream.

_____ Comb the section with a regular comb to ensure the hair is as smooth as possible and tangle-free.

_____ Heat the pressing comb to the desired temperature, then test it on a white cloth or tissue. If the fabric becomes discolored (scorched), allow the comb to cool for a few seconds and test again.

_____ Insert the pressing comb as close to the scalp as possible without risking scalp damage. The teeth should be pointing down, and the back of the comb should be up.

Natural Hair Styling

131. Number the steps in the procedure for creating a natural hairstyle using the coily method, from 1 to 11. One step has been numbered for you.

____3____ Apply medium-weight leave-in conditioner or prep cream to wet hair.

_____ Apply a styling foam or gel.

_____ Dry and style the hair depending on length.

_____ Use a detangling brush to stretch the coils, then rake fingers through the hair.

_____ Gather and separate the hair by opening and closing your fingers together. Do not touch, finger-style, or manipulate the coils after setting them in place. They must completely dry to avoid frizz.

_____ Have client sit upright. Detangle hair with a wide-tooth comb or detangling brush, depending on hair length and texture.

_____ Place clean neck strip on client and drape with cutting or styling cape.

_____ Apply curl-defining or curl-enhancing cream for coily and super coily textures and smooth the product all over.

_____ Palm coil and/or finger coil the hair until you see complete coil definition all over the head.

_____ With client reclined in shampoo chair, cleanse and condition the hair.

_____ Lightly dry hair around neckline with towel.

132. Match each type of hair texture with the description of products that are best for it.

Type of Hair Texture

a. All textures
b. Wavy and curly textures

Product

c. Very curly to coily textures
d. Tightly coiled to Afro/highly textured

_____ Light, water-based products with light humectant creams

_____ Heavy moisturizing products with butters and essential oils

_____ Hydrating and moisturizing, water-based (H_2O) products

_____ Combination of water-based products and moisturizing products with botanical/essential oils

133. Match the types of natural textured sets and styles with their descriptions.

a. Bantu knot or Nubian knot
b. Bantu knot-out style

c. Braid-out set
d. Flat twist
e. Glamour waves

f. Spiral rod set

Natural Textured Sets and Styles

Description

_____ This style involves individual braiding or cornrowing of the hair either wet or dry, then opening the braid to create a crimped, texture-on-texture effect with added volume.

_____ The hair is double-strand twisted or coil twisted and wrapped around itself to make a knot, which is then secured with bobby pins or elastic bands

_____ Hair is wrapped around a vertical rod, moving up the rod in a spiral pattern. Hair must completely dry, or the style will appear frizzy.

_____ Once dry, the flat twist set is untwisted and opened to create a wavy texture.

_____ Knots can be opened and released to create wavy and fuller loose curls.

_____ The hair is parted in several rows over the entire head. Each section is divided into two subsections and then twisted and interwoven to lie flat on the scalp.

134. What is the sponge used for when creating curly or coily hairstyles?

_____

_____

_____

135. How is the sponge used in the sponge technique?

_____

_____

_____

136. How are coil twists created using the finger coil technique? The comb coil technique?

_____

_____

_____

137. Which coil technique is also used to start locs?

_____

_____

_____

138. What is the procedure for the coil-out? Describe the result.

_____

_____

_____

139. What is another name for twist hairstyles?

_____

_____

_____

140. When starting a twist hairstyle with wet hair, what is the goal?

_____

_____

_____

141. What is a twist-out style? What is the resulting effect?

_____

_____

_____

FILL IN THE BLANK

Complete the sentences below using words from the word bank. Each word will be used once.

Word bank: Afro, at-home, botanical, butter, cutting, frizzy, hairline, hydrate, leave-in, maintenance, oil, overtwisted, pomade, regular, repair, sewing, steam, vitamins, weeks

142. After locs are started, the stylist should recommend that the client visit the salon for basic loc

_____—cleansing, _____ conditioning, and retwisting the locs—at least every

two to three _____ .

143. Stylists should advise clients about _____ maintenance between salon visits. This

includes telling them to _____ loc shafts with a liquid spray _____ conditioner;

moisturize scalp and locs with essential _____ sprays daily or as needed; and retwist

_____ locs around the _____ as needed with a loc butter, which is a creamy

_____ made with _____ oils, shea _____, and _____ .

144. When locs have not had _____ hair care or conditioning and oil steam treatments,

they become _____ or stressed, and end up weak, thin, and requiring _____

—typically, by wrapping _____ -textured human hair around the entire loc or area.

Alternative repairs include removing and _____ them back onto an individual braided

base or _____ the weak areas and starting over.

Indicate whether the statements below are true or false. For any false statements, explain why they are false.

145. Nubian coils and coil-out styles last two to three months and can easily start locking the hair if not combed out before four months.

     T   F   _____

146. As part of client aftercare, comb out Nubian coils, shampoo, and use conditioning steam treatments to keep the hair and scalp healthy.

     T   F   _____

147. Clients should retwist frizzy locs around the hairline using a leave-in conditioner.

     T   F   _____

148. Other client aftercare includes advising clients to wrap their locs while sleeping using a very large satin or silk scarf or bonnet to help prevent breakage, drying out, or lint attaching to the locs.

     T   F   _____

149. After locs have grown to approximately 5 inches (12.5 centimeters), they can be styled into braids, Bantu knots, cornrows, flat twists, or twists.

     T   F   _____

150. Match the four ways to cultivate locs with their descriptions. Each method will be used at least once.

a. Coil comb technique
b. Palm roll method

c. Braids or extensions
d. Sisterloc method

**Method of Cultivating
Locs**   **Description**

_____ Gentlest on the hair, and it works through all the natural stages of locking; this method takes advantage of the hair's natural ability to coil

_____ Interlocking method that instantly locs any textured hair—whether straight, relaxed, wavy, curly, coily, or highly textured—using a special tool to achieve the single loc

_____ Particularly effective during the early stages of locking while the coil is still open

_____ Offers the option to add a synthetic hair fiber, human hair fiber, or yarn to form a loc

_____ Involves applying gel to dampened subsections, placing the hair portion between the palms of both hands, and rolling in a clockwise or counterclockwise direction, forming the entire coil with each revolution as you move down the shaft

_____ Involves sectioning the hair for the desired loc size and single braiding the hair to the end

_____ Involves placing the comb at the scalp and, with a rotating motion, spiraling the hair into a coil

Understanding and Creating Curls

MATCHING

151. Match the terms related to a curl with their descriptions. Each term will be used twice.

a. Base   b. Stem   c. Curl

Curl Terms   Description

_____ The panel of hair on which the roller or barrel is placed

_____ The hair that is wrapped around to form a complete circle, which largely determines the size of the wave or curl

_____ Affects the volume

_____ Gives the hair direction and mobility

_____ Also known as a circle

_____ The hair between the scalp and the first turn of the hair

152. Label the parts of the curl.

153. Which relationship determines the shape of the curl?

_____

_____

_____

154. What are the three curl shapes?

_____

_____

_____

155. What curl shape does one turn create?

_____

_____

_____

156. What curl shape does one-and-a-half turns create?

_____

_____

_____

157. What curl shape does two-and-a-half turns create?

_____

_____

_____

MATCHING

158. Match the curl turn with the resulting curl shape.

CURL TURN	RESULTING CURL SHAPE	ANSWER
a.		
b.		
c.		

159. Complete the chart below, including making a sketch of each specific curl pattern.

CURL PATTERN	BEST FOR	DESCRIPTION	SKETCH OF CURL PATTERN
Spiral curl			
		Creates a finished appearance by turning the hair ends under or over with a curling iron	
		Creates volume and movement by forming curls from roots to ends	
Wave			

ROLE PLAY

160. Create an example of each curl base type, using your mannequin and rollers. Take a photo of each base type to show (1) the hair in the proper position for the intended base type and (2) the resulting curl.

    Share your photos with a classmate and ask each other to identify the base types in your photos. How accurate were each of you?

SHORT ANSWER

161. What are three other terms for backcombing?

    _____

    _____

    _____

162. What is another term for backbrushing?

_____

_____

_____

163. What is the purpose of backcombing? Backbrushing?

_____

_____

_____

164. What are two effects that you can create with directional teasing, using either a comb or a brush?

_____

_____

_____

MATCHING

165. Match the curl base types with their descriptions.

   a. Volume base   c. Half base
   b. Full base   d. Off base

Curl Base Type	Description
_____	Hold the strand straight up (90 degrees) from the head and roll the hair down
_____	Wrap the hair with medium tension
_____	Hold the hair at a 135-degree angle
_____	Hold the panel of hair 45 degrees from the base and roll the hair in a downward direction
_____	Achieves the least volume
_____	Placed very high on the base for maximum lift and volume
_____	Hold the hair at a 125-degree angle

_____ Created by sitting the styling tool completely off the base

_____ Created by sitting the styling tool halfway on its base and halfway behind the base

_____ Wrap the strand around the barrel with medium tension

_____ Achieves medium volume

_____ Sit in the center of the base, which provides strong curl with full volume

SEQUENCE

166. Number the steps for performing the backcombing technique, from 1 to 6.

_____ Smooth hair. To smooth hair that is backcombed, hold the teeth of a comb at a 45-degree angle pointing away from you and lightly move the comb over the hair's surface.

_____ Push comb down. Push the comb gently and firmly toward the scalp. Repeat this action, working up the section until achieving the desired volume.

_____ Section hair. Starting in the front, pick up a hair section no more than 1 inch (2.5 centimeters) thick and no more than 2 to 3 inches (5 to 7.5 centimeters) wide.

_____ Create a cushion. To create a cushion (base), the third time you insert the comb, use the same sliding motion but firmly push the hair down to the scalp. Slide the comb out of the hair.

_____ Insert comb. Insert the fine teeth of your comb into the hair at a depth of about 1 inch (2.5 centimeters) away from the scalp. Hold the hair you are teasing with tension.

_____ Repeat for volume. Repeat this process, working up the strand until the desired volume is achieved.

SHORT ANSWER

167. In your own words, list the five steps for backbrushing.

_____

_____

_____

Wet Sets

168. How wide should the hair section be when preparing to roll it?

_____

_____

_____

169. What is applied to the hair before rolling to achieve the amount of hold needed for a strong set?

_____

_____

_____

170. Where does rolling begin and how far does it go?

_____

_____

_____

171. According to the procedure for performing wet sets with rollers outlined in your text (Procedure 12-14), what should you avoid doing when wrapping the hair on the roller?

_____

_____

_____

172. What is a barrel curl?

_____

_____

_____

173. What is the most common roller set used today?

_____

_____

_____

174. What is the difference between styling a damp set and a dry set? What are dry sets used to create?

_____

_____

_____

175. Label the type of directional roller set depicted and describe what its purpose is.

IMAGE	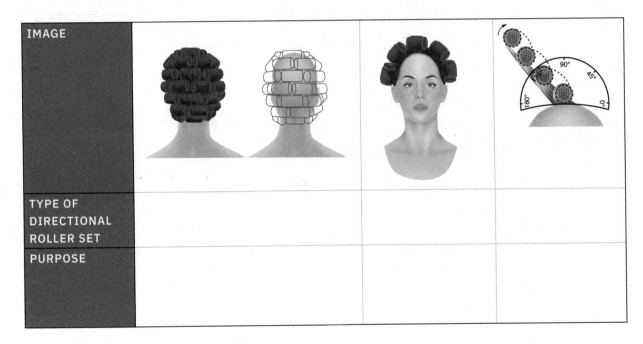		
TYPE OF DIRECTIONAL ROLLER SET			
PURPOSE			

176. Complete the sentences below using the words from the word bank. Each word will be used once.

Word bank: glamour, curvature, comb, modern, fingers, retro, lotion

To create finger waves, you use your _____, a styling _____, and styling

_____ or foam to shape and direct the hair into an S pattern. Finger waves add

_____, unique details, and shapes to _____ designs and can be used to create

_____ styles. Learning how to create them will teach you how to move and direct the hair

and style it to the _____ of the head.

SHORT ANSWER

177. What is finger-waving lotion, and what does it do?

_____

_____

_____

178. What are two ways to keep hair pliable as you progress in your finger-wave design?

_____

_____

_____

179. What are the three types of hair molding techniques?

_____

_____

_____

180. What type of hair is hair molding performed on?

_____

_____

_____

181. Describe the procedure for performing a textured mold.

_____

_____

_____

SEQUENCE

182. Number the steps for performing a basic flat mold, from 1 to 9.

_____ Proceed with a thermal service to style as desired.

_____ Place hair strips (wrapping strips) around the circumference of the head.

_____ Secure hair strips by tying or twisting them together.

_____ Allow hair to dry completely

_____ When hair is partially dry, remove the strips.

_____ Lay each section flat, working your way from the nape to the top of the head while laying each section over the last section.

_____ Place your client under a hooded dryer.

_____ Create the side part, then begin in the nape area using setting foam.

_____ Comb all hair to release the "mold."

LABELING

183. Label the type of wrap based on the information given.

Type of Wrap	_____	_____	_____	_____	_____
Description		Uses a blowdryer, flat iron, and "cling wrap"	Performed on highly textured virgin hair; uses rollers to stretch the curl pattern	Large rollers at the crown and apex, remainder of hair wrapped around the head	

184. Match each type of hair wrapping technique with its description/purpose. Each type will be used at least once.

a. Volume wrap
b. Roller wrap
c. Blow-out wrap
d. Doobie wrap
d. Silk press

Hair Wrap	Description
_____	Best for highly textured virgin hair, preferably hair that has a loose curl, is wavy, or does not require smoothing using a flat iron
_____	Can be used as nightly maintenance for all clients
_____	For clients who like the smoothness of a wrap but prefer more volume throughout the entire style
_____	Performed on highly textured virgin hair—all wave and curl patterns can benefit from this procedure if a straight look is desired
_____	Begin by setting the entire head on rollers using setting foam
_____	Apply a thermal protectant and a small amount of smoothing cream on the hair before setting in a straight pattern with jumbo rollers
_____	Used to achieve volume or attain height
_____	Wrap the hair around the head using the same steps as a wet wrap; if the hair is too short to stay in this position on its own, use duckbill clips to hold hair in place until all hair is wrapped and secured
_____	Best with naturally straight, wavy, or relaxed hair
_____	To style, use a boar-bristle round brush and a blowdryer to smooth the base area of the hair first
_____	Use rollers to stretch the curl pattern and a blowdryer and round brush to smooth the hair
_____	Remove the rollers and use a boar grooming brush or comb to perform a "dry" wrap, which involves placing the hair tightly around the contour of the head
_____	Begin by applying leave-in conditioner and thermal protectant to the client's hair; blowdry using techniques for thermal pressing; to complete the flat press, wrap the hair using the doobie "dry wrap" method and securely cover the entire head with cling wrap
_____	Comb out the hair by following the direction the hair is wrapped until all hair is hanging loose; use a feather comb to distribute hair in the final desired look and apply a light sheen or spray to complete it

185. What kind of curls do pin curls create?

_____

_____

_____

186. How should pin curls be arranged and formed to work best?

_____

_____

_____

187. What hair types can pin curls be used on?

_____

_____

_____

188. What is a shaping in terms of pin curls?

_____

_____

_____

189. Where on a shaping should you begin a pin curl?

_____

_____

_____

190. What types of waves and curls do open-center pin curls create?

_____

_____

_____

191. Describe the waves and curls produced by closed-center curls.

_____

_____

_____

192. What happens if you make pin curls with the ends outside the curl?

_____

_____

_____

MATCHING

193. Match each type of pin curl with its description.

    a. No-stem curl   b. Half-stem curl   d. Full-stem curl

Type of Pin Curl   **Description**

_____ Permits medium movement

_____ Curl is placed completely off the base

_____ Gives good hair control

_____ Produces a tight, firm, long-lasting curl

_____ Allows for the greatest mobility; gives as much freedom as the length of the stem permits

_____ Curl (circle) is placed half off the base

_____ Allows minimum mobility

_____ It is used to give the hair a strong, definite direction

_____ Placed directly on the base of the curl

194. Label the chart by drawing or sketching an open-center pin curl and a closed-center pin curl. Then draw the resulting waves for each type.

Type of Pin Curl	Open-center pin curl	Closed-center pin curl
Drawing of Pin Curl		
Drawing of Resulting Wave		

Complete the sentences below.

195. The finished result of a pin curl determines the stem's _____.

196. The terms *clockwise curls* and *counterclockwise curls* describe the _____ of the pin curls.

Curls formed in the _____ direction as the movement of a clock's hands are clockwise curls. Curls formed in the _____ direction are counterclockwise curls.

197. Label each type of pin curl base/foundation depicted below.

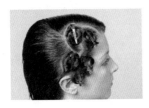 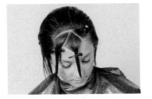 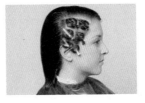 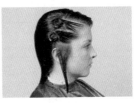

_____

Gives good direction and may be used at the hairline or in the nape

_____

Recommended along the front or facial hairline to prevent breaks or splits in the finished hairstyle

_____

Suitable for curly hairstyles without much volume or lift

_____

Usually recommended at the side front hairline for a smooth, upswept effect

198. Match each pin curl technique with its description. Each technique will be used at least once.

a. Ribboning
b. Carved curls
c. Pin curl waves
d. Ridge curls
e. Skip waves

Pin Curl Technique   Description

_____ Creates controlled and compacted ends and thus more precise finished pin curl styles

_____ Pin curls that are sliced from a shaping and formed without lifting the hair from the head

_____ Two rows of ridge curls that create a strong wave pattern with well-defined lines between the waves

_____ Involves forcing the hair between the thumb and the back of the comb to create tension

_____ Pin curls that are placed immediately behind or below a ridge to form a wave

_____ Use two rows of pin curls; one row is set clockwise and the second row is set counterclockwise

_____ Also known as sculptured curls

_____ This technique represents a combination of finger-waving and pin curls

SHORT ANSWER

199. What is the difference between a barrel curl and a curl created with a roller?

_____

_____

_____

200. What is another name for cascade curls? What effect do they have in hair design?

_____

_____

_____

201. What determines the amount of height in a comb out of pin curls?

_____

_____

_____

Special-Occasion Styles

SHORT ANSWER

202. Describe what a special-occasion style, or updo, is.

_____

_____

_____

203. What is a half updo? What is another name for it?

_____

_____

_____

204. What are the five key points you must consider with special occasion hairstyles?

_____

_____

_____

205. What is the foundation of the chignon knot?

_____

_____

_____

206. Before styling it into a chignon, how should you prepare hair that is very straight and silky?

_____

_____

_____

207. If the client's hair is extremely curly, what are two options for working with it in a chignon?

_____

_____

_____

208. What are two ways to form a bun?

_____

_____

_____

MATCHING

209. Match each type of foundational updo with its description.

    a. Ponytail   b. French pleat

Foundational Updo   **Description**

_____ Classic hairstyle that has been popular since the 1950s; also called a French twist or French roll

_____ Foundation for a chignon, bun, and knot, among other designs

_____ This style might use filler hair for support, also referred to as padding/forms

_____ The most used hairstyle because of its versatility

_____ Elegant style that can be adapted for any client; for example, they can be placed vertically, horizontally, or diagonally, and they can also be open or closed, tight or loose, small or large

_____ Can be styled casual, classic, or trendy

_____ Can include them as a component of a combination updo style

_____ Can be placed on various parts of the head

210. Place the steps for creating a chignon from Procedure 12-19 in your text in order, from 1 to 10. One step has been numbered for you.

_____ Apply appropriate styling product for hold. Blowdry the hair with styling brush for a smooth, sleek finish.

___4___ Brush hair into a low ponytail at the nape. Secure the ponytail with an elastic band, keeping the hair as smooth as possible. Use the side of the bristles to smooth the hair.

_____ Take the remaining section at the front and brush it over into a side sweep and then wrap around chignon. Finish with a strong hair spray. Add flowers or ornaments if desired.

_____ Place two bobby pins onto the band and spread them apart, one on each side. Place one bobby pin in the base of the ponytail. Stretch the band around the ponytail base. Place the second bobby pin in the base. Lock the two pins together.

_____ Fan out both sides by spreading the chignon with your fingers. Secure with hairpins, pinning close to the head. Use bobby pins if more hold is needed.

_____ Part a small section of hair from the underside of the ponytail, wrap it around the ponytail to cover the elastic, and secure with a bobby pin underneath.

_____ Drape client with neck strip and styling or cutting cape.

_____ Smooth out the ponytail and hold it with one hand, then begin backbrushing from underneath the ponytail with your other hand. Gently smooth the outside layer of the ponytail after backbrushing, using the sides of the bristles.

_____ Part the hair on desired side. On the heavy side, create a radial section from the back of your side part to the back of the ear.

_____ Roll the hair under and toward the head to form the chignon. Secure on the left and right undersides of the roll with bobby pins.

211. Now that you've practiced creating a variety of hairstyles (natural textured styles, wet sets, teasing, curls, special-occasion styles, etc.), it's time to design your own!

First, list the features that you plan to incorporate into your design. Will it include pin curls, teasing, a chignon?

Next, sketch pictures of the significant features of your design and how you will achieve them (such as starting with a dry set, sectioning in a particular way, using no-base curls).

Finally, practice your design on your mannequin—be sure to take before and after photos.

Then spend a few minutes reflecting on your design. What do you like about it? What could have gone better? What would you need to do first when trying newly designed hairstyles on a client?

DISCOVERIES AND ACCOMPLISHMENTS

In the space below, write notes about key concepts discussed in this chapter. Share your discoveries with some of the other students in your class and ask them if your notes are helpful. You may want to revise your notes based on good ideas shared by your peers.

Discoveries:

_____

_____

_____

_____

_____

_____

_____

List at least three things you have accomplished since you decided to enroll in school.

Accomplishments:

_____

_____

_____

_____

_____

_____

_____

1. Identify a reason why cosmetologists should study and have a detailed understanding of hairstyling.

   A) because hairstyling services are listed under a podiatry license and performing procedures that are listed under any podiatry license is a primary responsibility of cosmetologists

   B) because they are required to inform clients about the parts of the hair that will be affected by hairstyling

   C) because hairstyling is a crucial, foundational skill that allows them to show their creativity and deliver a client's desired specific outcome

   D) because they are licensed to diagnose, treat, prescribe, or work on unhealthy hair and perform any service required in the process

2. As a cosmetologist, which of the following should you most likely do during a natural hairstyling consultation?

   A) Determine whether a prospective client will be able to pay for a hairstyling service.

   B) Check if the client is fine with the use of a curette.

   C) Perform a detailed hair and scalp analysis.

   D) Prepare the tools that will be required during the hairstyling service.

3. Once you learn about your client's home care regimen during a consultation, you can give them instructions for preserving natural hairstyles with _____, which refers to using textured hairstyling techniques, usually performed at night, and then covering the hair with a satin or silk bonnet/scarf to preserve a long-lasting textured style.

   A) ruffing   C) sugaring

   B) co-styling   D) co-washing

4. In the context of the types of hairbrushes, identify a true statement about vent brushes.

   A) They create more natural styles because they do not force the hair into a particular shape.

   B) They are the best brush for smooth flat blowouts.

   C) They are designed for backbrushing hair.

   D) They are used to smooth edges and create "baby hair" after applying edge control.

continued

5. In the context of hairstyling tools, _____ are used to secure long hair.

    A) hair picks   C) butterfly clamps

    B) duckbill clips   D) croc clamps

6. Which of the following is a styling product that gives a soft luster and shine to the hair while developing textural definition?

    A) spritz   C) serum

    B) mousse   D) setting foam

7. In the context of styling products, _____ is an oily, greasy, or waxy styling aid that gives the hair a shiny and slick appearance, or a matte finish, and keeps the hair in place with either a light or strong hold.

    A) spritz   C) foam

    B) pomade   D) mousse

8. The technique of drying and styling damp hair in a single operation from beginning to end is called _____.

    A) thermal pressing   C) blowdry styling

    B) ratting   D) tempering

9. Which of the following guidelines should you follow when working with blowdryers?

    A) Never towel dry the hair partially or completely before blowdrying to prevent overstretching and damaging the hair.

    B) When working with chemically treated or damaged hair, avoid any tension by "combing" the hair with a brush.

    C) Never move the blowdryer in a constant back-and-forth motion, except when using the cool shot button.

    D) Always direct the hot air away from the client's scalp to avoid scalp burns.

10. In the context of the parts of a thermal iron, the _____ is the clasp or clamp that presses the hair against the rod of a thermal iron.

    A) base   C) shell

    B) prong   D) barrel

continued

11. Identify the most common type of iron used by consumers.

   A) the clipless iron

   B) the flat iron

   C) the wand iron

   D) the spring iron

12. Identify a true statement about professional flat irons.

   A) The plates are coated with highly polished materials, such as titanium, tourmaline, or ceramic, to ensure a smooth, snag-free glide.

   B) They include a spring-loaded clamp controlled by the thumb.

   C) The plate edges are always beveled under to softly cup the ends of the hair.

   D) They allow users to manually control the clamp's pressure.

13. Identify a guideline that you should follow while styling hair using a thermal iron.

   A) Use metal combs rather than plastic combs when styling hair.

   B) Test the iron's temperature by clamping it around a white cotton towel or tissue for five seconds before placing it on the hair.

   C) Use only cellulose acetate combs for thermal curling services as they are nonflammable.

   D) Never place a comb between the scalp and the thermal iron when waving or curling hair at the base of the head.

14. _____ is a technique of hair pressing that removes about 50 to 60 percent of the curl by applying the thermal pressing comb once on each side of the hair.

   A) Medium press

   B) Double press

   C) Soft press

   D) Hard press

15. Identify a rule for hair pressing.

   A) Recommend conditioning treatment masks twice a day to help strengthen and moisturize the hair and scalp.

   B) Consider using a pressing comb rather than a flat iron on high heat for fine hair texture.

   C) Use a moderately cold comb to press short hair on the temples and back of the neck.

   D) Adjust the temperature of the pressing comb to the texture and condition of the client's hair.

continued

16. Identify a difference between the coily method and the curly method.

    A) Unlike the coily method, the curly method can be created with a detangling brush, a wide-tooth comb, and the palm and fingers of your hand.

    B) The coily method is created with palm rolling and finger coil techniques, whereas the curly method is created with raking and scrunching techniques.

    C) Unlike the curly method, the coily method can be applied to loose and silky coily textures.

    D) The curly method is used with short, cropped styles, whereas the coily method is used with wavy hair that is chin length or longer.

17. _____ are a type of natural textured set and style where the hair is double-strand twisted or coil twisted and wrapped around itself to make a knot and secured with bobby pins or elastic bands.

    A) Flat twists   C) Bantu knots

    B) Glamour waves   D) Cornrows

18. _____ are separate networks of coily, textured hair that are intertwined and meshed together.

    A) Braids   C) Locs

    B) Cornrows   D) Plaits

19. _____ is a teasing technique used to build a soft cushion or to mesh two or more curl patterns together for a uniform and smooth comb out.

    A) Backcombing   C) Backbrushing

    B) Matting   D) French lacing

20. Which of the following gives the strongest curl and hold of any hair set?

    A) wrapping a wet roller set without tension

    B) wrapping a dry roller set with tension

    C) wrapping a dry roller set without tension

    D) wrapping a wet roller set with tension

continued

21. _____ is a setting technique done on very short to mid-length chemically relaxed hair that prepares the hair for a thermal service.

   A) Ruffing

   B) Ribboning

   C) Hair molding

   D) Hair pressing

22. In the context of curl mobility, the _____ curl is placed completely off the base and allows for the greatest mobility.

   A) half-stem

   B) mid-stem

   C) full-stem

   D) no-stem

23. Which of the following is described as a section of hair that is molded in a circular movement in preparation for the formation of curls?

   A) a stem

   B) a wave

   C) a base

   D) a shaping

24. In the context of pin curls that are especially effective in adding volume to the hair, _____ curls are pin curls with large center openings and are fastened to the head in a standing position on a rectangular base.

   A) cascade

   B) stand-in

   C) barrel

   D) ridge

25. In the context of the basic hairstyles that are the foundation of every updo, a _____ is the most commonly used hairstyle because of its versatility and is the foundation for a bun, chignon, and knot.

   A) fishtail braid

   B) French pleat

   C) ponytail

   D) cornrow

finished!

Practical Skills

Self-Evaluation Checklist

Regular self-assessment helps you to improve your technical skills and achieve success. After performing each procedure, review the procedure steps in the textbook and rate yourself as "Competent" or "Needs Work," and write in comments on how you were successful or where you can improve. Rating yourself helps you identify your strengths and weaknesses and develop your own plan for improvement.

CRITERIA	COMPETENT	NEEDS WORK	COMMENTS
PROCEDURE 12-1 PREPARING HAIR FOR STYLING			
Preparation			
Procedure			
Timing			
PROCEDURE 12-2 BLOWDRYING HIGHLY TEXTURED HAIR PRIOR TO THERMAL SETTING			
Preparation			
Procedure			
Post-Service			
Timing			
PROCEDURE 12-3 BLOWDRYING AND THERMAL SETTING TO PRODUCE FULL, SMOOTH HAIR			
Preparation			
Procedure			
Post-Service			
Timing			
PROCEDURE 12-4 BLOWDRYING SHORT, CURLY HAIR IN ITS NATURAL WAVE PATTERN			
Preparation			
Procedure			
Post-Service			
Timing			
PROCEDURE 12-5 DIFFUSING CURLY HAIR IN ITS NATURAL WAVE PATTERN			
Preparation			
Procedure			
Post-Service			
Timing			
PROCEDURE 12-6 BLOWDRYING STRAIGHT OR WAVY HAIR FOR MAXIMUM VOLUME			
Preparation			
Procedure			
Post-Service			
Timing			
PROCEDURE 12-7 BLOWDRYING BLUNT OR LONG-LAYERED, STRAIGHT TO WAVY HAIR INTO A STRAIGHT STYLE			
Preparation			
Procedure			
Post-Service			
Timing			

Practical Skills Self-Evaluation Checklist

CRITERIA	COMPETENT	NEEDS WORK	COMMENTS
PROCEDURE 12-8 MARCEL MANIPULATIONS (THERMAL CURLING)			
Preparation			
Procedure			
Post-Service			
Timing			
PROCEDURE 12-9 HOLLYWOOD WAVES (THERMAL WAVING)			
Preparation			
Procedure			
Post-Service			
Timing			
PROCEDURE 12-10 CURLY AND COILY METHODS			
Preparation			
Procedure			
Post-Service			
Timing			
PROCEDURE 12-11 DOUBLE-STRAND TWIST			
Preparation			
Procedure			
Post-Service			
Timing			
PROCEDURE 12-12 COIL COMB TECHNIQUE—NUBIAN COILS AND STARTING LOCS			
Preparation			
Procedure			
Post-Service			
Timing			
PROCEDURE 12-13 CULTIVATING AND GROOMING LOCS			
Preparation			
Procedure			
Post-Service			
Timing			
PROCEDURE 12-14 WET SET WITH ROLLERS			
Preparation			
Procedure			
Post-Service			
Timing			

Practical Skills
Self-Evaluation Checklist

CRITERIA	COMPETENT	NEEDS WORK	COMMENTS
PROCEDURE 12-15 HORIZONTAL FINGER-WAVING			
Preparation			
Procedure			
Post-Service			
Timing			
PROCEDURE 12-16 HAIR WRAPPING ON COARSE, COILY HAIR			
Preparation			
Procedure			
Post-Service			
Timing			
PROCEDURE 12-17 CURLING SHORT, RELAXED HAIR			
Preparation			
Procedure			
Post-Service			
Timing			
PROCEDURE 12-18 SILK PRESS			
Preparation			
Procedure			
Post-Service			
Timing			
PROCEDURE 12-19 CHIGNON			
Preparation			
Procedure			
Post-Service			
Timing			
PROCEDURE 12-20 CURLY CHIGNON UPDO			
Preparation			
Procedure			
Post-Service			
Timing			
PROCEDURE 12-21 FRENCH PLEAT OR TWIST			
Preparation			
Procedure			
Post-Service			
Timing			

Ch. 13: Braiding and Braid Extensions

Why Study Braiding and Braid Extensions?

SHORT ANSWER

1. What are three reasons cosmetologists should study and have a thorough understanding of braiding and braid extension styles?

   _____

   _____

   _____

2. Where did braiding originate?

   _____

   _____

   _____

Braiding Salons

3. Describe natural hairstyling, as practiced in braiding salons.

_____

_____

_____

4. In what two ways can having the ability to offer your clients different braid styles help you, as a stylist?

_____

_____

_____

5. Where are braiding salons typically found in the United States?

_____

_____

_____

6. What are three specific, important areas for you to evaluate during the client consultation for braiding, in addition to those assessed during a general hairstyling consultation?

_____

_____

_____

7. What are the three goals of conducting a client consultation?

_____

_____

_____

8. Even if a client knows exactly which type of braid style they want, what is the braider's/stylist's responsibility for guiding the client during the consultation?

_____

_____

_____

TRUE OR FALSE

Indicate whether the statements below are true or false. For any false statements, explain why they are false.

9. Most braided styles can be achieved in approximately an hour.

   T   F   _____

10. The more complex braided styles are not disposable hairdos to be casually brushed out.

   T   F   _____

11. With proper care, a braided hair design can last one to two weeks.

   T   F   _____

12. You don't want the client to reject your work and demand that the braids be removed because the investment in these complex styles is high for both the client and stylist.

   T   F   _____

13. If a client wants a braided hairstyle, there is no need to fill out a client intake form during the initial consultation because no chemicals will be involved in these types of natural hairstyles.

   T   F   _____

14. Giving your clients a thorough and detailed consultation is the best way to avoid miscommunication and ensure a positive outcome.

   T   F   _____

Complete the sentences below.

15. During the consultation, check the scalp to see if the client has the condition of _____, or other excessive, active, or abnormal hair loss.

16. Since the hair around the _____ is generally thinner and finer, never choose a style that pulls on the hair follicle or places excessive _____ in this or any _____ area.

17. Avoid offering services to a client with damaged hair so as not to further stress the hair _____.

RESEARCH

18. Contact various salons in your area and interview them by asking the following questions. Record the information below.

   - Contact information for salons:

   Salon 1: _____

   Salon 2: _____

   Salon 3: _____

   - Does your salon offer braiding or braid extensions as a service?

   Salon 1: _____

   Salon 2: _____

   Salon 3: _____

   - If yes, what braiding services do you offer?

   Salon 1: _____

   Salon 2: _____

   Salon 3: _____

   - What braids are the most popular in your salon?

   Salon 1: _____

   Salon 2: _____

   Salon 3: _____

- What is the average time it takes your stylists to complete a full head of cornrows?

  Salon 1: _____

  Salon 2: _____

  Salon 3: _____

- What is the price structure your salon charges for braiding services?

  Salon 1: _____

  Salon 2: _____

  Salon 3: _____

- Do you have any specific advice for a newly licensed professional with respect to offering braiding services?

  Salon 1: _____

  Salon 2: _____

  Salon 3: _____

Tools and Materials for Braiding and Extensions

LABELING

19. Identify each tool associated with performing braiding services shown below.

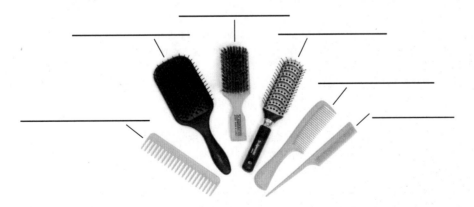

20. Match each tool used for braids and extensions with its description/function. Each tool will be used once.

a. Hooded dryer
b. Soft nylon brushes combined with boar bristle
c. Hackle
d. Steamer
e. Vent brush
f. Small rubber bands
g. Boar-bristle brush
h. Drawing board
i. Double-tooth comb
j. Long clips
k. Wide-tooth comb
l. Tail comb
m. Butterfly and small clips
n. Blowdryer with comb nozzle attachment
o. Square paddle brush/ detangling brush

Braids/Extensions Tool   **Description/Function**

_____ Used to secure hair ends

_____ Option for fine, soft hair, especially around the hairline and for smoothing or wrapping/molding wet textured hair

_____ Excellent for design parting, sectioning large hair segments, and opening and removing braids

_____ Used for separating hair into large sections

_____ Used to separate and hold hair into large or small sections

_____ Board of fine, upright nails through which human hair extensions are combed; used for detangling or blending colors and highlights

_____ Removes excess moisture before blowdrying the hair

_____ Larger spaced teeth allow textured hair to move between the rows of teeth without snagging

_____ Good for releasing tangles, knots, and snarls in short textured hair and long, straight, wavy, and curly hair

_____ Gently removes tangles in wet and wavy hair, dry and curly hair, and human hair extensions

_____ Flat leather pads with very close, fine teeth that sandwich human hair extensions

_____ Deeply hydrates, moisturizes, and conditions the hair with water vapor

_____ Loosens the curl pattern in textured hair for braiding styles, and dries, stretches, and softens textured hair

_____ Used for separating the hair; excellent for wet, curly hair

_____ Best for stimulating the scalp, smoothing dry textured hair, and removing dirt and lint from locs

RESEARCH

21. Using the Internet, catalogues from beauty supply shops, or cosmetology industry publications, look for different types of hair extensions you could use with your braiding clients: Remy, Kanekalon®, yak hair, nylon, rayon, and other natural or synthetic offerings you find.

    Then use the chart below, a separate sheet of paper, or follow the link to list your resources and create a quick reference guide to use the next time you're in the market for braiding and extension products. In turn, having this information ready will help you become a resource for your braiding clients.

+ BONUS
Visit: bonus.milady.com/cos-wb/toc

PRODUCT	COST	COLORS	PROS/CONS	BRAIDING STYLE
Remy				
Kanekalon®				
Yak hair				
Nylon				
Rayon				
Other				

SHORT ANSWER

22. What are the three common types of hair used in hair extensions?

    _____

    _____

    _____

23. What type of fiber is the "gold standard" for hair extensions?

    _____

    _____

    _____

24. What are five examples of synthetic fibers used in extensions?

_____

_____

_____

25. Describe Kanekalon®.

_____

_____

_____

Braiding the Hair

SHORT ANSWER

26. What is the first step in braiding?

_____

_____

_____

27. What are the benefits of blowdrying the hair? Which length benefits most from blowdrying?

_____

_____

_____

28. What is the main benefit of placing a client under the dryer to dry their hair? How long does it take?

_____

_____

_____

29. Complete the sentences below using words from the word bank. Not all words will be used.

Word bank: cream, frizzy, wet, dry, wax, foam, straight, textured, stiff, pomade, scalp, shrinkage, pliable, breakage

It is best to braid _____ hair when it's _____ to prevent _____ and

excessive _____ tension. If you are performing a braiding style that requires your

client's hair to be _____, apply a _____ or curl _____ and allow

for _____ when braiding. For _____ hair, very lightly coat the hair with a

_____, _____, or texturizing spray to make it more _____.

LABELING

30. Identify the type of foundational braid depicted in each image below.

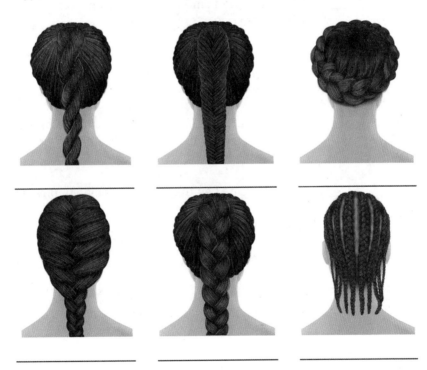

31. Match the foundational braid types with their descriptions. Each type will be used twice.

a. Rope   c. Halo   e. Single
b. Fishtail   d. Invisible   f. Cornrow

Foundational Braid	Description
_____	Best performed on nonlayered hair that is at least shoulder length
_____	Can be done on or off the scalp and with or without extensions; ideal for long hair; also works on shorter hair with long layers
_____	Narrow rows of visible braids that lie close to the scalp; created with a three-strand, on-the-scalp braiding technique
_____	Created with two strands that are twisted around each other; pick up and add hair to both sides before twisting the right side over the left
_____	Also known as plaits or visible braids, box braids, or individual braids
_____	Top crown is left smooth and neat, while cornrows are pinned around the head to create the effect
_____	Free-hanging, with or without extensions; executed using either an underhand or an overhand technique; can be used with all hair textures in various ways
_____	Two or three long, simple, inverted, thick cornrows created around the head; the extended long braids are then wrapped around the head and pinned
_____	can be done on hair that is all one length or on long layered hair
_____	Uses an overhand pick-up technique
_____	Also known as canerows
_____	Simple two-strand braid in which hair is picked up from the sides and added to the strands as they are crossed over each other

CREATE

32. Now it's time to practice some braids! Using modeling clay, Play-Doh (or make your own), or even something like bread dough if you like to bake, practice the six foundational braids above (rope, fishtail, halo, invisible, single, and cornrow). Roll multiple "strands" of hair and think about how many strands you need for braids using the pick-up technique, what braids look like when each

strand is a different thickness, and the different styles of tight and loose braids using the same technique. Take some notes below. Finally, design one braid of your choice (such as a six-strand single braid) and consider how mastering the foundational braids can allow you to create new designs and express your creativity!

33. What is a protective style? How do protective styles preserve hair health?

_____

_____

_____

34. If you are creating an invisible braid for a client whose hair is straight and layered, what can you do to help hold shorter strands in place?

_____

_____

_____

35. What are the four shapes into which partings or subsections can be formed when creating single box braids? What does the parting determine?

_____

_____

_____

36. Why should you show the extension fibers to the client during the consultation step?

_____

_____

_____

37. Explain how to use a drawing board to prepare extension fibers for easy access when integrating them into your client's braid.

_____

_____

_____

Complete the sentences below. Then draw the three steps of each braiding technique as described. The first one is given to you.

38. _____ technique is a braiding technique in which the _____ section goes under the middle strand, then the _____ section goes under the middle strand.

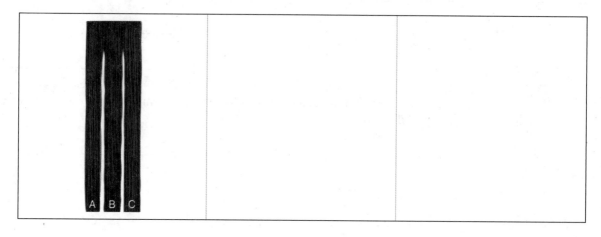

39. _____ technique is a braiding technique in which the first _____ section goes over the middle one, then the other _____ section goes over the middle strand.

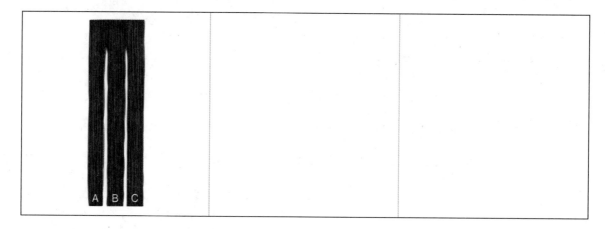

Indicate whether the statements below are true or false. For any false statements, explain why they are false.

40. To create a small invisible knot when performing single braids with human hair extensions, you would loop a small strand of hair around the braid and pull the hair strand through the loop.

    T   F   _____

41. An alternative method of incorporating the hair extension into a single braid is to continue braiding well past the desired hair length and secure it with an elastic band.

    T   F   _____

42. To secure the ends and create a bend or spiral on the ends of synthetic fibers, wrap the braid ends with a curling rod, then dip all the rodded ends into hot water for 10 to 15 minutes.

    T   F   _____

43. Other optional finishes for braid ends, such as singeing with a ceramic flat iron or hot gun (i.e., keratin glue hot tool used for fusion weaving), are advanced methods but require no special training.

    T   F   _____

SHORT ANSWER

44. What is the key to creating beautiful cornrows?

    _____

    _____

    _____

45. In what three specific ways will practicing cornrows on a mannequin help you improve your technique?

    _____

    _____

    _____

46. Why is it important to apply the correct tension and amount of extension material when using the feed-in method to create cornrows?

    _____

    _____

    _____

47. What are the benefits of using the feed-in method to create cornrows with extensions, even though it takes longer to perform than traditional cornrowing?

_____

_____

_____

MATCHING

48. Match each facial shape with the braid style or technique that would be most appropriate or flattering.

a. Oval   c. Round   e. Heart-shaped
b. Oblong   d. Square   f. Triangular

Facial Shape   **Flattering Braid Style**

_____   Requires a style with more width at the sides

_____   Minimized by allowing longer braids to frame the face

_____   Bring at least some braids forward to create the illusion of a narrower chin line

_____   Most braided styles suit this facial shape

_____   Use bangs or sweep braids across the forehead

_____   Benefits from a style with height, such as one in which braids are gathered high on top and secured below the crown in back

REFLECTION

49. Using YouTube or your favorite hair stylist on social media, watch three videos that demonstrate a different braiding or extension technique you learned in this chapter. The link below provides access to a chart that will guide your viewing experience and reflections. As you watch the videos, think about how, as a cosmetologist, you can use these foundational braiding and extension skills to create the perfect style for any client: adding color, designing updos for special events, daily looks, or something completely new. Take notes while you watch. What was similar or different in the video compared to your studies? Is this a braiding or extension technique you would want to perform on a client? Explain.

+ BONUS
Visit: bonus.milady.com/cos-wb/toc

50. For each facial shape shown below, design a flattering braid style or braided updo. Draw directly on the face outlines provided. For inspiration, look through magazines, the Internet, or even photos you've taken or appeared in. Use colors, arrows, and so on to point out any special features/effects. Also, feel free to draw a close-up of any important details or a particular area of your design.

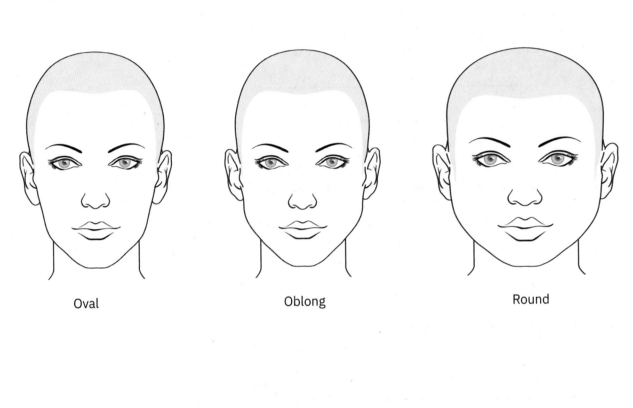

Oval   Oblong   Round

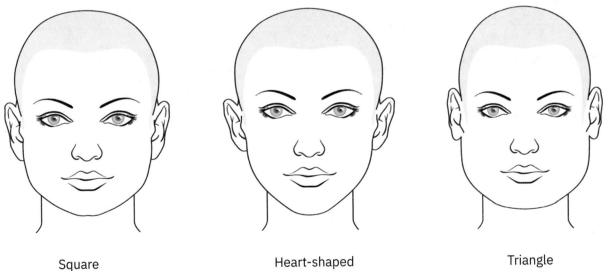

Square   Heart-shaped   Triangle

51. Describe what tree braiding is and explain how it differs from other techniques used for adding hair.

_____

_____

_____

52. What are the two main methods of applying loc extensions?

_____

_____

_____

53. What type of fiber is considered best for loc extensions?

_____

_____

_____

54. What is "faux" about faux locs?

_____

_____

_____

55. How are faux locs installed?

_____

_____

_____

DISCOVERIES AND ACCOMPLISHMENTS

In the space below, write notes about key concepts discussed in this chapter. Share your discoveries with some of the other students in your class and ask them if your notes are helpful. You may want to revise your notes based on good ideas shared by your peers.

Discoveries:

_____

_____

_____

_____

_____

_____

_____

List at least three things you have accomplished since you decided to enroll in school.

Accomplishments:

_____

_____

_____

_____

_____

_____

_____

1. Which of the following is the best way to avoid miscommunication with clients and ensure a positive outcome?

   A) giving the clients a brochure with instructions for a service

   B) asking the clients to sign a client intake form

   C) giving the clients a detailed and thorough consultation

   D) asking the clients to sign a service record card

2. There are three specific considerations for a braiding consultation. Identify one of them.

   A) Analyze whether a prospective client will be able to pay for a braiding service.

   B) Check if the client is fine with the use of a curette.

   C) Pay special attention to hair type, texture, and curl configuration.

   D) Prepare the tools that will be required during the braiding service.

3. During a braiding consultation, stylists should always check the scalp for _____, which refers to active, excessive, or abnormal hair loss.

   A) hirsutism   C) alopecia

   B) pityriasis   D) hypertrichosis

4. Which of the following tools is best for stimulating the scalp?

   A) a double-tooth comb   C) a tail comb

   B) a detangling brush   D) a boar-bristle brush

5. Identify the tool that gently removes tangles in dry and curly hair, wet and wavy hair, and human hair extensions.

   A) a boar-brittle brush   C) a vent brush

   B) a tail comb   D) a boar-bristle brush

continued

6. _____ are created with prefabricated synthetic hair that is added to individual braids or cornrows.

   A) Faux locs

   B) Bantu knots

   C) Rope braids

   D) Nubian knots

7. Which of the following tools is excellent for opening and removing braids, design parting, and sectioning large hair segments?

   A) a detangling brush

   B) a vent brush

   C) a tail comb

   D) a natural hairbrush

8. Identify a true statement about a vent brush.

   A) It should be used to gently remove tangles in dry and curly hair, wet and wavy hair, and human hair extensions.

   B) It is typically used for lifting and dividing textured hair.

   C) It should be used for design parting and opening and removing braids.

   D) It is typically used for cutting large sections.

9. Which of the following is used to deeply hydrate, moisturize, and condition the hair with water vapor?

   A) a paraffin bath

   B) a blowdryer with comb nozzle attachment

   C) a steamer

   D) a diffuser

10. Which of the following statements is true of long clips?

    A) They are used to secure hair ends.

    B) They are used for separating hair into large sections.

    C) They are used for creating finished looks and shapes.

    D) They are excellent for sectioning small hair segments.

continued

11. Identify a true statement about a hooded dryer.

A) It is best for stimulating the scalp before a hair service begins.

B) It is used to completely dry and finish braided styles.

C) It is highly ineffective in dry finishing locked and textured or braided styles.

D) It deeply hydrates, moisturizes, and conditions the hair with water vapor.

12. Which of the following is a board of fine standing nails through which human hair extensions are combed?

A) a drawing board   C) a hackle

B) a curette   D) a nipper

13. A _____ consists of flat leather pads with very close, fine teeth that sandwich human hair extensions.

A) drawing board   C) hackle

B) hair nipper   D) curette

14. Which of the following is an excellent quality synthetic fiber that is highly heat resistant and made specifically for braided styles?

A) remy hair   C) Kanekalon®

B) virgin hair   D) angora

15. Which of the following is the quickest and most effective way to prepare the hair for a braiding service as it will soften the hair, making it easier to comb and section?

A) blowdrying   C) air drying

B) steaming   D) twisting the hair

continued

16. Which of the following is a helpful tip that you should follow before, during, or after braiding a client's hair?

    A) Use a locking/twist comb rather than a wide-tooth comb.

    B) After shampooing the hair, towel blot the hair without tension or rubbing.

    C) Begin combing the hair at the center of the scalp and gently move toward the end of the hair strands.

    D) Avoid using pomades or serums on braided hair.

17. The _____ braid is created with two strands that are twisted around each other.

    A) halo

    C) rope

    B) single

    D) visible

18. Which of the following is a simple two-strand braid in which hair is picked up from the sides and added to the strands as they are crossed over each other?

    A) the rope braid

    C) the halo braid

    B) the fishtail braid

    D) the box braid

19. _____ braids are two or three long, simple, inverted, thick cornrows created around the head.

    A) Halo

    C) Rope

    B) Box

    D) Fishtail

20. Which of the following statements is true of the invisible braid?

    A) It uses an underhand pick-up technique.

    B) It can be done on or off the scalp.

    C) It can only be done with extensions.

    D) It is ideal for short, nonlayered hair.

continued

21. _____ braids are also known as inverted braids or French braids.

    A) Single   C) Rope

    B) Box   D) Invisible

22. _____ braids are free-hanging braids, with or without extensions, created using either an underhand or an overhand technique.

    A) Rope   C) Halo

    B) Fishtail   D) Single

23. Identify a true statement about cornrows.

    A) Cornrows usually last seven to nine weeks.

    B) Traditional cornrows are irregular and not contoured to the scalp.

    C) Consistent and even partings are essential for beautiful cornrows.

    D) Cornrows are best done on short, curly hair.

24. When a hairstylist cornrow braids a client's hair along with hair extensions, but the completed look mostly shows faux hair, the type of braids created are called _____ braids.

    A) tree   C) rope

    B) halo   D) fishtail

25. Identify a true statement about loc extensions.

    A) An example of human hair loc extensions is Kanekalon®.

    B) They are an ineffective way to start locs.

    C) Synthetic hair loc extensions are the most natural looking locked style.

    D) They create a natural-looking loc style with additional human hair or synthetic hair fibers.

finished!

Practical Skills
Self-Evaluation Checklist

Regular self-assessment helps you to improve your technical skills and achieve success. After performing each procedure, review the procedure steps in the textbook and rate yourself as "Competent" or "Needs Work," and write in comments on how you were successful or where you can improve. Rating yourself helps you identify your strengths and weaknesses and develop your own plan for improvement.

CRITERIA	COMPETENT	NEEDS WORK	COMMENTS
PROCEDURE 13-1 PREPARING TEXTURED HAIR FOR BRAIDING			
Preparation			
Procedure			
Timing			
PROCEDURE 13-2 HALO BRAIDS			
Preparation			
Procedure			
Post-Service			
Timing			
PROCEDURE 13-3 SINGLE BRAIDS WITH EXTENSIONS			
Preparation			
Procedure			
Post-Service			
Timing			
PROCEDURE 13-4 BASIC CORNROWS			
Preparation			
Procedure			
Post-Service			
Timing			

Ch. 14: Wigs and Hair Additions

⚑ TRACK MY PROGRESS!

Use this simple tracker to record your progress as you work through the activities in each learning objective.

COMPLETED	# OF CORRECT ANSWERS	OBJECTIVE
☐	_____/6	**LO 1** - Explain why cosmetologists should study wigs and hair additions.
☐	_____/3	**LO 2** - List the considerations for effective hair addition consultations.
☐	_____/20	**LO3** - Describe the different hair and fiber types used for hair additions and wigs.
☐	_____/32	**LO 4** - Outline several different methods of attaching hair extensions.
☐	_____/30	**LO 5** - Describe different types of wigs and hairpieces and how to care for them.
☐	_____/15	**LO 6** - Describe several types of hairpieces and their uses.

Why Study Wigs and Hair Additions?

SHORT ANSWER

1. Describe hair extensions. What is their purpose?

   _____

   _____

   _____

2. What is a wig? What is the purpose of a wig?

   _____

   _____

   _____

3. What materials do hair additions consist of?

_____

_____

_____

4. List three examples of the forms that hairpieces might take.

_____

_____

_____

5. What are two reasons it is important for cosmetologists to study and thoroughly understand wigs specifically?

_____

_____

_____

6. Overall, what is your duty, as a cosmetologist, during the consultation?

_____

_____

_____

Hair Addition Consultations

SHORT ANSWER

7. What are three ways that your clients' answers to your specific questions will help you work with someone who is considering hair additions or a wig?

_____

_____

_____

8. In addition to asking your client a number of specific questions about their interest in hair additions or a wig, what are three other, possibly uncomfortable, things you should mention and explain during the consultation? Why is it important for you, as the cosmetologist, to bring up these aspects?

_____

_____

_____

ROLE PLAY

9. Listed below are specific questions that cosmetologists should ask clients during a consultation for hair additions and wigs. For this exercise, pair up with a classmate. Together, use your textbook, the Internet, or professional beauty magazines to research the significance of each consultation question. (_Hint:_ Combine the topic of each question with search terms such as "hair extensions," "wigs," "hair loss," or "hair additions.") Then take turns being the client and cosmetologist. As the cosmetologist, ask the client the consultation questions from your text, take notes on their responses, and engage in a discussion that results in a recommendation for your client. As the client, prepare some authentic answers that a real client might provide—be specific and creative—and ask a few questions of your own.

CONSULTATION QUESTIONS FOR HAIR ADDITIONS AND WIGS	WHY DO YOU NEED TO ASK THIS?
Why do you want to wear hair extensions?	
Have you worn hair extensions before? Which types of extensions?	
If you have worn hair extensions or a wig, what did you like and dislike about them?	
How long do you plan to wear hair extensions?	
How much time do you expect to devote to caring for your extensions at home (daily, weekly)? Are you experiencing any hair loss?	
Are you taking any medication for hair thinning or hair loss?	
Do you have an outdoor vacation planned? Are you planning on spending time at the beach?	
Do you frequently swim in a chlorinated pool or soak in a hot tub?	

Hair Additions and Wig Fibers

10. Why is it important for stylists to know whether the human hair in extensions or wigs either has the cuticle or is cuticle-free?

    _____

    _____

    _____

11. What are the three categories of fiber used in hair additions and wigs?

    _____

    _____

    _____

12. What are two other terms for remy hair?

    _____

    _____

    _____

13. What is the source of remy hair, and what are three benefits of that source?

    _____

    _____

    _____

14. List at least three qualities/benefits of remy hair.

    _____

    _____

    _____

15. What is the source of cuticle-free hair? How is it collected?

_____

_____

_____

16. When does cuticle-free hair need to be replaced?

_____

_____

_____

17. What are three types of animal hair fibers?

_____

_____

_____

18. Which is the most desirable animal hair fiber? Why?

_____

_____

_____

19. Describe how to test whether a strand of hair is human fiber or synthetic fiber.

_____

_____

_____

20. Match each type of Remy hair with its description.

   a. Virgin European hair

   b. Virgin human hair
       from India

   c. Virgin Asian hair
       (Chinese hair)

Type of Remy Hair	Description
_____	Has a natural luster and bounce, and can be styled straight or curly
_____	Middle cost
_____	Average lengths range from 12 to 18 inches (30 to 46 centimeters)
_____	Silky, lightweight, lustrous, and durable; this hair type has a delicate wave that responds well to styling
_____	Most expensive and highest quality
_____	Most of this type of hair is naturally straight
_____	Costs about the same as Indian hair
_____	Medium luster, generally with some curl, and very fine

TRUE OR FALSE

Indicate whether each statement below is true or false. For any false statements, explain why they are false.

21. Extensions and wigs made of synthetic fibers are ideal for integrating with natural braids or locks; they can also be worn alone.

   T   F   _____

22. Extensions and wigs made of synthetic fibers are more expensive than human hair.

   T   F   _____

23. Kanekalon®, a synthetic fiber, is very durable but only vaguely resembles human hair.

   T   F   _____

24. Kanekalon® is the top synthetic hair fiber.

   T   F   _____

25. Most synthetic fibers are available in preset styles, such as coily textures, waves, and structured curls.

    T   F   _____

26. Synthetic hair color is fade-free, although the fiber breaks down much faster than remy hair.

    T   F   _____

27. Lower grades of synthetic hair are typically very dull, so shop wisely.

    T   F   _____

MATCHING

28. Indicate whether each feature of human, synthetic, or animal fibers listed below is a Pro (a benefit) or a Con (a disadvantage).

    a. Pro—Human fiber hair   c. Pro—Synthetic fiber hair   e. Pro—Animal fiber hair
    b. Con—Human fiber hair   d. Con—Synthetic fiber hair   f. Con—Animal fiber hair

Pro or Con of Which Type of Fiber?   **Feature of the Fiber**

_____   Can be color-treated using demipermanent, semipermanent, or temporary dyes

_____   Offers limitless colors and won't fade

_____   Depending on its natural texture, may frizz or lose its style when exposed to humidity, water-related activities, or perspiration

_____   Moves and behaves like the client's natural hair

_____   Blends well with human and synthetic hair

_____   Needs to be reset after shampooing

_____   Less expensive than human hair

_____   Is sometimes so shiny it does not look natural

_____   Can be heat-styled using warm to moderate temperatures with a blowdryer, curling iron, flat iron, or hot rollers

_____   Is not a stand-alone fiber (must be blended with another fiber hair)

_____   Most of these types of wigs, hairpieces, and extensions are precut and styled according to the latest trends

_____ Is naturally reflective and multicolored

_____ Provides permanent styles

_____ Generally reacts to heat in the same way as human hair

_____ Is more expensive than synthetic or animal fibers

_____ Does not accept regular hair dye

_____ Easy to maintain at home

_____ Cannot be restyled

_____ Splits, breaks, and fades in color

_____ Cannot be exposed to high heat

RESEARCH

29. Select a single type of hair addition—for example, braid, ponytail, or extensions—or a wig. Use the Internet or a beauty supply catalogue to compare costs, quantities/sizes, and so on for a human, synthetic, and animal fiber hair version of the hair addition or wig that you selected. Record your findings in the chart below, or follow the link for a PDF version. Which type was the best overall option for the type of hair additional you chose and why? Was surprised you most?

+ BONUS

Visit: bonus.milady.com/cos-wb/toc

HAIR ADDITION	HUMAN HAIR	SYNTHETIC HAIR	ANIMAL HAIR
Source (Store or Website)			
Origin of Manufacture			
Name/Brand			
Cost			
Sizes/Quantities			
Available Colors			
Recommendations for Use			
Maintenance Information			
Unique Features Advertised			

Hair Extension Methods

30. What are the four main methods for attaching hair extensions?

_____

_____

_____

31. Are hair extensions applied in thick, medium-width, or thin strands?

_____

_____

_____

32. Describe a weft.

_____

_____

_____

RANKING

33. Place the following general guidelines for performing professional hair augmentation services in order of highest importance (1) to lowest (4).

	Security of the hair additions so that they don't slip or fall out
	Safety for the client's own hair
	Style and fashion
	Client comfort when applying hair extensions by not pulling, pinching, or using excessive tension on the natural hair

Complete each item from the hair augmentation services checklist below.

34. Decide whether you are adding _____ or _____, or both.

35. With very _____ hair, ensure the _____ site does not show through.

36. With _____ hair, determine whether you are matching the _____ or adding another _____ pattern.

37. Know which final style you want to achieve and _____ or visualize the placement pattern.

38. As a general rule, stay _____ inch (2.5 centimeters) away from the _____ at the front, sides, and nape, and _____ inch (2.5 centimeters) away from the _____.

39. Curly hair appears _____ than _____ hair, even when they share the same density. This means you may not need to attach as many extensions on _____ hair.

SHORT ANSWER

40. What is another name for the braid-and-sew method?

_____

_____

_____

41. What determines how the hair in the hair extensions will fall once they are attached? What are four directions (or lines) in which you can position the hair extensions?

_____

_____

_____

42. What are two best practices for positioning the tracks? (*Hint:* One is for looks, and the other is to protect the hairline.)

_____

_____

_____

43. Describe the recommended tool to use for sewing on hair extensions. Why is it recommended?

_____

_____

_____

LABELING AND SEQUENCE

44. Label (or describe) each step of the braid-and-sew method depicted below. Then number each step from 1 to 6, beginning to end.

NUMBER	IMAGE	DESCRIPTION

NUMBER	IMAGE	DESCRIPTION

ROLE PLAY

45. For this activity, wrap a foam head with a tight stocking and grab a piece of cloth—a rag, old t-shirt, sock, anything will do—and gather a needle, thread, and a pair of scissors. Then prepare your needle and thread. Being very careful not to poke yourself, sew the piece of cloth (the "weft") onto the stocking covering the foam head, using lock, double lock, and overcast stitches. Be sure to take photos of the finished stitches. Do they look like the photos in the textbook? What could you do to improve your stitches in the future?

Indicate whether each statement below is true or false. For any false statements, explain why they are false.

46. When applied correctly, tape-in extensions are lightweight and do not stress the hair, making them ideal for thin and chemically damaged hair.

    T   F   _____

47. Tape-in extensions provide length and fullness, but the application process is very time-consuming.

    T   F   _____

48. Quality tape-in extensions have a medical-grade adhesive to enhance longevity.

    T   F   _____

49. When applying tape-in extensions, it's recommended that you avoid sandwiching the section of natural hair between two of them.

    T   F   _____

50. Once removed, the adhesive is replaced, and tape-in extensions can be reapplied on the same client.

    T   F   _____

51. Tape-in extensions can be worn for one to two weeks.

    T   F   _____

52. Some tape-in hair extension companies require taking a certification course before ordering their products, and many offer online training.

    T   F   _____

SHORT ANSWER

53. In your own words, briefly describe how hair extensions are attached when using the fusion bonding method.

    _____

    _____

    _____

54. How long do the attachments usually last when applied using the fusion bonding method? How does this compare with other attachment methods?

_____

_____

_____

55. Describe the role of the keratin-based tip in the fusion bonding method.

_____

_____

_____

56. What are three reasons that clients might prefer having extensions that have been attached using the fusion bonding method?

_____

_____

_____

57. What is another way to refer to the linking method of attaching hair extensions?

_____

_____

_____

58. What is the recommended minimum length for natural hair when using the linking method to attach hair extensions to it?

_____

_____

_____

59. Place the steps of the linking method in order, from 1 to 8.

	Properly remove the links using a removal tool.
	Use a hook to pick up a small amount of natural hair from a parting.
	Move the link up the hair strand to the scalp.
	Reuse the extensions on the same client as desired.
	Pinch the link flat with a special pair of pliers.
	Insert a thin hair extension into the link.
	Position the link slightly off base to ensure mobility and avoid scalp tension.
	Feed the natural hair through a link.

MATCHING

60. Indicate whether each description of the four attachment methods listed below is a Pro (a benefit) or a Con (a disadvantage).

a. Pro—Braid-and-sew
b. Con—Braid-and-sew
c. Pro—Tape-in
d. Con—Tape-in
e. Pro—Fusion bonding
f. Con—Fusion bonding
g. Pro—Linking
h. Con—Linking

Pro or Con of Which Attachment Method?   **Description of Attachment Method**

_____ Uses lightweight bonds that wear comfortably

_____ Not appropriate for clients with extremely damaged hair, baby fine hair, or poor scalp hygiene

_____ Can be reused

_____ Flexible and has natural movement

_____ Requires only a specialized needle and thread

_____ Time-consuming and expensive service

_____ Preferred for hair recovering from severe damage

_____ Does not use an adhesive

_____ Can be a highly lucrative service

_____ Lie flat for a natural and seamless look and feel

_____ Visible when hair is tightly pulled into a ponytail or top knot

_____ Causes added scalp and hair tension

_____ Easily removed by gently breaking the bond and sliding it out of the client's hair

_____ Can be reused

_____ Apparent if not properly cut and blended

_____ Very safe technique

_____ Faster drying times than the weft method because there is less bulk

_____ Can be done quickly

_____ Can damage clients' existing hair if applied with too much tension

_____ Must avoid contact with haircolor or lightening products if using copper cylinders

_____ Adhesive may dissolve in chlorinated pools and saltwater, causing slippage if poor quality

_____ Creates the illusion of dimension through color selection

_____ More expensive (which limits the pool of clients who choose this service)

_____ Offers styling versatility

_____ Prone to shedding

_____ Requires a longer appointment to perform the service

_____ Less detectable for greater styling versatility

_____ Preserves natural hair's integrity when applied properly (links are coated with silicone to help prevent hair damage)

61. For each topic below, list the specific instruction that stylists should give their clients regarding care for their hair extensions.

TOPIC	CARE INSTRUCTIONS FOR CLIENTS WITH HAIR EXTENSIONS
Bathing	
Conditioning the hair	
Sitting in saunas or using steam showers	
Washing the hair	
Sleeping	
Brushing the hair	
Styling	
Maintenance appointments	
Swimming	

Wigs

MATCHING

62. Match each type of wig with its description. Each type will be used seven times.

    a. Cap wigs   b. Capless wigs

Type of Wig:
Cap or Capless   **Description**

_____ Constructed with an elasticized, mesh-fiber base to which the hair is attached

_____ Have a cap, but the wefts of hair are less dense and are sewn in with vertical lace strips, resulting in a lot of open space

_____ Closed framework

_____ Machine-made from human or artificial hair

_____ Available in several ready-to-wear sizes, as well as custom-made units that require special fittings

_____ Excellent for clients who want to frequently change their hairstyle, desire the convenience of wearing a wig, are transitioning to natural hair, or have thin hair

_____ Hair fibers attached by various methods, including lace front wigs, which create the illusion of natural hair growth along the hairline and allow for styling away from the face

_____ Also known as open caps

_____ Allow scalp ventilation, help prevent excess perspiration, and are extremely light and comfortable

_____ Hair fibers attached by various methods, including 100 percent hand-tied, monofilament caps (one strand of hair is attached at a time) that allow each hair to move freely for the most natural look

_____ Open framework

_____ Hair fibers attached by various methods, a combination of machine-attached wefts with hand-tied hair at the parting and crown

_____ Generally a less expensive type of wig

_____ Best for clients with extremely thin hair, or no hair at all

SHORT ANSWER

63. Are wigs a modern invention?

_____

_____

_____

64. Why do people today wear full and partial wigs?

_____

_____

_____

65. How can you demonstrate sensitivity toward clients who have experienced hair loss due to a serious illness or medical treatment such as chemotherapy?

_____

_____

_____

LABELING

66. Identify which image depicts a cap wig and which one depicts a capless wig.

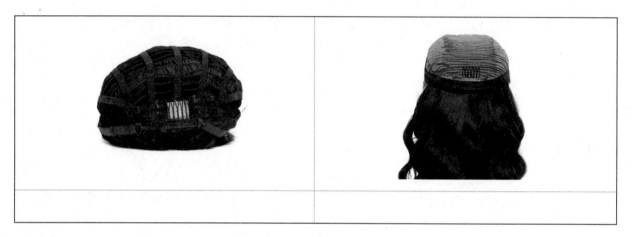

MATCHING

67. Match each type of wig construction with its features.

   a. Hand-tied

   b. Machine-made

Type of Wig Construction	Feature
_____	Made by inserting one to two strands of hair at a time into mesh foundations and knotting them with a needle
_____	Most favorable characteristic is their bounce-back quality; even after shampooing, the style returns
_____	Sewn in specific directions, offering no brushing or styling versatility
_____	Also known as hand-knotted wigs
_____	Commonly made with synthetic fibers

_____ Least expensive option

_____ Can be combed in almost any direction because the hair has
no definite direction

_____ Have a natural, realistic look and are wonderful for styling

_____ Made by feeding wefts through a sewing machine, then
stitching them together to form the wig's base and shape

_____ Most closely resemble human hair growth, with flexibility at
the roots

SHORT ANSWER

68. What are T-pins used for?

_____

_____

_____

69. Name two types of wig and hairpiece adhesives. What is a special feature of some adhesives?

_____

_____

_____

70. What salon item is used to make, service, store, and/or display a wig?

_____

_____

_____

71. If the salon permits, what item should you retail to clients who wear hair attachments or
replacements?

_____

_____

_____

72. Complete the sentences below using the words from the word bank. Each word will be used once.

    Word bank: tip, flexible, bristles, less, base, rounded, shears, plastic, length, knotting, coating, boar

    A _____ brush made from 100 _____ is the most desirable wig brush. A soft,

    pliable, _____-bristle brush with _____ tips is also acceptable. If even one

    _____ is missing, replace the brush. To avoid damaging the _____, never brush

    or comb the hair at the wig's _____.

    _____ measuring tape is used to measure clients for wigs and hairpieces or to measure a

    wig's _____ while on a wig block.

    To avoid significantly dulling your quality haircutting _____, use _____

    expensive ones specifically for wigs, add-on hair, synthetic hair, and human hair that has an

    appearance-enhancing _____.

SHORT ANSWER

73. What is the most common size of wig? How many people wear that size?

    _____

    _____

    _____

74. How can you ensure the accuracy of your measurements when using a measuring tape?

    _____

    _____

    _____

75. What are three things that should always be done at the time of purchase when selecting a wig?

    _____

    _____

    _____

76. Pair up with a classmate and take turns being the client and cosmetologist. As the cosmetologist, measure your client for a wig sizing and fill out the measurements in the table below. Then refer to the measurements given in Table 14-1 in your textbook to determine the best size wig for your client for each measurement. What would you recommend if your client is between sizes, or if certain measures match up with different sizes of wigs? As the cosmetologist, be sure to give your best recommendation to your client and explain why.

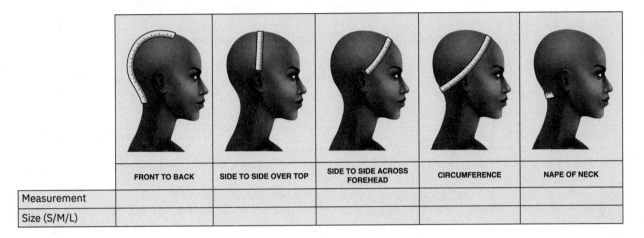

	FRONT TO BACK	SIDE TO SIDE OVER TOP	SIDE TO SIDE ACROSS FOREHEAD	CIRCUMFERENCE	NAPE OF NECK
Measurement					
Size (S/M/L)					

_____

_____

_____

77. Number the steps for placing a wig on a client's head, from 1 to 5.

	Place the wig on your client's head.
	Smooth the hairline's perimeter away from the face using a fine-tooth comb or mascara wand.
	Securely pin the client's brushed, flattened hair close to the head.
	Brush the client's natural hair straight back all around the front hairline and distribute it as evenly as possible.
	To ensure that natural hair does not show around the front hairline, apply a small amount of gel or hairspray to a fine-tooth comb or a clean, disposable mascara wand.

78. Where on the head should the wig settle overall? Where in the front? Where in the back?

_____

_____

_____

79. How can you use the wind test to check how realistic a wig is around the hairline? In what way can that help your client?

_____

_____

_____

80. What are two ways that you can assist your client when placing the wig?

_____

_____

_____

TRUE OR FALSE

Indicate whether each statement below is true or false. For any false statements, explain why they are false.

81. The more solid the wig's haircut shape, the more natural the hair will look.

T   F   _____

82. It's recommended that you follow the basic wet haircutting methods—blunt, layered, and graduated—using the same sectioning and elevations as on a real head of hair.

T   F   _____

83. For the most realistic results, cut the wig and style it while it is on the wig block.

T   F   _____

84. The goal of cutting a wig is to make it look realistic, which can be done by blunting the ends.

    T   F   _____

85. One way to achieve a more natural look in the wig is to use your fingers and palms to create less structured styles on layered hair.

    T   F   _____

REFLECTION

86. Think about your practice with wet and dry wig cutting, and review the photos you took during the procedure. Write a few sentences in which you respond to the following questions:

    • Overall, how did it go?
    • Which type of cutting did you think was easier? Why?
    • Which type turned out better (more realistic) for your "client"?
    • Did the results match the diagram you sketched for your design? If not, what could you have done differently?
    • What did you enjoy about the dry cutting? The wet cutting?

FILL IN THE BLANK

87. For each topic listed below, describe the appropriate guideline specific to caring for a wig.

TOPIC	GUIDELINES FOR WIG CARE
General handling	
Brushes and brushing	
Cleaning	
Storage	
Styling tools	

TOPIC	GUIDELINES FOR WIG CARE
Shampooing and conditioning	
Blowdrying	
Combs and combing	
Maintenance appointments	
Drying process	

88. What are three ways that you can offer to provide private wig consultations for clients who have experienced hair loss due to chemotherapy treatments for cancer?

_____

_____

_____

89. What is another term for a silicone wig? Is it actually considered a wig?

_____

_____

_____

90. What is a benefit of a silicone wig?

_____

_____

_____

91. Your text describes the Look Good Feel Better program that helps patients with cancer deal with hair loss. Visit its website and explore some of the organization's programs, volunteer information, and blog posts.

    While you're visiting the site, ask yourself how you, as a cosmetologist, might be able to participate in their programs. Is there a particular program or workshop that interests you? Did you find a helpful article or blog post? How will you share this resource with your clients who are experiencing hair loss due to illness?

    When you've finished examining the site, write a few sentences about what you found interesting or helpful. Briefly describe how you plan to apply this information in your work and, if you decided to volunteer or attend a workshop, describe what motivated you to do so. You may also find it interesting and inspiring to meet with a classmate or two and discuss your findings and impressions of the site.

Hairpieces

SHORT ANSWER

92. What is a wiglet? A bandeau? A cascade?

    _____

    _____

    _____

93. What are three other examples of fashion hairpieces?

    _____

    _____

    _____

94. What are three ways to attach fashion hairpieces?

    _____

    _____

    _____

95. List three ways that the hair can be prepared before attaching a temporary hairpiece to it.

_____

_____

_____

96. Why is an integration hairpiece not a good solution for clients with complete hair loss?

_____

_____

_____

97. What are two benefits of integration hairpieces over a wig?

_____

_____

_____

98. A client with pattern baldness comes in looking for a way to wear an authentic-looking hairpiece but is not interested in wearing a wig. What would you recommend for them and why?

_____

_____

_____

CREATE

99. Imagine that a client comes into your salon with severely thinning hair and wants to find a temporary solution for a wedding they are attending. The client wants an updo that looks like their natural hair. Thinking about the types of hairpieces (such as fashion hairpieces, integration hairpieces, and toupees), what solution would your offer your client, especially if they feel self-conscious about their hair loss or wearing a hairpiece in general?

_____

_____

_____

Once you've decided on your hairpiece of choice, find images online or in beauty magazines as inspiration for how to personalize and design a style for your client and their special occasion. Draw the design below, showing how you will integrate the client's natural hair and the hairpiece into the style. Remember, just because a client cannot have their natural hair styled alone does not mean that you need to be less creative when giving them the perfect look.

TRUE OR FALSE

Indicate whether each statement is true or false. For any false statements, explain why they are false.

100. Toupees can be applied for temporary or semipermanent use.

    T   F   _____

101. A wig specialist removes and reattaches semipermanent toupees every two to three months.

    T   F   _____

102. Quality toupees are machine-made and composed of human hair.

    T   F   _____

103. Integration hairpieces are made with hair that matches the client's existing hair color and texture.

    T   F   _____

104. Integration hairpieces add substantial density but are heavy as a result.

    T   F   _____

105. Professional toupees are custom-made hairpieces that match the balding area, the client's hair texture and surrounding thickness, and the existing hair color.

    T   F   _____

106. Use the Internet or beauty supply catalogue to identify a popular hairpiece, wig, and toupee manufacturer. Explore their offerings and use the chart provided below or by following the link to record your findings. Which products would you consider recommending to clients with thinning hair or pattern baldness? Keep this sheet with you as a reference as you complete your cosmetology degree and after your license. Once you start interacting with clients who are anxious about their thinning hair or wearing hairpieces, you can refer to a top manufacturer and recommend solutions with confidence.

+ BONUS

Visit: bonus.milady.com/cos-wb/toc

	HAIRPIECE MANUFACTURER	WIG MANUFACTURER	TOUPEE MANUFACTURER
Name of Manufacturer			
Advertising Slogan or Motto			
Range of Products			
Price Range			
Services Offered			
Training Programs			
Specialty/Area of Expertise			
Where Can You Buy Their Products?			
What Makes Them a Top Manufacturer (in your opinion)?			

DISCOVERIES AND ACCOMPLISHMENTS

In the space below, write notes about key concepts discussed in this chapter. Share your discoveries with some of the other students in your class and ask them if your notes are helpful. You may want to revise your notes based on good ideas shared by your peers.

Discoveries:

_____

_____

_____

_____

_____

_____

_____

List at least three things you have accomplished since you decided to enroll in school.

Accomplishments:

_____

_____

_____

_____

_____

_____

_____

1. An artificial head covering that consists of a network of interwoven hair fibers is called a _____.

   A) fabric wrap

   B) wig

   C) well

   D) stress strip

2. Why should cosmetologists have a thorough understanding of wigs and hair additions?

   A) The market for products and services related to supplemental hair is limited to a specific consumer group.

   B) Wigs are an important grooming aspect for those with extreme hair loss, including patients with cancer undergoing chemotherapy.

   C) Hair addition, extension, and custom wig clients are seldom committed to regular maintenance appointments.

   D) Hair additions facilitate the grow-out phase and address hair loss, generating a reduced income for stylists.

3. Which of the following questions or statements should be considered a starting point by cosmetologists when conducting a hair consultation for hair extensions?

   A) Are you planning to consult us for medical diagnosis on hair thinning or hair loss?

   B) You have a scalp disorder called scabies.

   C) Are you experiencing any hair loss?

   D) We can improve the appearance of certain scalp and hair conditions that are medical disorders.

4. When conducting a thorough hair consultation before suggesting or offering any hair extension, a cosmetologist should _____.

   A) not hesitate to offer information, ask questions, and take notes

   B) not lay out the budget required for the selected hair addition

   C) assure clients that the appearance of certain hair conditions that are medical disorders can be improved

   D) diagnose, prescribe, treat, and/or work on unhealthy hair

5. Identify a true statement about remy hair.

   A) It is the lowest quality of hair for extensions, wigs, and hairpieces.

   B) It is synthetic hair without an intact cuticle layer.

continued

C) Virgin human hair from India is the most expensive and highest quality Remy hair.

D) Most remy hair is virgin hair, meaning it was free of hair-altering chemicals at collection time.

6. In the context of hair addition and wig fibers, which of the following is an advantage of human fiber hair?

A) It does not need to be reset after shampooing.

B) It is generally more durable than synthetic hair.

C) It is less expensive than animal fibers.

D) It does not split, break, or fade in color.

7. In the context of hair addition and wig fibers, a disadvantage of synthetic fiber hair is that it _____.

A) is more expensive than human hair

B) does not accept regular hair dye

C) does not offer permanent styles

D) fades and offers a limited range of colors

8. In the context of hair addition and wig fibers, a disadvantage of animal fiber hair is that it _____.

A) does not blend well with human and synthetic hair

B) is not naturally reflective or multicolored

C) is not a stand-alone fiber

D) does not react to heat in the same way as human hair

9. The first factor to be emphasized by cosmetologists when they practice a professional approach to all hair augmentation services is _____.

A) client comfort when applying hair extensions

B) safety for the client's own hair

C) security of the hair additions so they do not fall out or slip

D) the fashion and style of the hair additions

10. When providing hair augmentation services, cosmetologists should _____.

A) stay 3 inches away from the hairline at the front, sides, and nape

B) ensure the attachment site of hair extensions is not visible through very thin hair

C) understand that straight hair appears thicker than curly hair

D) not use the braid-and-sew method to attach hair extensions

continued

11. Which of the following statements is true about the braid-and-sew hair extension method?

   A) It requires only a specialized thread and needle.

   B) It is considered a very unsafe technique.

   C) It is appropriate even for clients with extremely damaged hair.

   D) It is also known as the fusion bonding method.

12. An advantage of tape-in hair extensions is that they _____.

   A) do not cause added scalp and hair tension

   B) are not prone to shedding

   C) are invisible when hair is tightly pulled into a ponytail

   D) lie flat for a seamless and natural look and feel

13. The fusion bonding hair extension method _____.

   A) is less expensive than other hair extension methods

   B) requires a longer appointment than other hair extension methods

   C) is highly detectable, reducing styling versatility

   D) uses heavyweight bonds

14. A disadvantage of the linking hair extension method is that it _____.

   A) does not offer styling versatility

   B) is time-consuming and expensive

   C) uses an adhesive

   D) does not preserve natural hair's integrity when applied properly

15. Identify an accurate statement about cap wigs.

   A) They are also known as open caps.

   B) They are generally less expensive than capless wigs.

   C) They are made with an elasticized, mesh-fiber base to which the hair is attached.

   D) They are ineffective for clients with extremely thin hair, or no hair at all.

16. Capless wigs are _____.

   A) wigs that lack a cap

   B) hand-tied, or hand-knotted, wigs

   C) generally less expensive than cap wigs

   D) extremely heavy

continued

17. Relating to the types of wig construction, hand-tied wigs are _____.

   A) constructed by inserting one to two hair strands at a time into mesh foundations and knotting them with a needle

   B) made by feeding wefts through a sewing machine, then stitching them together to form the wig's base and shape

   C) the least expensive option for wig construction

   D) known for having an artificial, unrealistic look

18. Identify an accurate statement about machine-made wigs.

   A) They are made by inserting a hair strand into mesh foundations and knotting it with a needle.

   B) They are more expensive than hand-tied wigs.

   C) They do not have bounce-back quality, especially after shampooing and conditioning.

   D) They do not offer brushing or styling versatility.

19. Which of the following guidelines should be followed when using tools for caring for wigs and hair additions?

   A) Use good quality haircutting shears to cut a wig made of synthetic hair or human hair with an appearance-enhancing coating.

   B) Do not use T-pins to secure wigs and hairpieces to a wig block.

   C) Do not use a boar brush as a wig brush.

   D) Take care of extensions, wigs, and hairpieces by using wig-specific shampoo or gentle shampoo and light conditioner.

20. Which of the following is a wig care guideline?

   A) When using heat on human hair, set the styling tool to high.

   B) Do not blowdry a synthetic wig unless the manufacturer certifies the fibers as heat tolerant.

   C) Do not use a wide-tooth comb to comb and detangle the wig hair when damp.

   D) Shampoo frequently worn wigs and hairpieces at least twice a week.

continued

21. Identify an accurate statement about fashion hairpieces.

    A) They are typically permanent additions.

    B) They include half-wigs, wiglets, falls, bandeaus, chignons, ponytails, cascades, bangs, braids, clip-in hair wefts, fillers, and full heads of clip-in hair extensions.

    C) They are only worn by clients with pattern baldness.

    D) They are also known as integration hairpieces.

22. Integration hairpieces are _____.

    A) known for reducing hair density

    B) not suitable for severely thinning hair

    C) not suitable for complete hair loss

    D) typically heavy

23. Which of the following statements is accurate about integration hairpieces?

    A) They are generally made with hair that differs from the existing hair color and texture of the client.

    B) They typically reduce hair density.

    C) They have openings in the base through which the client's own hair is pulled, resulting in a completely natural look.

    D) They are suitable for complete hair loss.

24. Identify an accurate statement related to hairpieces.

    A) Most toupees lack a fine-net base.

    B) Integration hairpieces are suitable for complete hair loss.

    C) Professional toupees look artificial and seldom match the client's existing hair color and balding area.

    D) A wig specialist removes and reattaches semipermanent toupees every five to six weeks.

25. Which of the following statements is accurate about a toupee?

    A) Permanent toupees are generally removed and reattached by a wig specialist every five to six weeks.

    B) Toupees are least common among clients with pattern baldness.

    C) Quality toupees are made of machine-made synthetic hair.

    D) Professional toupees match the balding area, the client's hair texture and surrounding thickness, and the existing hair color.

finished!

TRACK MY PROGRESS!

Use this simple tracker to record your progress as you work through the activities in each learning objective.

COMPLETED	# OF CORRECT ANSWERS	OBJECTIVE
☐	_____/4	LO 1 - Explain why cosmetologists should study chemical texture services.
☐	_____/14	LO 2 - Define the different chemical formulations used for relaxing hair.
☐	_____/20	LO 3 - Describe hydroxide relaxers and the various types and strengths that are available to relax hair.
☐	_____/17	LO 4 - Define ammonium thioglycolate (thio) relaxers and how to use them.
☐	_____/3	LO 5 - Describe the tools and supplies that are used for relaxing hair.
☐	_____/22	LO 6 - Outline the safety guidelines and precautions for chemical relaxer services.
☐	_____/3	LO 7 - Explain how to conduct a thorough chemical relaxer consultation.
☐	_____/8	LO 8 - Safely perform virgin and retouch chemical services.
☐	_____/17	LO 9 - Define permanent waving and different types of waving solutions that are used to perform these services.
☐	_____/12	LO 10 - Explain the importance of selecting the right type of permanent wave solution for each client and processing the hair correctly.
☐	_____/10	LO 11 - Describe the tools and supplies that are used for permanent waves.
☐	_____/18	LO 12 - Describe the various permanent wave patterns, placements, and results.
☐	_____/9	LO 13 - Outline the safety guidelines and precautions for permanent wave services.
☐	_____/4	LO 14 - Explain how to conduct a thorough permanent wave consultation.
☐	_____/24	LO 15 - Safely perform permanent wave services.

Why Study Chemical Texture Services?

SHORT ANSWER

1. What are three reasons cosmetologists should study and have a thorough understanding of chemical texture services?

_____

_____

_____

2. In general, what do chemical texture services allow you to change for your clients? How does this benefit them?

_____

_____

_____

3. What are the two broad categories of texture services?

_____

_____

_____

FILL IN THE BLANK

4. Complete the chart below.

TEXTURE SERVICE	FUNCTION	WORKS BEST FOR ...
Keratin-based smoothing treatment (semipermanent)		
	Adds wave or curl to the hair; also used to loosen curls	
		Clients who want to permanently rearrange their coils to a looser curl pattern
	Removes curl or wave, leaving hair smooth or straight	

Chemical Relaxers

5. What are the two general types of chemical hair relaxers commonly used by cosmetologists?

_____

_____

_____

6. What is the main protein that makes up hair fibers?

_____

_____

_____

7. Which two types of bonds determine a person's individual hair texture and curl pattern?

_____

_____

_____

8. Which type of bond breaks when the hair is wet and then naturally reforms as the hair dries?

_____

_____

_____

9. Which type of bond must be broken by chemical hair relaxers (not water) to create a permanent change in the hair?

_____

_____

_____

10. Describe in general terms how chemical hair relaxers work to create a permanent change in the hair.

_____

_____

_____

Indicate whether each statement below is true or false. For any false statements, explain why they are false.

11. Coarse, highly textured hair with a strong, compact cuticle layer requires a high-acid chemical solution.

    T   F   _____

12. Porous, damaged, or chemically treated hair requires a less alkaline solution.

    T   F   _____

13. On a pH scale, relaxers are above 7 pH.

    T   F   _____

14. The pH of hair is 7 (neutral).

    T   F   _____

15. When a chemical relaxer is applied to hair, it can increase the hair's acidity up to pH 14.

    T   F   _____

LABELING

16. Using the word bank, indicate on the pH scale where certain hair types, chemical relaxers, and characteristics fall. Neutral pH (7) has been provided for you.

    Word bank: a. Coarse hair   c. Porous hair   e. Hair and scalp   g. Thio relaxer
                   b. Acidic   d. Alkaline   f. Hydroxide relaxer

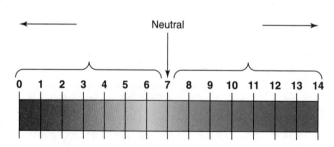

17. Three different clients come into your salon, each asking for a chemical relaxer treatment on their hair. The first client has very coily, highly textured hair, and is looking for a smooth, straight look. The second client wants to keep some texture in their hair and has never tried a relaxer treatment before. The third client has looser curls and is concerned about the scalp irritation they received from a previous relaxer treatment but also wants to make sure their hair stays straight. Based on Table 15-1 in your textbook, which type of relaxer would you recommend for each client? Name the active ingredient for each type of relaxer.

Client 1: _____

Client 2: _____

Client 3: _____

18. A client comes into your salon with coarse, highly textured hair and wants the least damaging relaxer treatment. Having done some research on the Internet, your client asks for an ammonium sulfite, low-pH relaxer. Considering both your client's hair type and the professional products at the salon, what would you tell your client about the service they requested?

_____

_____

_____

Hydroxide Relaxers

Indicate whether each statement below is true or false. For any false statements, explain why they are false.

19. Sodium hydroxide, potassium hydroxide, lithium hydroxide, and guanidine hydroxide are all types of hydroxide relaxers that can shrink the hair down to half its normal diameter.

   T   F   _____

20. Hydroxide ions, the active ingredient in all hydroxide relaxers, are very strong alkalis with pH 13.

   T   F   _____

21. Hydroxide relaxers break disulfide bonds the same way as the reduction reaction of thio-based relaxers.

   T   F   _____

22. The disulfide bonds broken by hydroxide relaxers can never be reformed.

    T   F   _____

23. In lanthionization, the process by which hydroxide relaxers permanently straighten hair, the relaxers remove one of the two bonded sulfur atoms from a disulfide bond and convert it into a lanthionine bond.

    T   F   _____

SHORT ANSWER

24. What is another term for sodium hydroxide relaxers?

    _____

    _____

    _____

25. What should you do if you notice pronounced redness or irritation on the client's skin or scalp during a lye relaxer treatment?

    _____

    _____

    _____

MATCHING

26. Match the type of relaxer—lye or no-lye—with its description.

    a. No-lye   b. Lye

    No-Lye or Lye?   **Description**

    _____ Causes the hair to feel and look dry after repeated usage

    _____ Uses sodium hydroxide

    _____ Chosen by most stylists for use in the salon

    _____ Will not penetrate the residue caused by calcium buildup

    _____ Popular for clients when relaxing their hair at home

_____ Excellent choice for clients with sensitive scalps

_____ Uses lithium hydroxide and potassium hydroxide

_____ Causes a line of demarcation if used on clients who use another relaxer at home

_____ Leaves a buildup of calcium residue

_____ Causes the hair to soften and swell, leaving soft, pliable hair

_____ Use this type of relaxer on a client who is using a no-lye relaxer at home

SHORT ANSWER

27. What is the purpose of base cream? What is its texture?

_____

_____

_____

28. Which type of relaxer is formulated as either base or no base?

_____

_____

_____

29. Which type of relaxer—base or no base—includes a protective base in it that melts at body temperature, causing it to settle on the scalp?

_____

_____

_____

30. When using a no-base relaxer, where else should you apply base cream? What if your client has a sensitive scalp?

_____

_____

_____

31. What will happen if the base cream contacts the hair you are relaxing?

_____

_____

_____

32. Do metal hydroxide relaxers require mixing before application?

_____

_____

_____

MATCHING

33. Match each hydroxide relaxer strength (concentration of hydroxide) with its description. Each strength will be used twice.

a. Mild   b. Regular   c. Super

**Hydroxide
Relaxer Strength   Description**

_____ Used for straightening coarse, highly textured hair

_____ Formulated for fragile hair (needs to be handled with care)

_____ Most commonly used strength

_____ Formulated for fine hair (fewer disulfide bonds to break) and color-treated hair (porous) hair

_____ Formulated for healthy hair with wavy to coily textures

_____ Formulated for maximum concentration

SHORT ANSWER

34. Why should you do a strand test before a hydroxide relaxer service?

_____

_____

_____

35. What steps should you take after applying relaxer to a client's hair and before placing that client under a hooded dryer? Why?

_____

_____

_____

36. What happens when hair is 100 percent relaxed? What is the maximum percentage that hair can be safely relaxed?

_____

_____

_____

37. When performing a relaxer touch-up on a client's new growth area, what should you do to the rest of the hair?

_____

_____

_____

SEQUENCE

38. Number the steps of the process for neutralizing a hydroxide relaxer application, from 1 to 5.

_____ Rinse the hair thoroughly with warm (not hot) water.

_____ Repeat application of the neutralizing shampoo multiple times to thoroughly remove all relaxer residue.

_____ Sufficiently process the hydroxide hair relaxer for your client.

_____ If desired, apply a normalizing lotion to lower the hair and scalp's pH level.

_____ Perform the neutralization step (called hydroxide neutralization), which is an acid–alkali neutralization reaction achieved by applying a neutralizing (acid-balanced) shampoo.

Thio Relaxers

Indicate whether each statement below is true or false. For any false statements, explain why they are false.

39. Thio relaxers use a two-part process, reduction and oxidation, to break the disulfide bonds in the hair and reform them to a more relaxed texture.

    T   F   _____

40. Potassium thioglycolate, or PTG, is the active ingredient in thio relaxers.

    T   F   _____

41. Viscosity refers to the concentration of a thio relaxer.

    T   F   _____

42. Thio relaxers are best for clients who wants to keep some texture in their hair, while hydroxide relaxers are better if a client desires completely straightened hair.

    T   F   _____

SEQUENCE

43. Number the steps of the process for reduction and oxidation of thio relaxers, 1 through 6.

    _____ Thio solution breaks the disulfide bond by adding a hydrogen atom to each of its sulfur atoms.

    _____ The sulfur atoms attach to the hydrogen atom, breaking their attachment to each other.

    _____ The disulfide bonds are rebuilt by removing the hydrogen atoms added by the thio solution.

    _____ The disulfide bonds join the sulfur atoms in two adjacent polypeptide chains.

    _____ A neutralizer, such as hydrogen peroxide, starts the oxidation process.

    _____ The neutralizer rebonds the hair and locks the new shape into place.

44. What must you assess during the client consultation for relaxer services? Why?

_____

_____

_____

45. What is the pH of water (H_2O)? Does it play a role in neutralization?

_____

_____

_____

46. What are three risks of being distracted or trying to multitask while performing relaxer services?

_____

_____

_____

47. What will happen if you apply thio relaxer to hair that has been treated with a hydroxide relaxer?

_____

_____

_____

TRUE OR FALSE

Indicate whether each statement below is true or false. For any false statements, explain why they are false.

48. Ammonium sulfate, ammonium sulfite, and ammonium bisulfite are sometimes used as the active ingredient in low-pH relaxers.

    T   F   _____

49. Low-pH relaxers are not recommended for use on color-treated hair.

    T   F   _____

50. Ammonium sulfate, sulfite, and bisulfite relaxers are compatible with hydroxide relaxers.

    T   F   _____

51. The active ingredients ammonium sulfate, sulfite, and bisulfite are all compatible with ATG relaxers.

    T   F   _____

SHORT ANSWER

52. Describe the results of using keratin-based smoothing treatments.

_____

_____

_____

53. How long do keratin-based smoothing treatments last?

_____

_____

_____

54. What is the main problem with the active ingredients used in most keratin smoothers, according to which two government regulatory bodies?

_____

_____

_____

55. Your text recommends visiting two websites to investigate more about keratin-based smoothing treatments and their ingredients, including www.cancer.gov and www.osha.gov/formaldehyde /hazards Explore them and take some notes about your findings. Then answer the following questions:

- According to the websites you visited, what are four or five health risks associated with keratin smoothing treatments (for either cosmetologists or clients)?
- What are the recommended safety precautions for offering keratin smoothing treatments? In what ways do they differ from other general precautions you would take when performing relaxer services?
- What are you required to tell clients who request these treatments?
- Will you offer keratin smoothing treatments to your clients? Why or why not?

Relaxer Tools and Supplies

DOS AND DON'TS

56. For each statement related to using the tools and supplies for relaxer services, indicate whether it is something you should do (Do) or something you should not do (Don't).

Do or Don't?	When Using Tools and Supplies for Relaxer Services
_____	Allow the teeth of a wide-tooth comb to make contact with the scalp
_____	Follow the manufacturer's directions for base creams
_____	Comb relaxer through the hair
_____	Use an applicator brush, hard rubber tail comb, or styling comb to clear the relaxer with the back or tail of the comb to test the hair relaxation progress
_____	Use a wide-tooth comb to spread the conditioner after removing the relaxer
_____	Use metal clips when working with the relaxer
_____	Use a comb to section the hair at the scalp
_____	Apply a base cream, when using milder strength and no-lye relaxers, to the exterior hairline area only
_____	Apply a base cream, when using professional strength products, to the front and back hairline (exterior), inside of the head form (interior), and ears

57. Match each tool or supply used in relaxer services with its description.

a. Applicator brush, tail comb, or styling combs
b. Base cream
c. Chemical cape

d. Conditioner
e. Disposable gloves
f. Neck strips
g. Plastic clips

h. Plastic/glass bowl
i. Timer
j. Towels
k. Wide-tooth comb

Relaxer Tool or Supply   **Description**

_____ Use to detangle and smooth the hair without pulling prior to the service

_____ Use to protect your client and when double-draping

_____ Use to track the total processing time and processing steps

_____ Must be worn to protect your hands from skin damage, chemical absorption, and possible contact dermatitis

_____ Use after removing the relaxer from the hair; the type will be based on your client's hair condition

_____ Use to apply the relaxer

_____ Use to dispense and hold the relaxer

_____ Use for added skin protection around the hairline, the nape, and the top and back of the ears; also use on the scalp for sensitive skin

_____ Must be used to protect your client from direct contact with the cape

_____ Use to protect your client throughout the relaxer service

_____ Use to keep the hair sectioned

RESEARCH

58. Use the Internet or beauty supply catalogues, or visit a drug store or beauty supply store, to investigate base and no-base relaxers—specifically, you will determine what the individual manufacturers' directions are for using a base cream with the products you identify.

Identify two "base relaxers" and two "no-base relaxers." Read about the products and either use the table or follow the link below to access a PDF chart that you can use to record your findings.

+ BONUS

Visit: bonus.milady.com/cos-wb/toc

FEATURES	BASE RELAXER #1	BASE RELAXER #2	NO-BASE RELAXER #1	NO-BASE RELAXER #2
Name/Brand				
Source (Store/Website)				
Cost/Size				
Advertised Benefits				
Manufacturers' Directions for Using Base Cream with the Product				
Warnings/Precautions				
Offers a "Kit" or "Set"? (if so, list the contents)				
Professional or Home Use?				

Chemical Relaxer Safety Guidelines

SHORT ANSWER

59. List the five ways that stylists can minimize risks before they perform chemical texture services.

_____

_____

_____

60. What information should you record about the chemical services you perform for your clients?

_____

_____

_____

61. If skin redness, itching, or similar irritation occurs after performing a patch test for chemical texture services, what does this tell you? Can you perform the chemical service for your client?

_____

_____

_____

62. If a client experiences no reaction from the patch test, do you need to note that on the client's service record card?

_____

_____

_____

63. Number the steps for a patch test, from 1 to 7.

_____ Check for scalp redness, hair elasticity, and the smoothness of all three strands. If redness or irritation is present, or the hair appears damaged, do not perform the service.

_____ Separate a strand in each area.

_____ Run a neutralizing shampoo (hydroxide relaxer) or neutralizer (thio relaxer) through the test strands. Rinse thoroughly.

_____ Record the results on the service record card.

_____ Apply the relaxer at the base of each test strand, allowing it to make contact with the scalp.

_____ Select three test areas on the head.

_____ Leave the relaxer on the scalp for three minutes. Examine the skin. If there is no skin redness, apply the relaxer to each entire strand and smooth the test areas with the back of a comb or the handle of a brush applicator. Keep the relaxer on the scalp for two additional minutes.

64. What is a possible consequence of failing to conduct a metallic salts test on a client's hair before performing chemical texture services?

_____

_____

_____

65. Describe the solution used to test hair strands for metallic salts.

_____

_____

_____

66. How many hair strands should you immerse in the metallic salts test solution? For how long?

_____

_____

_____

67. After conducting the metallic salts test, what does it mean if the hair strands lightened slightly?

_____

_____

_____

68. What are three potential outcomes of a metallic salts test that would indicate you should not proceed with the chemical texture service?

_____

_____

_____

69. What two things does the hair analysis tell you about the relaxer that should be used on the client's hair?

_____

_____

_____

70. At what point should you evaluate the scalp's condition when a client is requesting chemical texture services?

_____

_____

_____

71. To be considered healthy, what five characteristics should be absent from the scalp?

_____

_____

_____

72. For each statement about safety tips and guidelines for performing chemical relaxer services, indicate whether it is something you should do (Do) or something you should not do (Don't).

Do or Don't?	Safety Tips and Guidelines for Performing Chemical Relaxer Services
_____	Apply relaxer to hair that has not been shampooed for one week
_____	Perform a relaxer service if the hair has been treated with henna
_____	Use only plastic or glass bowls and plastic clips when relaxing hair
_____	Trim the ends of the hair
_____	Decline a relaxer service if the hair has been treated with metallic dyes, which are chemically incompatible with relaxers
_____	Establish a treatment program to restore the hair's strength and elasticity before scheduling a relaxer service
_____	Change the client's neck strip and towel when they become wet or come in contact with the relaxer solution
_____	Overlap base cream when applying it to hair that will be relaxed
_____	Wear protective gloves when performing every relaxer service
_____	Relax lightened (bleached) hair
_____	Apply a hydroxide relaxer to hair that has been relaxed with a thio relaxer and vice versa
_____	Apply a relaxer formulation appropriate for the client's hair texture and condition
_____	Use metal bowls or clips when relaxing hair
_____	Relax hair to the point that it is completely straight
_____	Use your gloved fingers to smooth the relaxer through the hair

_____ Follow manufacturer and instructor directions for rinsing out the relaxer and neutralizer

_____ Use the teeth of a comb to smooth relaxer through the hair

_____ Use two different relaxer types

_____ Apply to the midshafts, then the root area, then the hairline, and finally the ends when performing a virgin relaxer

_____ Touch the scalp when separating the hair in sections

_____ Use your fingers, the tail of a tail comb, or an applicator brush to separate the hair in sections

_____ Relax hair up to 75 percent of its original wave

_____ Perform both a permanent or demipermanent haircolor service and a relaxer service in the same day

_____ Rinse the relaxer and neutralizer out of the hair with warm water

_____ Rinse with cool water if the scalp appears irritated

_____ Flush the client's eye with cool water if the relaxer or neutralizer solution gets in it; if irritation persists, recommend that the client seek medical attention

_____ Keep partially used relaxer products after the service

_____ Apply a semipermanent haircolor the same day as the relaxer service if desired

_____ Perform a lightener (bleach) service on relaxed hair

TRUE OR FALSE

Indicate whether each statement below is true or false. For any false statements, explain why they are false.

73. Hair becomes rough, dull, and prone to breakage when it has a damaged cuticle.

    T   F   _____

74. Although healthy, a cuticle will not be able to protect the hair from damage.

    T   F   _____

75. Even though hair may have a very high level of porosity, it is still able to safely absorb chemical texture services.

T   F   _____

76. Porosity is the hair's ability to stretch and return to its original length without breaking.

T   F   _____

77. The degree of the hair's elasticity indicates the strength of the side bonds in the cortex.

T   F   _____

78. Sodium hydroxide and thio relaxers are chemically incompatible and can cause severe damage—even hair loss—when mixed or overlaid on the hair.

T   F   _____

SEQUENCE

79. Number the steps for conducting the relaxer strand test, from 1 to 5.

_____ Separate each strand from the rest of the hair, apply the relaxer as directed, and monitor the relaxation process.

_____ Check the test strands at five-minute intervals until the process is complete.

_____ Midway through the recommended processing time, lift each test strand, gently stretch and release the strand, and observe the curl reversion. (You can also do this step by using the back of a comb to remove the relaxer and then observe the curl reversion.)

_____ Select a strand at the back, and one on each side of the head.

_____ Ask yourself: Is the hair halfway there? Almost there?

REFLECTION

80. Many types of tests and analyses should be conducted when preparing to perform a chemical relaxer service, and it is helpful to create a chart for quick reference. Follow the link below to complete a chart that will help you organize and summarize the important points of each kind of test. Keep the completed chart with you to ensure you are giving every client excellent service.

+ BONUS

Visit: bonus.milady.com/cos-wb/toc

PRE-SERVICE RELAXER TEST	PURPOSE OF TEST	WHEN TO PERFORM	REQUIRED MATERIALS	TIME NEEDED	DECLINE SERVICE IF ...
Patch test					
Strand or skin sensitivity test					
Metallic salts test					
Hair analysis					
Scalp analysis					
Relaxer strand test					

Chemical Relaxer Consultation

81. Partner with a classmate to practice your consultation technique for a client who is requesting a chemical relaxer service. You will take turns playing the roles of stylist and client, making sure to ask the questions specific to chemical relaxer services in your text. Before you meet for this activity, independently prepare for each role as described below. Afterward, work with your classmate on what you each did well, and think about ways to make sure a consultation goes even better the next time.

    As the stylist:

    - Familiarize yourself with the client consultation questions for chemical relaxer services

    - Imagine how you would ask the questions in your own words; keep a list handy and practice

    - Prepare responses to the client's possible answers—this includes being able to explain why you're asking the question or even declining the service, as well as any follow-up comments or questions that might help facilitate the consultation

    As the client:

    - Prepare responses to the stylist's consultation questions about a proposed chemical relaxer treatment for you—with real or fictional/creative responses, including how you might respond to the stylist declining services for you

SHORT ANSWER

82. What are the three main goals of conducting a client consultation for chemical relaxer services?

    _____

    _____

    _____

83. In addition to the client intake form, what else should you have ready when you consult with your client? Why?

_____

_____

_____

Relaxer Application

84. Do the requirement to follow safety guidelines and the steps outlined in this section apply to both virgin and retouch relaxer services?

_____

_____

_____

85. What characteristic of your client's hair will determine the strength of the chemical relaxer solution?

_____

_____

_____

86. What characteristic of your client's hair will help you determine the application of the chemical relaxer and the length of time required for application and processing?

_____

_____

_____

87. Why is it important to determine your client's wave pattern?

_____

_____

_____

MATCHING

88. Match each type of relaxer with the description of its neutralizing process and guidelines. Both types might apply to the same description.

a. Hydroxide relaxer   b. Thio relaxer

Type of Relaxer   **Description of Neutralizing Process and Guidelines**

_____ Requires multiple applications of a neutralizing shampoo

_____ When neutralizing this type of relaxer, avoid leaving too much moisture in the hair before working the neutralizer through the hair with your fingers to ensure even saturation

_____ When neutralizing this type of relaxer, you have the option of first applying a normalizing lotion to lower the pH

_____ Follow the manufacturer's guidelines and your instructor's directions regarding neutralizing the hair

_____ When neutralizing this type of relaxer, first gently blot the hair until it is damp

SEQUENCE

89. Number the steps of the procedure for performing a virgin relaxer application, from 1 to 23. Some steps have been numbered for you.

_____ Perform the strand test following manufacturer's guidelines. Proceed with the application if the strand test results are favorable.

_____ Apply to porous ends in back right quadrant. Continue applying to porous ends in the back left, front right, and front left quadrants.

_____ Thoroughly rinse the relaxed hair with warm water and blot excess water from the hair.

_____6_____ Put on gloves.

_____ Drape the client for a chemical service.

_____ Dispense a small amount of relaxer into an applicator bowl.

_____ Smooth each subsection using the back of a hard rubber comb, tail of a comb, applicator brush, or your gloved fingers to smooth each subsection.

_____ Section hair into four quadrants. Clip and secure the sections out of the way.

_____ If the hair fails the patch test or any of the tests conducted during the hair and scalp analysis, decline to perform the service.

_____ Apply barrier cream around hairline and over the ears according to manufacturer's directions.

_____ Thoroughly rinse the neutralized hair.

_____ Perform the hair and scalp analysis.

____17____ Check for even results according to timing determined by preliminary strand test.

_____ Condition the hair according to manufacturer's directions.

_____ Dispense relaxer into applicator bowl.

_____ Follow the neutralizing steps for either hydroxide relaxer or thio relaxer.

_____ If there is any relaxer remaining in the hair, repeat the shampooing steps as needed until all product is removed from the hair.

_____ Apply to midshaft in back right quadrant. Continue applying to midshaft in back left, front right, and front left quadrants.

_____ Perform patch test 24 to 48 hours before relaxer appointment.

_____ Dry the scalp. (Thio relaxers may or may not recommend that hair, but not the scalp, be shampooed before the service.)

_____ Apply to scalp in back right quadrant. Continue applying to scalp in back left, front right, and front left quadrants.

____12____ Use the information gathered during the consultation to determine where to begin the application of the relaxer service and determine the timing.

_____ Check the hair for residual relaxer, using all of your senses.

90. Complete the sentences below using words from the word bank. Some words will be used more than once, and others will not be used.

   Word bank: 1.25, overprocessing, underprocessing, 0.25, scalp, nape, retouch, last, first, growth, chemical, 0.6, new, old, 0.5

   For hair that has received a _____ relaxer service, use a relaxer _____

   application. This type of application includes only the _____ growth. Start the

   _____ relaxer application _____ to _____ inch (_____

   to _____ centimeters) away from the _____. To avoid _____ and

   _____ irritation, apply the relaxer closest to the scalp during the _____ few

   minutes of processing.

REFLECTION

91. Now that you've practiced the procedures for virgin and retouch relaxer applications, consider what you knew about these services before you began this section compared to what you've studied. Write a few sentences in which you reflect on and answer the following questions:

   • Can you picture yourself performing the relaxer application procedures confidently during your examination?

   • Which relaxer application steps or techniques do you excel at?

   • Are there relaxer application steps, tests, or techniques that you're uncertain about?

   • During your examination, how do you plan to demonstrate your thorough understanding of the safety precautions and guidelines that are required for relaxer procedures?

   • Overall, how can you make your relaxer application flawless for the examination?

   When you're finished, meet with a classmate and discuss your responses. As you do so, look for opportunities to fill in each other's gaps and help each other master the relaxer application techniques and specifics.

Permanent Waving

92. Briefly describe what permanent waving is. What is another term for permanent waving?

_____

_____

_____

93. What are the two perm solution categories? How are they similar to each other?

_____

_____

_____

94. Which perm solution category is stronger, therefore making it more suitable for coarse and moisture-resistant hair? What is its active ingredient?

_____

_____

_____

95. Which perm solution category is more ideal for fine, color-treated, and fragile hair? What is its common active ingredient?

_____

_____

_____

96. Of the two perm solution categories, which one contains the same active ingredient as thio relaxers? How does it differ when it's in a perm solution?

_____

_____

_____

97. Match each perm wave type with its features and descriptions. More than one type might have the same feature or match a description.

a. Alkaline   c. Acid-balanced   e. Low-pH
b. True acid   d. Ammonia-free

Type of
Permanent Wave   **Features and Descriptions**

_____ Recommended for coarse, thick, or nonporous hair types

_____ Process with heat and process more slowly than alkaline waves

_____ pH 9.0–9.6

_____ Produce firmer curls than true acid waves; recommended for porous or damaged hair types

_____ pH 6.5–7.0

_____ pH 7.0–9.6

_____ Active ingredient: glyceryl monothioglycolate (GMTG)

_____ Recommended for porous to moisture-balanced hair types

_____ pH 4.5–7.0

_____ Active ingredient: ammonium thioglycolate (ATG)

_____ Active ingredients: ammonium sulfate, ammonium sulfite, and ammonium bisulfite

_____ pH 7.0

_____ Active ingredient: aminomethylpropanol (AMP) and monoethanolamine (MEA)

_____ Process without heat

_____ Process does not require a hair dryer's heat

_____ Does not provide a firm curl on coarse hair; recommended for moisture-balanced, fine, or damaged hair types

_____ Does not produce as firm a curl as alkaline waves do; recommended for extremely porous or very damaged hair types

Indicate whether the statements below are true or false. For any false statements, explain why they are false.

98. The perm solution's strength is primarily determined by the reducing agent's concentration and the alkalinity degree, which temporarily alter the hair.

    T F _____

99. Most acid waves also contain ATG, just like an alkaline wave.

    T F _____

100. Acidity increases as alkalinity decreases.

    T F _____

101. A true acid wave, having a pH below 7.0 (which is neutral on the pH scale), will cause hair to shrink because pH 5.0 for hair is considered neutral.

    T F _____

102. Although acid waves' low pH seem ideal, repeated exposure to GMTG is known to cause allergic reactions and skin sensitivities in hair stylists and clients.

    T F _____

103. An exothermic chemical reaction absorbs heat from its surroundings, while an endothermic chemical reaction produces heat.

    T F _____

104. Ammonia-free means damage-free.

    T F _____

105. Thio substitutes (such as cysteamine or mercaptamine) are not technically ATG, but they are still thio compounds.

    T F _____

106. Ammonium sulfate, ammonium sulfite, and ammonium bisulfite are ATG alternatives. As a group, they are known as ammonia-free waves.

    T F _____

107. Accidentally mixing the activator tube's contents with the neutralizer instead of the perm solution will cause a violent chemical reaction that can cause injury, especially to the eyes.

    T F _____

108. Your text mentions that permanent wave solutions' ingredients, strength, and pH differ among manufacturers and vary considerably, even within the same category. As a result, it recommends that you always check the manufacturer's instructions and the product's Safety Data Sheet (SDS) for accurate, detailed information. For this activity, select two different types of perm solutions and locate the SDS for each one. Examine the package and the SDS. Then, use the chart below or follow the link to a PDF that you will use to record your findings and answer the following questions:

1. How did the advertised features and information from the SDS for each perm solution compare to the information listed in Table 15-2 of your text?

2. In what ways was the information listed in the SDS the same or different for each perm solution you examined?

3. Did you find the SDSs helpful?

+ BONUS

Visit: bonus.milady.com/cos-wb/toc

FEATURES	PERM SOLUTION #1	PERM SOLUTION #2
Name/Brand		
Advertised Features		
Type of Hair Intended For		
Contents of Package		
Manufacturer's Directions for Use		
Safety Guidelines on Package		
Safety Guidelines on SDS		
pH Level		
Active Ingredient		

Perm Selection and Processing

SHORT ANSWER

109. Is there a difference between hair that has been treated with a semipermanent color and permanent "color-treated" hair, in terms of perm solutions?

_____

_____

_____

110. What are three possible consequences of performing a perm service on lightened (bleached) hair?

_____

_____

_____

111. What should you do when a client requests a perm on their lightened hair?

_____

_____

_____

112. How should you apply perm solution to coarse hair? Why?

_____

_____

_____

FILL IN THE BLANK

113. Complete the sentences below using words from the word bank. Some words will be used more than once, and others will not be used.

   Word bank: underprocessed, strength, 30, coarse, smell, overprocessed, hydrogen, pH, 15, fine, coarse, thick, strong, weak, concentration, disulfide, 10, 5

   A permanent wave solution's _____ is based on its reducing agent's _____.

   A _____ solution, which releases many _____ atoms, may be perfect for

   _____ hair but too harsh and damaging for _____ hair. If a mild perm solution

   is used on _____ hair, there may not be enough _____ ions to break the

   necessary number of _____ bonds, no matter how long the perm is processed. If the

   hair is _____ after 10 minutes, a stronger solution should have been used. If your client's

   hair is _____, it probably happened within the first 5 to _____ minutes, and a

   weaker perm solution should have been used.

Indicate whether these statements are true or false. For any false statements, explain why they are false.

114. Properly processed perms should break and rebuild approximately 10 percent of the hair's disulfide bonds.

    T   F   _____

115. A thorough saturation with a stronger (more alkaline) solution will break more disulfide bonds, which automatically translates into more curl.

    T   F   _____

116. Underprocessed hair is the opposite of overprocessed hair.

    T   F   _____

117. Hair is considered underprocessed if too many disulfide bonds are broken, resulting in insufficiently softened hair that typically has a very weak curl or is even straight.

    T   F   _____

118. If the hair is underprocessed, further processing will make it curlier.

    T   F   _____

119. If hair is overprocessed, further processing will make it straighter and incur even more damage.

    T   F   _____

DRAW

120. In the boxes below, draw two pictures: one that shows overprocessed hair and one that shows underprocessed hair. Indicate the location of the hair ends and scalp in your drawings.

Overprocessed		Underprocessed	

Permanent Wave Tools and Supplies

121. What is the most common type of perm rod?

_____

_____

_____

122. What does the perm rod's size determine? What does the perm rod's shape determine?

_____

_____

_____

123. Which two types of rods come in different lengths to accommodate different sections of the head? Provide an example of how this can be beneficial.

_____

_____

_____

124. What are end papers? What are two other terms for them?

_____

_____

_____

125. What are the three functions of end papers?

_____

_____

_____

126. Complete the chart below by filling in the tool or supply used in the permanent waving service or its description.

Tool or Supply Used for Permanent Waving	Description
_____	Apply around the client's hairline to keep the permanent solution from dripping down the client's face
Tail comb	_____
Roller picks	_____
_____	Must be worn to protect your hands from skin damage, chemical absorption, and possible development of contact dermatitis
_____	Use to track the total processing time and processing steps
_____	Use to protect your client and when double-draping
Neck strips	_____
Plastic tail comb	_____
_____	Use to protect your client throughout the perm service
_____	Some manufacturers recommend applying this after rinsing out the perm solution and before applying the neutralizer
_____	Use if the perm manufacturer indicates that it is necessary before the service; be sure to avoid irritating the client's scalp
Protective barrier cream	_____
_____	Use the appropriate size and shape of this as determined by your client's final desired curl
Conditioner	_____
_____	To prevent the neutralizing solution from running onto the client's shoulders and back, or dripping onto the floor, use this to capture the solution
Spray bottle	_____
_____	These are necessary to control the hair's ends when winding the hair on the perm rods
Plastic clips	_____

127. Match each type of perm rod with its description. All perm rod types will be used at least twice.

    a. Concave   c. Soft bender
    b. Straight   d. Loop

Type of Perm Rod   **Description**

_____ Produce a tighter curl on the curl's center, and a looser curl on the strand's sides

_____ Soft foam rods that have a flexible wire inside that allows them to bend into almost any shape

_____ Produce a uniform curl shape along the strand's entire width

_____ Rod is secured by fastening the ends together after the hair has been wrapped

_____ Recommended when clients want a hybrid combination of soft waves and curls for volume, texture, and beach waves

_____ Have a smaller diameter in the center, increasing to a larger diameter on the ends

_____ Also known as a circle rod

_____ Usually about 12 inches (30.5 centimeters) long with a uniform diameter along the rod's entire length

_____ Equal in diameter along their entire length or curling area

128. Identify each type of rod depicted below.

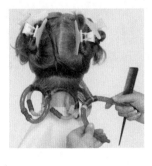 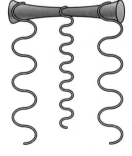 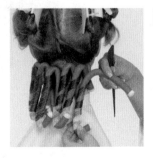 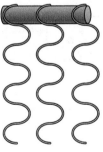

_____   _____   _____   _____

129. Match each type of end paper wrap with its description. Each type of wrap will be used at least once.

    a. Double flat wrap   b. Single flat wrap   c. Bookend wrap

Type of End Wrap Description

_____ Similar to the double flat wrap but uses only one end paper placed over the top of the base panel of hair

_____ Uses one end paper folded in half over the hair ends

_____ One end paper placed under and another placed over the hair's base panel (subsection) that's being wrapped; both papers extend past the hair ends

_____ Eliminates excess paper and can be used with short rods or very short hair lengths

_____ Provides the most control over the hair ends and helps keep them evenly distributed over the rod's entire length

_____ When using this wrap, avoid placing the hair in the paper's fold to give hair room to swell

130. Label each type of end paper wrap depicted below.

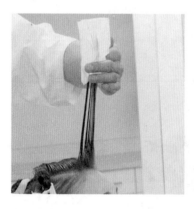 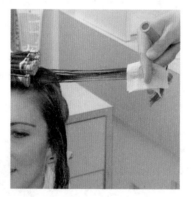 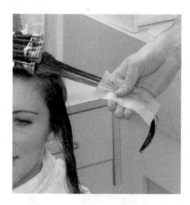

_____   _____   _____

Permanent Wave Designs

131. How do you start each perm wrap?

_____

_____

_____

132. What is a base section? How many rods are normally placed in a base section?

_____

_____

_____

133. What should you do with panels that you are not working on? Why?

_____

_____

_____

134. What is the best comb to use for perm panels and base sections? How is it used?

_____

_____

_____

135. What are three possible outcomes of wrapping the hair with too much tension? What is the ideal tension when wrapping for perms?

_____

_____

_____

136. Match each type of base placement used for perm rods with its description. Each type will be used at least twice.

    a. On-base placement   b. Half off-base placement   c. Off-base placement

**Type of Placement
for Perm Rods**   **Description**

_____ This placement minimizes stress and tension on the hair.

_____ Caution should be used with this type of placement because the additional stress and tension can break the hair.

_____ This type of base placement creates the least amount of volume and results in a curl pattern that begins farthest away from the scalp.

_____ Hair is wrapped 45 degrees beyond perpendicular to its base section, and the rod is positioned on its base

_____ This type of placement may result in greater volume at the scalp area, but any increase in volume will be lost as soon as the hair begins to grow.

_____ Hair is wrapped at 45 degrees below the base section's center.

_____ Hair is wrapped at a 90-degree angle to its base section.

137. Match each wrapping technique with its description. Each type will be used at least three times.

    a. Croquignole   b. Spiral

**Wrapping
Technique**   **Description**

_____ Hair is wrapped around the rod, with each new layer of hair on top of the previous layer, increasing the curl's size (diameter) with each new overlapping layer

_____ Wraps the hair around the rods vertically until it fills each rod's length like stripes on a candy cane

_____ Wraps the hair from the ends toward the scalp in overlapping concentric layers

_____ Causes the curl's size (diameter) to remain constant along the strand's entire length and produces a uniform curl from the scalp to the ends

_____ When wrapping rods using this technique, the hair might partially overlap the preceding layers

_____ Longer, thicker hair increases the effects of this technique

_____ Produces a tighter curl at the ends and a larger curl at the scalp

138. What does base direction refer to in terms of the rod position?

_____

_____

_____

139. What does base direction refer to in terms of wrapping the hair?

_____

_____

_____

140. In which direction should the hair be wrapped to minimize the amount of stress to the hair and result in higher quality curls?

_____

_____

_____

141. Label the base direction for each wrap depicted below.

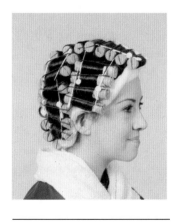

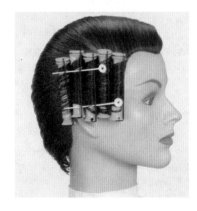

_____   _____

142. Match each wrapping pattern with its description. Each wrapping pattern will be used at least three times.

   a. Basic wrap
   b. Bricklay wrap

   c. Spiral wrap
   d. Double-rod wrap

Wrapping Pattern   **Description**

_____ All rods within panel move in the same direction and are positioned on equal-sized bases

_____ Useful for extra-long hair

_____ Produces a uniform curl from scalp to end, with the permed hair naturally falling in ringlets or corkscrew curls

_____ Also known as a straight set wrap

_____ Uses the spiral wrap technique in which hair is wrapped in vertical, or near-vertical, sections

_____ Base sections offset from each other row by row, to prevent noticeable splits and blend the hair's flow

_____ Hair is wrapped on one rod from the scalp to midway down the hair shaft, and another rod is used to wrap the remaining hair in the same direction

_____ Different patterns of this technique use different starting points (front hairline, occipital area, or crown) that affect the hair's directional flow

_____ All base sections are horizontal and are the same length and width as the perm rod

_____ Also known as a piggyback wrap

_____ Longer hair (past the shoulder) benefits most from this effect

_____ Allows for more even curl from root to end in extra-long hair and better processing solution penetration

_____ Can be used with various combinations of panels, base sections, and directions; wrapping techniques; and perm rod placements

143. How can you protect the hair outside the perm section when performing a partial perm?

_____

_____

_____

144. Where should you wrap the cotton rope (coil) when performing a partial perm?

_____

_____

_____

145. Describe how to make a smooth transition from the perm section to the nonperm section in a partial perm.

_____

_____

_____

146. What is the purpose of a soft curl perm?

_____

_____

_____

147. What steps are required to produce the Jheri curl?

_____

_____

_____

148. Can hair treated with hydroxide relaxers be treated with soft curl perms? Why or why not?

_____

_____

_____

Permanent Wave Safety Guidelines

149. Why is it important to study and understand the safety guidelines for perms, even though they are not as strong as chemical relaxers?

_____

_____

_____

150. List the three tests that you must conduct before beginning any perm service.

_____

_____

_____

151. Describe the results of a patch test that will allow you to proceed with the perm.

_____

_____

_____

152. In your own words, briefly describe how you would conduct a general analysis of the hair's health before performing a perm. What would you look for? What might indicate that you should decline to perform the perm service?

_____

_____

_____

153. What are two types of hair you should use when creating test curls for a perm service?

_____

_____

_____

154. List the six goals of creating test curls for a perm service.

_____

_____

_____

SEQUENCE

155. Number the steps for performing test curls, from 1 to 16. Some steps have been numbered for you.

_____ Apply perm solution to the wrapped curls.

___4___ Gently shampoo and towel dry the hair.

_____ Perform a patch test 24 to 48 hours before the service.

_____ Drape the client for a shampoo service.

_____ Check each test curl for proper curl development by unfastening the rod and unwinding the curl two to three turns.

_____ Redrape for a chemical service.

___14___ Apply neutralizer and process according to the manufacturer's directions.

_____ Wrap a coil of cotton around each rod.

_____ Gently dry the hair and evaluate the final results.

___9___ Set a timer and process the perm solution according to the manufacturer's directions.

_____ Gently move the rod toward the scalp and check the wave pattern.

_____ Curl development is complete when a firm S is formed.

_____ When the desired curl has been formed, rinse with warm water for at least five minutes, then blot thoroughly.

_____ Wrap one rod on different areas of the head (top, side, and nape).

_____ If the test curl results are satisfactory, proceed with the perm, but do not reperm these preliminary test curls.

_____ Perform hair and scalp analysis, elasticity, porosity, and metallic salts tests on day of service. If hair fails any of these tests or analyses, do not perform the perm service.

156. For each statement about safety tips and guidelines for performing permanent waving services, indicate whether it is something you should do (Do) or something you should not do (Don't).

Do or Don't?	Safety Tips and Guidelines for Performing Permanent Waving Services
_____	Apply protective cream around the hairline, the neck's nape, and the ears, and apply cotton all around the hairline
_____	Review the client's intake form and service record card each time before performing a chemical service
_____	Step away from or leave the client during a perm process
_____	Wear gloves when performing a perm service
_____	Carefully check the hair condition and the curl quality
_____	Thoroughly flush the eye with cool water if perm solution drips into the client's eye
_____	Remove the cotton after the solution application is complete and no longer dripping
_____	Perform a perm service on lightened (bleached) hair
_____	Wrap the hair with the appropriate rod size for the desired curl size
_____	Have a perm design in mind and know how you are going to achieve it
_____	Perform an oxidative haircolor service within two weeks after a perm service
_____	Prebook clients for a perm check and strengthening conditioning treatment
_____	Skip the client consultation for a repeat client who perms their hair regularly
_____	Perform a patch test 24 to 48 hours before a service, as well as a metallic salts test, and porosity and elasticity tests
_____	Take a test curl before the service and throughout the processing phase
_____	Shampoo the scalp before a perm service
_____	Rinse the hair with a gentle warm water stream for the recommended time, and rinse longer if there is lingering odor in the hair
_____	Blot the hair, reapply the cotton, replace the towel used in the double drape, and check for skin redness before applying the neutralizer
_____	Use a perm bib to catch dripping neutralizer solution
_____	Apply a nonoxidative semipermanent or temporary haircolor (if desired) right after the perm service

157. Now that you've studied the safety guidelines and tests required before performing perm services, including creating test curls, consider what you knew about perm services before you began this section compared to your understanding now. Write a few sentences in which you reflect on and answer the following questions:

    • Can you picture yourself performing the test curl procedure confidently during your examination?

    • What parts of the procedure do you perform the best? Which parts are you uncertain about?

    • During your examination, how do you plan to demonstrate your thorough understanding of the safety precautions and guidelines that are required for perm procedures?

    • Overall, how can you make your perm service flawless for the examination?

    When you're finished, meet with a classmate and discuss your responses. As you do so, look for opportunities to fill in each other's gaps and help each other master the perm techniques and specifics.

Permanent Wave Consultation

SHORT ANSWER

158. List three goals of the consultation you conduct with a client who is requesting perm services.

    _____

    _____

    _____

159. When discussing the client's goals for the perm they are considering, why is it helpful to review examples shown in photos and images?

    _____

    _____

    _____

160. What should you do if a client insists on a perm style that is not suitable for their hair texture, even after you've explained why you don't recommend it?

    _____

    _____

    _____

161. Listed below are the specific questions that cosmetologists should ask clients during a permanent wave consultation. For this activity, partner with two other classmates. Together, use your textbook or the Internet, or consult professional beauty magazines to research the importance of each consultation question. Add the reasons for asking each consultation question to the table. Then you will each take turns recording a video of the other two members of your group as they play the roles of client and cosmetologist in a permanent wave consultation. Record a one- to two-minute video of each pair, for a total of three videos. Be sure to leave time at the end of your consultation to state that you will either (1) proceed with the perm service or (2) decline but offer an alternative service instead.

The point is to conduct a compact but realistic consultation, focusing on what you think the most important questions might be, and to respond appropriately, politely, and efficiently to your client/stylist. The role of the recorder is to serve as both coach and witness.

When you're finished with your videos, your group should carefully watch all three of them together, pausing them where needed, and discuss how you think you did. Be thoughtful, kind, and helpful.

PERMANENT WAVE CONSULTATION QUESTIONS	REASON FOR ASKING
1. Are you currently taking any medications?	
2. Have you had a perm in the past? How long ago did you receive this service? Did you experience any adverse reactions like inflamed skin or a rash?	
3. What do you like least about your current hair texture? What do you like most?	
4. Do you want to add more body to your hair?	
5. What is your main goal for receiving a perm? Are you looking to achieve curls or waves, or just add body and lift to your hair?	
6. Are you willing to style your hair each day? Do you want to wear your hair smooth or curly? Are you willing to commit to styling rituals?	
7. Have you ever been an overall blonde or had blonde highlights in your hair? How long ago?	
8. Have you ever experienced hair loss? Are you experiencing any hair thinning? Have you been diagnosed with any form of alopecia?	
9. Have you ever had a henna treatment? If you have, how recently?	
10. What type of haircolor is on your hair right now?	
11. Describe your hair care regimen at home. Which hair care products are you using? How often do you shampoo and deep condition your hair?	
12. Are you open to using the products and home care regimen that I recommend for your hair?	

PERMANENT WAVE CONSULTATION QUESTIONS	REASON FOR ASKING
13. Are you committed to having regular salon treatments and occasional trims, including a light trim on the day of your service?	
14. Are you aware of the potential risks of having a perm service?	
15. Are you planning to spend time at the beach soon? Do you regularly swim in the ocean or a pool, or participate in outdoor activities? Are you able to abstain from these activities for at least 48 to 72 hours?	
16. May I analyze your scalp and hair today?	

Permanent Wave Application

DRAW

162. For each view of the head provided below, draw a picture of the panels and rod placement used for creating the basic wrap. Feel free to use colors and label any areas that you might be having difficulty illustrating.

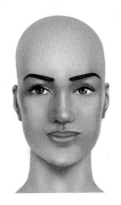 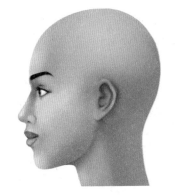 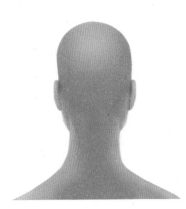

SHORT ANSWER

163. When dividing the hair into panels for the basic wrap, what determines the width of the panels?

_____

_____

_____

164. Describe how to roll the hair, including the base placement, for a basic wrap.

_____

_____

_____

165. When applying the perm solution to the rods, how should you direct the client to sit as you move through different areas of the head? How should you apply perm solution to the most resistant area?

_____

_____

_____

166. When checking for curl development during the perm service, should you check the same rod or different ones each time?

_____

_____

_____

167. How should you place the neutralizer bib?

_____

_____

_____

DRAW

168. For each view of the head provided below, draw a picture of the panels and rod placement used for creating the bricklay wrap. Feel free to use colors and label any areas that you might be having difficulty illustrating.

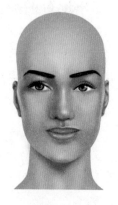 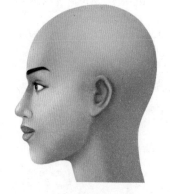 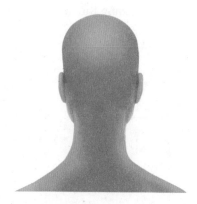

169. What angle do you roll the hair to in a bricklay wrap?

_____

_____

_____

170. In a bricklay wrap, where do you position the rod?

_____

_____

_____

171. Once you have established your bricklay wrap, to what part of the head do you continue to part out rows?

_____

_____

_____

172. How far down do you extend the rows as you continue wrapping the bricklay wrap?

_____

_____

_____

173. After wrapping the sides and top area back to the crown, where do you move on the head to complete the bricklay wrap? Why might you need to change the length of the rods as you work?

_____

_____

_____

174. For each view of the head provided below, draw a picture of the panels and rod placement used for creating the spiral wrap. Feel free to use colors and label any areas that you might be having difficulty illustrating.

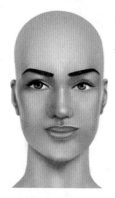 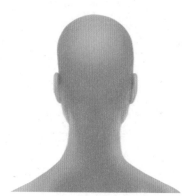

175. Number the steps of the process to perform a perm service using a spiral wrap, from 1 to 19. Some steps have been numbered for you.

_____ Place picks under all rod bands.

_____ Begin wrapping at the opposite side from the side where the first row began and move in the direction opposite the direction established in the first row.

_____ Perform a patch test 24 to 48 hours before the service.

____5____ Perform strand tests per the directions of the manufacturer.

_____ Perform a shampoo service before the service if directed by the manufacturer.

_____ Section out the third row above and parallel to the second row, and follow the same wrapping procedure, alternating the rows from left to right as you move up the head.

_____ Section out a fifth panel from ear to ear in the nape area.

_____ Put on gloves, apply perm solution, process accordingly, rinse solution, apply neutralizer, rinse neutralizer, remove rods, condition, and then style the hair.

_____ Spiral the hair and roll to the scalp; position the rod half off-base, and secure it by fastening the ends of the rod together.

_____ Continue wrapping using the same technique, in the same direction, until the first row is completed.

_____ Part the hair into four panels, by parting from the center of front hairline to center of the nape, and from ear to ear.

_____ Complete wrapping.

_____ Section out the first row along the hairline in the nape area, and comb the remaining hair up and secure out of the way.

_____ Section out the second row above and parallel to the first row.

_____ Perform hair and scalp analysis, elasticity, porosity, and metallic salts tests on day of service.

___15___ Continue wrapping with the same technique, in the same direction, until the second row is completed.

_____ Redrape the client for a chemical service.

_____ Follow the same procedure to wrap the second row, but begin wrapping each rod at the opposite end established in the first row.

___9___ Part out the first base section and begin rolling the hair.

SHORT ANSWER

176. Describe how to part the hair into the five panels that are used in the spiral wrap.

_____

_____

_____

177. Why do you alternate the rows from left to right as you move up the head when using the spiral wrap?

_____

_____

_____

178. For each view of the head provided below, draw a picture of the panels and rod placement used for creating the double-rod (or piggyback) wrap. Feel free to use colors and label any areas that you might be having difficulty illustrating.

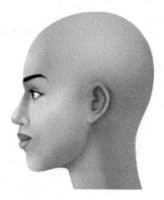 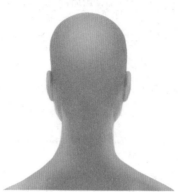

SEQUENCE

179. Number the steps of the procedure for performing a perm service using the double-rod wrap, from 1 to 13. Some steps have been numbered for you.

_____ Roll the rod up to the base area, letting the loose ends follow as you roll.

_____ Perform hair and scalp analysis, elasticity, porosity, and metallic salts tests on day of service.

____6____ Start in the bottom/back section below the occipital bone. Make the parting the same size as the rod.

_____ Put on gloves, apply perm solution, process accordingly, rinse solution, apply neutralizer, rinse neutralizer, remove rods, condition, and then style the hair.

_____ Perform a patch test 24 to 48 hours before the service.

_____ Insert roller picks to stabilize the rods and eliminate any tension caused by the bands.

_____ Wrap the end of the strand one revolution around the rod while holding it to one side.

_____ Perform a shampoo service before the service if directed by the manufacturer.

_____ Perform strand tests per the directions of the manufacturer.

____10____ Place end papers on the ends of the strand, position the rod, and roll from the ends toward the base.

_____ Secure the end rod on top of the base rod with a roller pick.

_____ Place the base rod in the middle of the subsection.

_____ Redrape the client for a chemical service.

180. In your own words, briefly describe the two different chemical processes that are used for a soft curl perm.

_____

_____

_____

181. After a soft curl perm service is completed, what should you recommend that your client use for moisture retention?

_____

_____

_____

182. How long should clients wait to shampoo their hair after receiving a soft curl perm?

_____

_____

_____

183. At what point can you allow the rearranger to touch the scalp? Why?

_____

_____

_____

184. Once the thio wrap lotion has been applied and the hair has been rolled, explain the circumstances under which you can use a hooded dryer for processing.

_____

_____

_____

185. Partner with a classmate to practice explaining to each other how to perform perm services using all four wraps—basic, bricklay, spiral, and double-rod. For soft curl perms, divide the service into two parts: the relaxer portion and the perm portion.

- Divide them up so that you are each explaining two different patterns and one aspect of soft curl perms.

- Review the Procedures (15-4 through 15-8) in your text and keep them handy.

- Gather the various rods, equipment, and your mannequins. (No need to use the perm solutions)

- Pretend that your partner does not know anything about perm services or the wraps.

- Explain to your partner exactly how to perform the perm service for the two wraps that you chose.

- During your explanation:

  - Be very specific

  - Demonstrate as needed while you narrate your process

  - Follow the same sequence set out in your text

- During your partner's explanation:

  - Watch and listen carefully to ensure that they follow the procedures in your text

  - Kindly let them know if they miss a step or explain/demonstrate something in the wrong order

When you're both finished, turn to the chart and respond to some reflection questions about perms on your own. How did watching your partner explain a technique make you more confident? Where can you fill in each other's gaps and help each other master the perm techniques and specifics? The point is to build your confidence with the procedures, practice talking and explaining while you are working, and to increase your proficiency with each type of perm service.

REFLECTION QUESTIONS	PERM WITH BASIC WRAP	PERM WITH BRICKLAY WRAP	PERM WITH SPIRAL WRAP	PERM WITH DOUBLE-ROD WRAP	SOFT CURL PERM
Can you picture yourself performing this perm and wrapping pattern confidently during your examination?					
What parts of the procedure do you perform the best?					
What parts of the procedure are you uncertain about?					
During your examination, how do you plan to demonstrate your thorough understanding of the safety precautions and guidelines that are required for this procedure?					
Overall, how do you plan to make your perm service flawless for the examination?					

DISCOVERIES AND ACCOMPLISHMENTS

In the space below, write notes about key concepts discussed in this chapter. Share your discoveries with some of the other students in your class and ask them if your notes are helpful. You may want to revise your notes based on good ideas shared by your peers.

Discoveries:

_____

_____

_____

_____

_____

_____

_____

List at least three things you have accomplished since you decided to enroll in school.

Accomplishments:

_____

_____

_____

_____

_____

_____

_____

1. Why should cosmetologists study chemical texture services?

   A) because they are required to inform clients about the parts of the hair that will be affected by a texture service

   B) Because chemical texture services have the potential to damage the hair and cosmetologists should therefore study them to perform these services safely

   C) because they are licensed to diagnose, treat, prescribe, or work on unhealthy hair and perform any service required in the process

   D) because chemical texture services are listed under a podiatry license and performing procedures that are listed under any podiatry license is a primary responsibility of cosmetologists

2. Identify the two categories of chemical relaxers commonly used by cosmetologists.

   A) ammonium sulfate relaxers and cysteamine relaxers

   B) mercaptamine relaxers and monoethanolamine relaxers

   C) hydroxide relaxers and ammonium thioglycolate relaxers

   D) aminomethylpropanol relaxers and glyceryl monothioglycolate relaxers

3. Your client has healthy brown hair with a wavy texture. Which of the following types of hydroxide relaxers should you use to straighten their hair?

   A) weak-strength relaxers   C) mild-strength relaxers

   B) super-strength relaxers   D) regular-strength relaxers

4. Which of the following relaxers uses reduction and oxidation to break the disulfide bonds and then reform them to a more relaxed hair texture?

   A) lye relaxers   C) sodium hydroxide relaxers

   B) thio relaxers   D) no-lye relaxers

5. Which of the following relaxer products is used for added skin protection around the hairline, the nape, and the top and back of the ears and is also used on the scalp for sensitive skin?

   A) a conditioner   C) a normalizing lotion

   B) a base cream   D) a styling cream

continued

6. You should perform a patch test at least two days before a scheduled chemical texture service to ensure that _____.

   A) the relaxer is the right strength

   B) the scalp is free of blemishes, abrasions, rashes, infections, or noticeably thin or balding areas

   C) the hair is healthy enough to undergo a relaxing service

   D) the client is not allergic to the chemical texture product you plan to use for the service

7. A chemical relaxer consultation is key to _____.

   A) discovering if the client is fine with the use of a curette

   B) diagnosing, treating, and working on unhealthy hair

   C) discovering whether there are red flags that must be addressed before agreeing or declining to perform the service

   D) informing clients about the parts of the hair that will be affected by the service

8. Which of the following statements is true of a virgin relaxer service?

   A) It includes the strand without the porous ends.

   B) It includes only the new growth.

   C) It begins on the midshaft.

   D) It starts 0.25 to 0.5 inch away from the scalp.

9. Which of the following is used for hair that has received a chemical relaxer service?

   A) a mask   C) a lacquer

   B) a virgin relaxer application   D) a relaxer retouch application

10. _____ is a two-step process to create body or curl in the hair.

   A) Thermal waving   C) Palm coiling

   B) Permanent waving   D) Marcel waving

continued

11. Identify a difference between acid perm solutions and alkaline perm solutions.

    A) Acid perm solutions produce far more cuticle layer swelling than alkaline perm solutions.

    B) The active ingredient in acid perm solutions is ammonium thioglycolate (ATG), whereas the active ingredient in alkaline perm solutions is glyceryl monothioglycolate (GMTG).

    C) Acid perm solutions are stronger than alkaline perm solutions.

    D) Acid perm solutions are ideal for fine, color-treated, and fragile hair, whereas alkaline perm solutions are suitable for coarse and moisture resistant hair.

12. Identify a true statement about low-pH waves.

    A) They use an ingredient such as mercaptamine or cysteamine as the primary reducing agent.

    B) They are strong and provide a firm curl to coarse hair.

    C) They are perms that use sulfates, sulfites, and bisulfites as an alternative to ammonium thioglycolate.

    D) They have a neutral pH value of 7.0.

13. In permanent waving, most of the processing occurs within the first _____ after the hair shaft is penetrated.

    A) two minutes   C) 30 to 60 seconds

    B) 5 to 10 minutes   D) 30 minutes

14. Which of the following is a characteristic of overprocessed hair?

    A) It results from the use of a mild perm solution.

    B) It can be made curlier with further processing.

    C) It is usually curlier at the scalp and straighter at the ends.

    D) It occurs when too few disulfide bonds are broken.

15. Identify a function of the neutralizing bib in a permanent wave service.

    A) to protect clients from direct contact with the chemical cape

    B) to control the hair's ends when winding the hair on the perm rods

    C) to prevent the neutralizer solution from touching the perm rods

    D) to prevent the neutralizer solution from running onto the client's shoulders and back

continued

16. _____ are the most common perm rod type and produce a tighter curl on the strand's ends and center and a looser curl on the strand's sides.

    A) Loop rods   C) Concave rods

    B) Straight rods   D) Soft bender rods

17. _____ are thin, absorbent papers that control the hair's ends when winding the hair on the perm rods.

    A) Gauze squares   C) End wraps

    B) Cotton puffs   D) Curettes

18. The term _____ refers to the angle at which the rod is positioned on the head: horizontally, vertically, or diagonally.

    A) base panel   C) base section

    B) base placement   D) base direction

19. A client wants a perm but does not want all their hair to be curled. They only want volume and lift in some areas and prefers a hairstyle with curls along the perimeter with a sleek crown. Which of the following types of perms should you suggest to the client?

    A) a spiral perm   C) a partial perm

    B) a bricklay perm   D) a soft curl perm

20. Identify a true statement about a soft curl perm.

    A) It is also known as a spiral perm.

    B) It includes a chemical process that uses a neutralizer to loosen the curly texture.

    C) It is used to restructure very curly hair into a larger curl pattern.

    D) It is performed on hair that has been treated with hydroxide relaxers.

21. Which of the following guidelines should you follow to safely perform a permanent wave service?

    A) Never apply a nonoxidative semipermanent or temporary haircolor right after a perm service.

    B) Never blot the hair before applying the neutralizer.

    C) Analyze the elasticity, porosity, and general health of the hair before starting a perm service.

    D) Always perform a perm service on lightened or bleached hair.

continued

22. Identify a permanent wave safety tip.

    A) Perform an oxidative haircolor service right after a perm service.

    B) Gently shampoo the scalp, not the hair, before a perm service.

    C) Do not apply any cream around the hairline, the neck's nape, and the ears.

    D) Perform a test curl before a perm service and throughout the processing phase.

23. You should not perform an oxidative haircolor service for at least _____ after a perm service.

    A) six hours   C) four days

    B) two weeks   D) one week

24. Which of the following should you most likely do during a professional perm consultation with a client?

    A) You should determine whether the client's hair is in the anagen phase, catagen phase, or telogen phase of the hair growth cycle.

    B) You should diagnose a hair disease or disorder.

    C) You should determine whether the client is committed to a home care regimen and periodic appointments to maintain the perm's quality and the hair's health.

    D) You should check if the client has the means to pay for the permanent wave service.

25. While performing a perm service on long hair, a hairstylist wraps the client's hair in vertical sections, enabling the permed hair to naturally fall in corkscrew curls. The style creates a uniform curl from scalp to end. Which of the following wrapping techniques does the hairstylist use in this scenario?

    A) a perm using the double-rod wrapping pattern

    B) a perm using the basic wrapping pattern

    C) a perm using the spiral wrapping pattern

    D) a perm using the bricklay wrapping pattern

finished!

Practical Skills
Self-Evaluation Checklist

Regular self-assessment helps you to improve your technical skills and achieve success. After performing each procedure, review the procedure steps in the textbook and rate yourself as "Competent" or "Needs Work," and write in comments on how you were successful or where you can improve. Rating yourself helps you identify your strengths and weaknesses and develop your own plan for improvement.

CRITERIA	COMPETENT	NEEDS WORK	COMMENTS
PROCEDURE 15-1 VIRGIN HAIR RELAXER			
Preparation			
Procedure			
Post-Service			
Timing			
PROCEDURE 15-2 RELAXER RETOUCH			
Preparation			
Procedure			
Post-Service			
Timing			
PROCEDURE 15-3 PRELIMINARY TEST CURL FOR A PERMANENT WAVE			
Preparation			
Procedure			
Post-Service			
Timing			
PROCEDURE 15-4 PERMANENT WAVE USING A BASIC WRAP			
Preparation			
Procedure			
Post-Service			
Timing			
PROCEDURE 15-5 PERMANENT WAVE USING A BRICKLAY WRAP			
Preparation			
Procedure			
Post-Service			
Timing			
PROCEDURE 15-6 PERMANENT WAVE USING A SPIRAL WRAP			
Preparation			
Procedure			
Post-Service			
Timing			
PROCEDURE 15-7 PERMANENT WAVE USING A DOUBLE-ROD WRAP			
Preparation			
Procedure			
Post-Service			
Timing			
PROCEDURE 15-8 SOFT CURL PERM (CHEMICAL CURL REFORMATION)			
Preparation			
Procedure			
Post-Service			
Timing			

ch. 16: Haircoloring

TRACK MY PROGRESS!

Use this simple tracker to record your progress as you work through the activities in each learning objective.

COMPLETED	# OF CORRECT ANSWERS	OBJECTIVE
☐	___/6	LO 1 - Explain why a thorough knowledge of haircoloring is needed for a successful cosmetology career.
☐	___/12	LO 2 - Explain how the hair's structure, texture, density, and porosity affect haircolor.
☐	___/18	LO 3 - Define the role of levels and tones in formulating haircolor.
☐	___/17	LO 4 - Explain primary, secondary, and tertiary colors, and their contributions to tone and intensity.
☐	___/31	LO 5 - Compare and describe the categories of haircolor.
☐	___/18	LO 6 - Detail the roles of hydrogen peroxide and ammonia in a haircolor formula.
☐	___/27	LO 7 - Explain the role and action of hair lighteners.
☐	___/12	LO 8 - Detail the steps for an effective haircolor consultation.
☐	___/13	LO 9 - List the five key questions to ask when formulating a haircolor.
☐	___/33	LO 10 - Outline the steps of haircolor application, from a preliminary strand test to a single process and a double process with lightener.
☐	___/31	LO 11 - Describe the techniques for highlighting.
☐	___/21	LO 12 - Explain the special haircoloring techniques for gray hair.
☐	___/16	LO 13 - Describe common haircoloring challenges and potential solutions.
☐	___/2	LO 14 - Describe the safety precautions to follow during the haircolor process.

Why Study Haircoloring?

SHORT ANSWER

1. What are three reasons a client might request haircoloring services?

   _____

   _____

   _____

2. Why is haircoloring potentially one of the most lucrative services that a stylist can offer?

   _____

   _____

   _____

3. How often do clients with colored hair typically visit the salon?

   _____

   _____

   _____

4. What is the difference between the terms *hair color* and *haircolor*?

   _____

   _____

   _____

5. What are the five reasons cosmetologists should have a thorough understanding of haircoloring?

   _____

   _____

   _____

6. On the chart below you will list five things about hair color and haircoloring services that you expect to learn in this chapter. (*Note:* The chart already includes one learning goal related to safety that all hair colorists are expected to set for themselves, in addition to the five that you will list.) Then, in the chart, explain how you plan to achieve the safety goal and each of the five goals you listed. Your lists should be specific and realistic. If necessary, conduct research on the Internet, on beauty blogs, or in professional beauty magazines to refine your plan.

As you work through the material in this chapter, keep your goals and plans in mind, and look for opportunities to execute your plans. At the end of this chapter, you will review your goals and reflect on how your plan turned out.

I EXPECT TO LEARN … ABOUT HAIR COLOR AND HAIRCOLORING SERVICES	TO ACHIEVE THIS GOAL, I PLAN TO …
I expect to learn about the chemicals, related procedures, and other precautions required to safely perform haircoloring services.	
1.	
2.	
3.	
4.	
5.	

Hair Color and Structure

7. What are the two general aspects of your client's hair that you must identify before you begin any haircoloring service for them? Why is this step crucial?

_____

_____

_____

8. What is another name for contributing pigment? What does it refer to?

_____

_____

_____

9. What is the purpose of also evaluating hair density and hair porosity when your client is requesting haircoloring services?

_____

_____

_____

10. When evaluating your client's hair specifically for haircolor services, what is important to keep in mind about a client's hair texture?

_____

_____

_____

MATCHING

11. Match the parts that make up the hair's structure with their descriptions. Each hair part will be used at least twice.

   a. Medulla   b. Cortex   c. Cuticle

Part of Hair Structure   **Description**

_____ Outermost layer; protects interior cortex

_____ Part of the hair structure that gives hair strength and elasticity

_____ Innermost layer

_____ Middle layer

_____ Part of the hair structure that plays no role in haircolor

_____ Contributes up to 20 percent of overall hair strength

_____ Melanin present in this part of the hair structure determines the natural hair color

12. Match each type of hair texture with its description. Each texture will be used at least once.

   a. Fine-textured   b. Medium-textured   c. Coarse-textured

Type of Hair Texture	Description
_____	Tightly packed melanin
_____	Takes longer to process
_____	Colors faster, looks darker
_____	Average reaction to haircolor
_____	Loosely grouped melanin

TRUE OR FALSE

Indicate whether the statements below are true or false. For any false statements, explain why they are false.

13. If hair has low porosity, this means that the cuticle is tight, and it allows chemicals to easily penetrate.

   T   F   _____

14. Hair with average porosity—also called medium porosity—has a slightly raised cuticle and has little to no difficulty absorbing or retaining moisture.

   T   F   _____

15. Hair with average porosity requires above-average processing time.

   T   F   _____

16. Color can process more quickly in hair that has high porosity.

   T   F   _____

17. Hair with high porosity is characterized by a lifted cuticle, allowing chemicals to easily penetrate.

   T   F   _____

18. Although hair with high porosity takes color quickly, it tends to hold color longer.

   T   F   _____

Hair Levels and Tones

19. What is the role of science and art in working in professional haircolor services? Which should be learned first, and why?

_____

_____

_____

20. What do colorists use the level system for?

_____

_____

_____

21. Describe the scale of hair levels.

_____

_____

_____

22. How do haircolor charts help colorists? What are two other terms for a haircolor chart?

_____

_____

_____

23. Why is it important to understand generic haircolor charts as well as a specific manufacturer's haircolor chart?

_____

_____

_____

24. Practice determining hair level by doing the following:

    1. Look at your own hair and determine what you think its level number is—keep it to yourself for now.

    2. Meet with four or five classmates and work together to arrange your group from darkest to lightest hair—no one should reveal what they think their own level number is yet.

    3. For each person, the group should then decide together what that person's level number is (without that person's input).

    4. When the group has agreed on a level number for each person, everyone should reveal what they originally thought theirs was.

    5. Discuss any differences in level numbers and come to an agreement about each person's (this time, with everyone's input, including your own).

    6. Arrange yourselves into the final sequence, darkest to lightest.

Were there differences between what each person thought their level number was compared to what the group determined? Did it change how your group ultimately arranged itself according to level numbers? How did you make the final determinations and line-up?

SHORT ANSWER

25. You are looking at a standard color chart and see 6.RVv. What do the letter and number components mean? Use 6.RVv to explain below.

   _____

   _____

   _____

26. In a situation where a manufacturer uses the same letter for different colors in its haircolor chart, what are some possible colors that the letter *G* might stand for? How can you make sure you know which colors a manufacturer's chart is referring to?

   _____

   _____

   _____

27. What are two resources that professional manufacturers might offer to assist in selecting haircolors?

   _____

   _____

   _____

28. Label the parts of the haircolor chart and identify the complete name of each haircolor indicated below.

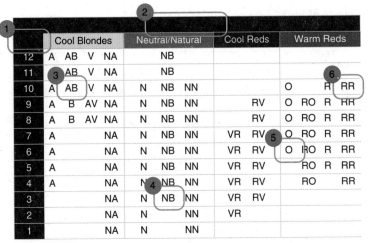

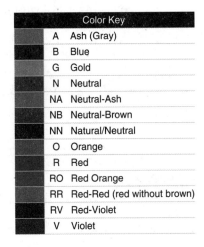

Note that information in this chart may change by haircolor manufacturer.

_____

_____

_____

_____

_____

_____

Indicate whether each statement below is true or false. For any false statements, explain why they are false.

29. Even if you are familiar with the light cast by artificial light, you will not be able to effectively check your haircolor results.

    T   F   _____

30. Fluorescent light casts a flat, cool color that enhances blues and greens.

    T   F   _____

31. For best results, use the artificial light provided in the salon during your hair analysis whenever possible.

T   F   _____

32. Halogen light casts a warm, amber light that enhances red and orange tones.

T   F   _____

33. Proper lighting and wall color are essential to your haircolor results, especially in a small space.

T   F   _____

LABELING

34. Label each hair color shown below with the type of lighting that is illuminating it.

    a. Halogen   b. Fluorescent   c. Incandescent

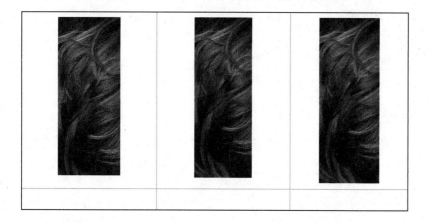

FILL IN THE BLANK

35. Complete the sentences below.

_____ hair has lost much of its _____. Only _____ hair is devoid of pigment.

_____ people become completely gray-haired, even though _____ loss is generally

progressive throughout a person's lifetime. Beyond assessing the hair level, gray hair requires

special attention in terms of the _____ of _____ and where the _____ hair is

the densest on the head.

36. Use the Internet or beauty supply catalogues, or visit a beauty supply store, to find three different haircolor charts and/or swatches. Review them and record your findings in the chart below or by following the link for a PDF version. When you're finished, state which haircolor chart seems the most useful and explain why. Also, describe two similarities and describe two differences among all three charts.

+ BONUS

Visit: bonus.milady.com/cos-wb/toc

FEATURES	HAIRCOLOR CHART #1	HAIRCOLOR CHART #2	HAIRCOLOR CHART #3
Name/Brand			
Price (or Free?)			
Location of Levels on Chart			
Range of Level Numbers (Lightest to Darkest)			
Location of Colors/Tones			
Range of Colors/Tones Displayed			
Color Key? (Yes/No)			
Lettering Used for Colors (provide three examples)			
Lettering for Primary Pigments (provide three examples)			
Lettering for Secondary Pigments (provide three examples)			
Swatches Provided? (Yes/No)			
Other Information Included with Haircolor Chart/Swatch System			

Color Theory

37. What is the law of color?

_____

_____

_____

38. What does a color wheel illustrate?

_____

_____

_____

39. Match each primary color with its description and/or effects. Each primary color will be used three times.

   a. Blue   b. Red   c. Yellow

   Primary Color   **Description or Effect**

   _____ The only cool primary color

   _____ Like red, can add warmth to colors if predominant

   _____ Adding this to yellow colors will make them appear darker

   _____ Weakest primary color

   _____ Strongest primary color

   _____ Adding this to blue-based colors will make them appear lighter

   _____ Adding this to other colors results in lighter and brighter colors

   _____ Can bring depth or darkness to any color

   _____ Medium-strength primary color

40. What is meant by the term *primary colors*?

_____

_____

_____

41. Which colors are created from the primary colors?

_____

_____

_____

42. What is the resulting color, according to traditional color theory, if all three primary colors are present in equal proportions?

_____

_____

_____

43. What is meant by the term *secondary colors*?

_____

_____

_____

44. What is meant by the term *tertiary colors*?

_____

_____

_____

45. Which categories of color make up natural-looking haircolor? Which category is always considered the dominant color in those combinations?

_____

_____

_____

46. If you combine green and blue to form a tertiary color, what is the formal name of the new resulting color? Put another way, which color is the dominant one in that pair?

_____

_____

_____

47. Add the primary, secondary, and tertiary colors to the color wheel below using markers or colored pencils, then label each one of them.

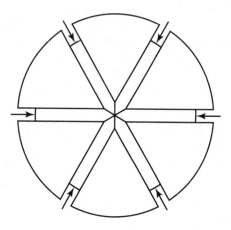

48. List the three pairs of complementary colors.

_____

_____

_____

49. What is meant by the term *complementary colors*? How are complementary colors arranged on the color wheel?

_____

_____

_____

50. What effect do complementary colors have on each other? How can understanding the relationships between the complementary colors ensure that you properly assist your client in achieving their haircoloring goals?

_____

_____

_____

51. What is tone, and what role does tone play in formulating haircolor for a client?

_____

_____

_____

MATCHING

52. Match each type of tone with its description. Each type of tone will be used three times.

    a. Warm tones   b. Cool tones   c. Neutral tones

    Type of Tone   **Description**

    _____ Tones that are blue, green, and violet

    _____ Might be described as sandy or tan

    _____ Tones that are gold, orange, red, and yellow

    _____ Some stylists might describe these tones as smoky or ash

    _____ Reflect more light, making them look lighter than their actual level

    _____ Flatter all skin tones

    _____ Tones that are neither cool nor warm

    _____ Absorb more light, making them look deeper than their actual level

    _____ Some haircolor manufacturers use words such as *auburn*, *amber*, *copper*, *strawberry*, and *bronze* to describe these tones

CASE STUDY

53. For this exercise, partner with a classmate to analyze the color of their hair (including tones) using hair swatches or a haircolor chart. Record your assessment in the chart below.

    Then, briefly describe the expected or intended result of changing your partner's hair color and tone. Be sure to consider your partner's eye color and skin tone. Determine two options from the chart (color, tone, and level) that would be flattering on your classmate, and one that you would not recommend if your partner were your client.

As you analyze the colors and discuss these choices with your partner, be sure to be sensitive, kind, and open-minded—just as you would be when consulting with a client. The point of this activity is to analyze color according to professional color theory and with the eyes of a professional who is being trusted to assist a client with their beauty goals. It's also a good opportunity to practice analyzing the relationships between different color combinations and tones.

Hair Color	
Hair Level	
Hair Tone	
Eye Color	
Skin Tone	
Effect of Changing Hair Color to Blonde	
Effect of Changing Hair Color to Brunette	
Effect of Changing Hair Color to Black	
Effect of Changing Hair Color to Red	
Effect of Changing Hair Level	
Effect of Changing Hair Tone to Warm	
Effect of Changing Hair Tone to Neutral	
Effect of Changing Hair Tone to Cool	
Best, Most Flattering, Recommended Changes to Hair Color, Hair Tone, and Level	

Types of Haircolor

MATCHING

57. Match each haircoloring product classification with its description. More than one classification might match a description.

a. Temporary
b. Semipermanent
c. Demipermanent
d. Permanent
e. Natural-based
f. Metallic

Haircoloring Product Classification   **Description**

_____ Lasts one to three shampoos.

_____ Mixed with a low-volume developer

_____ Tones pre-lightened hair

_____ Progressive haircolor built up over multiple applications

_____ Contains an alkaline agent and is mixed with developer

_____ Lasts three to eight shampoos, depending on the formula

_____ Plant-based dyes with very limited shades; most just stain the cuticle; some can penetrate the cortex with developer provided by the manufacturer

_____ Lays on the hair's surface

_____ Can lighten and deposit haircolor at the same time

_____ Adds a variety of color results, ranging from subtle to bold

_____ Can neutralize unwanted tones

_____ Rarely used in salons and generally regarded as an at-home haircolor product

_____ Permanently changes existing haircolor

_____ Has no ammonia (or other alkalizing agents) or developer

_____ Lasts 12 to 24 shampoos

_____ Glosses natural or color-treated hair for added shine and richness

_____ Can build up and interfere with other chemical services

_____ Creates bright or natural-looking haircolor changes

_____ Lasts four to six weeks

_____ Color lasts four to six weeks; metallic salts deposited by progressive haircolors can stay in the hair for up to two years

_____ Generally replaces ammonia with another alkalizing agent

_____ Can be a great introduction to haircolor services, or a low-commitment option for self-expression

_____ Refreshes faded haircolor

_____ Can create subtle or bold results

_____ Covers gray

54. What are the two classifications of oxidative haircolor?

_____

_____

_____

55. What are the two classifications of nonoxidative haircolor?

_____

_____

_____

56. In what setting are natural-based hair dyes and metallic dyes typically used?

_____

_____

_____

TRUE OR FALSE

Indicate whether each statement below is true or false. For any false statements, explain why they are false.

58. To identify whether a client is allergic to a product, the U.S. Food, Drug, and Cosmetic Act requires that a patch test be given 24 to 48 hours prior to each application of haircolor that is formulated with aniline derivative dyes.

   T   F   _____

59. Temporary (or nonpermanent) haircolor has small pigment molecules that only deposit a coating of haircolor on the cortex, which may be removed by shampooing the hair.

   T   F   _____

60. It is not possible for temporary haircolors to fill the hair with lost color molecules before a color correction service.

   T   F   _____

61. Traditional semipermanent haircolor lasts one to six months, depending on how frequently the hair is shampooed, the level and intensity of the haircolor, and the pigment concentration.

   T   F   _____

62. Traditional semipermanent haircolors are used right out of the bottle.

   T   F   _____

63. Semipermanent haircolor lightens the hair, so it requires maintenance of new growth, also called regrowth, the part of the hair shaft between the scalp and previously colored hair.

   T   F   _____

FILL IN THE BLANK

64. For each form of haircolor listed below, provide a brief description of its intended purpose. Be sure to include if the product is temporary (T) or semipermanent (S)

FORM OF HAIRCOLOR	INTENDED PURPOSE
Hair mascara and colored powder	
Colored mousses and gels	
Dimensional haircolor	
Color-enhancing shampoos and conditioners	
Spray-on haircolor	
Natural hair colors	
Colored rinses	
Delicate traditional pastels	
Colored glosses	
Nontraditional haircolors	
Colored waxes	

SHORT ANSWER

65. What are the two types of demipermanent haircolor?

   _____

   _____

   _____

66. What is the intended result of using demipermanent haircolors?

_____

_____

_____

67. How have demipermanent haircolors been used in recent years? What is the purpose of that application method?

_____

_____

_____

68. What are four ways that permanent haircolors are used on gray hair?

_____

_____

_____

69. Why are permanent haircolors able to lighten and deposit color simultaneously, and in a single process?

_____

_____

_____

70. What is another name for dye precursors? What chemical do they combine with to form large color dye molecules once they are within the cortex?

_____

_____

_____

71. Why are permanent haircoloring products considered the best for covering gray hair?

_____

_____

_____

72. Does permanent haircolor require a patch test 24 to 48 hours before the service?

_____

_____

_____

MATCHING

73. Match each type of demipermanent with its description.

    a. Acidic   b. Alkaline   c. Both acidic and alkaline

Type of Demipermanent   **Description**

_____ Generally in the pH 6.7 range

_____ Can shift undertones, lift natural hair color up to a half level, and deposit more opaque color for depth and coverage

_____ Because this type of demipermanent is more alkaline than hair (which is pH 4.5–5.5), will slightly swell and open the cuticle to deposit color between the cuticle and the cortex layers

_____ Requires a patch test 24 to 48 hours before the haircolor service

_____ Also known as no lift or deposit-only colors

_____ Used with dedicated 10-volume developers

_____ Generally in the pH 8.0 range

_____ Can blend gray with the existing color; minimize brassy tones; and deposit a veil of sheer, rich color

_____ Most commonly formulated with an ammonia substitute, such as monoethanolamine (MEA) or calcium carbonate

_____ Type of demipermanent that will swell the cuticle layer to a greater degree than the other type of demipermanent and deposit color in the outer margins of the cortex

_____ Available in gel, cream, or liquid formulations

_____ Can also be used as a finishing gloss for most haircolor services

74. For each image below, label which type of haircoloring molecular action is depicted.

a. Temporary
b. Semipermanent

c. Demipermanent
d. Permanent

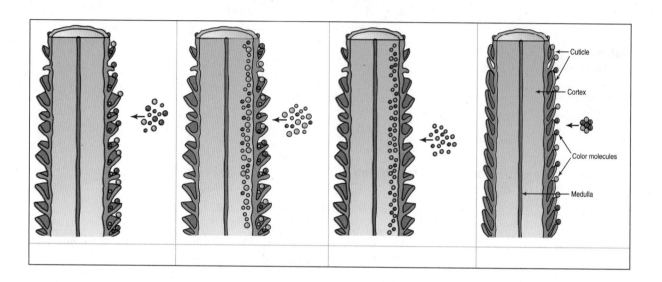

Indicate whether each statement below is true or false. For any false statements, explain why they are false.

75. Even though natural-based and metallic haircolors generally are not used in the salon, you should still be familiar with these products because you will occasionally have clients that use these haircolors at home.

T   F   _____

76. If your client has applied natural haircolor products or those containing metallic salts to their hair, they will be relieved to learn that most traditional haircolor products can be applied over these products.

T   F   _____

77. Another term for *natural-based haircolors* is *vegetable-dye haircolors*.

T   F   _____

78. Henna, a permanent natural haircolor, uses developer and can lighten natural hair color.

    T   F   _____

79. If the henna haircolor is anything except burnished red-orange, any such colors have been mixed with, or entirely replaced by, other substances that may or may not be safe for humans; in addition, those ingredients may not be listed on the product label.

    T   F   _____

SHORT ANSWER

80. What is the ingredient in metallic haircolors that changes hair color gradually? What is another term for metallic hair color?

    _____

    _____

    _____

81. What will happen if you apply an oxidative haircolor to hair that contains metallic salts? How can you determine if hair contains metallic salts?

    _____

    _____

    _____

82. What are the five goals that color fillers accomplish?

    _____

    _____

    _____

83. What are three possible conditions of the hair that should prompt you to consider pretreating it with a filler?

    _____

    _____

    _____

84. Complete the following sentences using the words from the word bank. Some words will be used more than once.

    Word bank: color, scalp, damaged, balanced, evenly, three, 9, one, 10, toned, conditioner, equalize, uniform, extend

    Color fillers _____ porosity and deposit color molecules in _____ application to provide a _____ contributing pigment. Regardless of why the hair needs to be filled before applying a haircolor, the goals are always to provide a layer of _____ contributing pigments that support the desired finished haircolor. As a general rule, if you are going _____ levels or more darker, or are dealing with level _____ or _____ blonde that needs to be _____, use a _____ filler.

    _____ fillers recondition and _____ porosity on _____ hair. They condition, strengthen, and help _____ haircolor longevity and make the haircolor formulation cover hair _____ from _____ to ends.

Hydrogen Peroxide and Ammonia

85. What is mixed with haircolor formula to achieve oxidation?

    _____

    _____

    _____

86. What is included in haircolor formula during the manufacturing process to achieve alkalinity?

    _____

    _____

    _____

87. Which feature of ammonia can cause changes to the hair's texture and curl pattern when used in haircoloring and lightening services?

_____

_____

_____

88. What is a developer, and what is the most popular one used in salons?

_____

_____

_____

MATCHING

89. Match each form of developer with its description. Each form will be used twice.

   a. Clear liquid developers   b. Cream developers   c. Dedicated developers

   Form of Developer   **Description**

   _____ Created by haircolor companies to be used with their proprietary haircolor products

   _____ Thicker consistency for use in a bowl-and-brush application

   _____ Require application control to avoid dripping in the client's eyes

   _____ Include conditioning agents to support the hair's integrity

   _____ Might contain specific ingredients not intended to be mixed with certain products, requiring stylists to give extra attention to product labels

   _____ Easy to apply the product from an applicator bottle

TRUE OR FALSE

Indicate whether each statement below is true or false. For any false statements, explain why they are false.

90. In haircolor products, the lower the developer volume, the greater the lift; the higher the volume, the less lift is achieved.

   T   F   _____

91. Volume measures the concentration and strength of hydrogen peroxide.

   T   F   _____

92. Most permanent haircolor products use 10-, 11-, 12-, or 13-volume hydrogen peroxide for targeted lift and haircolor development.

   T   F   _____

93. Developer volumes in lighteners strengthen the chemical reaction and can severely damage the hair.

   T   F   _____

94. In lightener products, the lift is determined by the developer used, and the speed is determined by the lightener itself.

   T   F   _____

95. Ammonia is an acidic agent that lowers the pH of the hair colorant.

   T   F   _____

96. Using ammonia to alkalize the hair colorant opens the cuticle to allow dye molecules to enter the cortex where haircoloring takes place.

   T   F   _____

97. Ammonia helps the peroxide action of dispersing the melanin that resides within the cortex.

   T   F   _____

98. Common low-odor alkalizing agents for haircolor, such as ethanolamine (commonly called monoethanolamine or MEA), are less damaging to the hair than ammonia.

   T   F   _____

SHORT ANSWER

99. Which three parts of the respiratory system are prone to possible negative health risks associated with mixing and applying hydrogen peroxide, ammonia, and even ammonia-free products?

   _____

   _____

   _____

100. What are two safety precautions for applying haircolor or lighteners? What is an additional precaution for stylists who have asthma or other breathing conditions?

_____

_____

_____

101. Why is it important to always follow the manufacturer's directions for haircolor and lightening products? What are two possible consequences of not following the manufacturer's directions?

_____

_____

_____

FILL IN THE BLANK

102. Complete the chart below.

DEVELOPER VOLUME	PERCENTAGE OF PEROXIDE	USES OF PEROXIDE AT THIS DEVELOPER VOLUME AND AMOUNT OF LIFT
		Up to four levels of lift (lightening) with standard high lift haircolor; provides maximum lift in a one-step color service; can be used with lightener for strong lift when bleaching hair but is not recommended for most hair due to possible damage
		Standard volume; provides two levels of lift; used to achieve most results with permanent haircolor; used for complete gray coverage due to gray hair's resistance; also used with lightener for a standard lift when bleaching hair
Higher Volumes		
		Used to deposit haircolor or, when little or no lift is desired, to enhance a client's natural hair color; also used with lightener for gently lifting when bleaching hair
30 volume		

Lighteners

103. Match each form of lightener with its description. More than one form might match a description.

a. Oil
b. Cream
c. Powder
d. Clay

Form of Lightener	Description
_____	Some brands of this form of lightener, if specified by the manufacturer, considered on-scalp lighteners
_____	Strong and fast-acting lightener formulated to lift the hair anywhere from four to seven levels (and some brands claim up to nine levels)
_____	Forms an outside shell to keep the product moist and active for the maximum amount of time
_____	Has conditioning agents for applying to the scalp with less irritation
_____	Used for foil-free, freehand painting techniques like balayage because they do not expand or run
_____	On-scalp lightener
_____	Off-scalp lightener
_____	Has the texture of toothpaste
_____	Most common form of hair lightening products
_____	Has dedicated developers that typically require 20 volume or less for scalp application
_____	Most lighteners in this form expand (swell) and spread out as they process, especially under heat or in a foil; the stronger the chemical reaction, the more swelling occurs
_____	Can lighten hair by three to five levels
_____	Off-scalp versions of this form contain persulfate salts (sodium persulfate) for quicker and stronger lightening, but also tend to dry out quicker than other lightener types

104. What are two other terms for lightener?

_____

_____

_____

105. When lightener is applied to the hair, where does the oxidation process occur?

_____

_____

_____

106. How does the pH of lighteners compare to that of permanent haircolor?

_____

_____

_____

107. Which two components are mixed together in the mixing ratio? What are typical mixing ratios when making lighteners?

_____

_____

_____

108. What three main factors determine the mixing ratio that you use when preparing lightener for a client?

_____

_____

_____

109. What are the risks of free-pouring or failing to measure, especially when completing an application through the full head?

_____

_____

_____

110. Describe how a lightener with a thicker consistency will dry.

_____

_____

_____

TRUE OR FALSE

Indicate whether each statement below is true or false. For any false statements, explain why they are false.

111. Contributing pigment refers to the unrefined cool tones revealed during the lightening process.

T   F   _____

112. The level system and contributing pigment are directly related to each other.

T   F   _____

113. Sometimes it's necessary to lighten a level higher than the desired result to get past the unwanted tone of natural contributing pigment.

T   F   _____

114. Taking contributing pigment into account, if the hair is a level 5 and your goal is to lighten it to a level 8, you must decolorize the hair to orange.

T   F   _____

115. There is no limit to how much you can lighten a client's hair if it is healthy.

T   F   _____

116. You should always be monitoring the health of a client's hair during a lightening service.

T   F   _____

117. Activators are liquid monomers added to powder lighteners to increase their lightening ability.

    T   F   _____

118. The amount of change that hair goes through during lightening is affected by the amount of contributing pigment in the hair, the strength of the lightening product, the volume of the developer, and the time the product is processed.

    T   F   _____

SHORT ANSWER

119. What should you do at the first sign of even minor damage during a lightening process? Why?

    _____

    _____

    _____

120. What is the term for the first step in the double-process haircoloring? What happens in that step?

    _____

    _____

    _____

121. What happens in the second step of the double-process haircoloring?

    _____

    _____

    _____

122. When is the double-process haircolor most effective? What is a benefit of this process?

    _____

    _____

    _____

123. Match the various options for toning pre-lightened hair with their descriptions. Each option will be used twice.

   a. Traditional toners
   b. Acidic demipermanent dyes
   c. Temporary and semipermanent haircolors
   d. Toning shampoos

Options for Toning Prelightened Hair	Description
_____	Used on pre-lightened hair to achieve pale blonde shades on level 9 (light blonde) and level 10 (lightest blonde)
_____	Popular products for toning accent pieces and vivid shades because they do not contain developers and will not lift the surrounding hair during the toning process
_____	Permanent haircolors mixed with a low-volume developer (usually 10 volume)
_____	Toners that close down the cuticle because of their pH and make the hair feel smoother after a lightening service
_____	Although considered temporary color, option that can deposit subtle to dramatic color
_____	Available in fashion shades such as light pink, baby blue, or peach, and applied as toners over prelightened level 10 hair for true color results
_____	Will not lift the existing hair color, making them great for highlighting services; known for their haircolor longevity
_____	Work as toner both in the salon and for client use at home

TRUE OR FALSE

Indicate whether each statement below is true or false. For any false statements, explain why they are false.

124. After pre-lightening, toners can be used to remove the exposed harsh undertones of the hair, neutralize or enhance tones as needed, and further lighten the hair.

   T   F   _____

125. Though most toners are formulated as semi- or demipermanent color, permanent color can be used as toners if the manufacturer allows it.

 T   F   _____

126. Although all-over pre-lightened hair should be toned to give it a definitive shade, such as pearl blonde, it is not recommended that you tone heavily highlighted hair.

 T   F   _____

127. Toners are intended exclusively for blonde hair.

 T   F   _____

128. The hair must be fully lightened before selecting a toner; choosing a toner before the hair has lightened can result in improper selection.

 T   F   _____

129. Hair color always appears lighter and warmer when wet, so you may need to dry the hair first to select the toner and follow the manufacturer's directions for application.

 T   F   _____

Haircolor Consultation

SHORT ANSWER

130. In addition to the responses your client provides, what are two nonverbal sources of information that you should pay attention to?

_____

_____

_____

131. In your own words, what is the overall goal of the client consultation?

_____

_____

_____

132. Is it necessary to conduct a client consultation before every haircolor service?

_____

_____

_____

133. Is brushing your client's hair before the haircolor service recommended? Why or why not?

_____

_____

_____

SEQUENCE

134. Number the overall steps in the haircolor consultation, from 1 to 13. Step 1 has been numbered for you.

_____ Move to an area with proper lighting and white or neutral walls (if possible) to conduct the consultation so that you can accurately determine the client's current hair color.

_____ Finish the haircolor service and ask them to prebook their next appointment before departing the salon.

_____ If one of the options you have offered your client is a corrective situation, then let them know what you can accomplish in one day and, if necessary, how many additional visits it would take to achieve the results they want; above all, be honest and do not promise more than you realistically can deliver.

_____ As you begin the consultation, pay attention to the client's skin and eye color (as they indicate color palette and overall abundance of melanin), hair condition and length, and the amount of gray in their hair.

_____ Have the client sign the salon's release statement.

_____ During the consultation, encourage the client to talk by asking questions that require more than a yes or no answer.

_____ During the service, (a) educate and inform the client about home care and rebooking, (b) let them know what steps you are doing as you complete them to reassure that you are completing the service as planned, (c) notify them immediately if something needs changing, (d) recommend the types of shampoo and conditioner needed to maintain the haircolor, and (e) let the client know how long it will be before they need to come back for another service.

_____1_____ On the client intake form, note the type of haircolor service the client wants.

_____ For the haircolor options that you have offered your client, review the procedure and application techniques required to achieve the targeted color, total service cost, and follow-up maintenance; have an economical backup solution ready.

_____ Finish inputting the client's haircolor information based on the haircolor service you ultimately completed for them that day.

_____ Gain client approval.

_____ After gathering all pertinent information, recommend at least two different haircolor options and always offer clients more than what they ask for.

_____ Start the haircolor service.

FILL IN THE BLANK

135. Follow the link or use a separate piece of paper to complete the chart listing the types of questions you should ask during a client consultation for haircolor services: lifestyle, time devoted to salon visits, budget, beauty goals, hair history, and medical history. For each type of question, list at least three (preferably open-ended) questions you would ask and write a brief explanation of why you would ask those questions.

+ BONUS

Visit: bonus.milady.com/cos-wb/toc

SHORT ANSWER

136. What are three kinds of vision impairment that your clients might have?

_____

_____

_____

137. What is the benefit of asking clients who are visually-impaired how they describe cool or warm tones, or certain colors?

_____

_____

_____

138. What is another technique you can use to express the dimensions (or range) of haircolor when consulting with clients who are visually impaired?

_____

_____

_____

139. What kinds of words and phrases should you use to convey haircoloring benefits to your clients? Provide two examples.

_____

_____

_____

140. Explain the purpose of a release statement. Does it protect the cosmetologist?

_____

_____

_____

CREATE

141. Your text stresses the importance of being able to visually convey the intended results of a haircolor service for your client—and to understand your client's expectations. An effective way of doing that is to build an image gallery that's organized according to color and style options.

    For this exercise, consult the table below that lists natural hair colors (brown, blonde, red, and black). For each color, identify or create at least 10 terms or phrases that can be used to describe the range, tones, and intensity that might be found among those hair colors. For inspiration, consult beauty catalogues, wallpaper and paint descriptions, car colors, fabric or clothing catalogues, or even kitchenware collections or art supply websites. Use these to broaden your color vocabulary but also to get a sense of how colors are marketed and how you can communicate what the color is to your clients.

    Once you've completed your list, use the Internet or beauty magazines to find images of at least five of the hair colors you listed in each column (for a total of 20 images) and use them to build your visual gallery or personal portfolio of different haircolors and haircolor placement, including highlights. You can also follow the link below to keep a digital record of your personal portfolio.

+ BONUS

Visit: bonus.milady.com/cos-wb/toc

BROWN	BLONDE	RED	BLACK
Rich chocolate brown	Soft buttery blonde	Spicy coppery red	Jet-set jet black
1.			
2.			
3.			
4.			
5.			
6.			
7.			
8.			
9.			
10.			

Haircolor Formulation

FILL IN THE BLANK

142. Complete the sentences below using words from the word bank. Some words will be used more than once.

    Word bank: level, gray, mixed, tone, formulating, contributing, natural, undertones, previously

    Haircolor formulation is of top importance when creating a successful haircolor that delivers the client's

    desired result. You must always ask yourself these five basic questions when _____ a haircolor:

    • What is the _____ level? What is the percentage of _____ hair?

    • What is the level and _____ of the _____ colored hair?

    • What is the client's desired _____ and _____ ?

    • Will _____ pigments (_____) be revealed?

    • What haircolors should be _____ to get the desired result?

143. Number the main steps of the hair strand test, from 1 to 5.

_____ Frequently check the test strand to ensure it is processing as you anticipated.

_____ Process it the same way as your planned formula.

_____ If the test strand meets your approval, proceed with your haircolor application.

_____ Mix a small amount of the formula you are planning to use on a hair strand separated by a foil to ensure it does not bleed onto other areas of the hair.

_____ Remove the haircolor with a damp towel.

SHORT ANSWER

144. What are the two methods you can use to apply permanent and demipermanent haircolors?

_____

_____

_____

145. Which application method is best for products with thicker viscosity? Which is best for products with thinner viscosity?

_____

_____

_____

146. Should the haircolor mixing bowl and whisk be metallic or nonmetallic?

_____

_____

_____

147. After the formulation has been mixed in the bowl, which tool is used to apply the haircolor to the hair?

_____

_____

_____

Indicate whether each statement below is true or false. For any false statements, explain why they are false.

148. Because formulation has a set ratio of color to developer, there is no need to measure.

    T   F   _____

149. Measuring with a scale is the most precise way to measure.

    T   F   _____

150. The drawback of measuring with a scale is that when you mix very small amounts, it will not prevent product waste.

    T   F   _____

151. Resting the measuring cup or bottle on a flat, even surface will result in better accuracy.

    T   F   _____

SHORT ANSWER

152. Why should you leave air space in the applicator bottle after filling it?

    _____

    _____

    _____

153. In what order do you add developer and haircolor to a bowl? To an applicator bottle?

    _____

    _____

    _____

154. What is the typical ratio for most permanent high lift blonde haircolors?

    _____

    _____

    _____

How to Apply Haircolor and Lighteners

Complete the sentences below.

155. Before applying haircolor that is formulated with _____ dyes, the U.S. Food, Drug, and

     _____ Act requires that within _____ hours of the scheduled service, a

     _____ test be performed.

156. A _____ test will help determine whether your client may have _____ or

     _____ to the haircolor mixture.

157. Perform a _____ test by creating the haircolor formula and applying it to a few small

     _____.

158. The _____ test determines how the hair will _____ to the haircolor formula

     and how _____ the formula should be left on the hair.

159. Number the steps for performing the temporary haircolor service, from 1 to 14. One step has been
     numbered for you.

     _____ Help client to recline comfortably on the shampoo bowl. Thoroughly shampoo the hair,
     then rinse. Repeat shampoo if necessary.

     _____ Blend color with your gloved hands then comb through hair with wide-tooth comb. Apply
     additional color as necessary.

     _____ Drape client for a shampoo service.

     _____ Towel dry the shampooed hair.

     _____ Spray leave-in conditioner into hair if needed.

_____ Apply barrier cream to avoid staining the client's skin.

_____ Section hair with tail of applicator brush or tip of applicator bottle.

___6___ Put on gloves.

_____ Perform hair and scalp analysis.

_____ Towel-blot excess product.

_____ Thoroughly saturate and apply as neatly as possible, following the client's natural hairline.

_____ Blowdry hair to lock in color and help lessen color transfer to client's clothing.

_____ Work very carefully around outer perimeter to ensure no line of demarcations are created.

_____ If product is thin, have client recline at shampoo bowl and use the applicator bottle technique. If product is of thicker viscosity, a bowl and brush maybe used and client may sit up or lay back for comfort.

TRUE OR FALSE

Indicate whether each statement below is true or false. For any false statements, explain why they are false.

160. The application process for a semipermanent haircolor is very different from a demipermanent haircolor application, with a rinse after the desired processing time.

    T   F   _____

161. Semipermanents are deposit-only, so haircolor can build up on the hair with repeated applications.

    T   F   _____

162. Haircolor applied on top of existing color will not necessarily result in a deeper haircolor and won't alter the tone.

    T   F   _____

163. Number the steps in the procedure for performing a demipermanent haircolor application, from 1 to 15. Two steps have been numbered for you.

_____ Part hair into four sections from ear to ear and from front center of forehead to center of nape.

_____ Work color through rest of hair shafts to the ends until hair is fully saturated.

_____ Based on manufacturer's directions, determine if application will be on dry hair or if hair should be shampooed and towel dried.

___11___ Set timer to process.

_____ Put on gloves.

_____ Remove any stains from around hairline with shampoo or stain remover.

___2___ Perform hair and scalp analysis.

_____ Apply protective cream around hairline and over ears.

_____ Drape client for a chemical service.

_____ Outline the partings with color product.

_____ When processing is complete, massage color into a lather and rinse thoroughly with warm water.

_____ Take ½-inch (1.25-centimeter) partings and apply color to new growth or scalp area in all four sections, working with horizontal subsections, starting at nape of rear quadrant and repeating on other back quadrant.

_____ Shampoo colored hair and condition as needed.

_____ When you reach the front, take vertical sections and apply product so hair lies away from the face.

_____ Check haircolor every five minutes as it is processing to ensure you are not overdepositing color on porous hair.

SHORT ANSWER

164. What type of application is used in a single-process haircoloring service?

_____

_____

_____

165. What are two terms for applying haircolor to new growth?

_____

_____

_____

166. What is the difference between a glaze and a gloss? What role do these products play when applying haircolor to new growth or refreshing faded ends?

_____

_____

_____

167. What will happen if you pull permanent color through to the ends during a retouch? What should you use instead to refresh faded ends?

_____

_____

_____

168. What is a line of demarcation? What causes it?

_____

_____

_____

Indicate whether each statement below is true or false. For any false statements, explain why they are false.

169. The procedure for single-process color on virgin hair is performed on damp, freshly shampooed hair.

T   F   _____

170. The first application to the subsections in all four quadrants is made to the midshafts of the hair. This is followed by application of haircolor to the scalp in all four quadrants.

T   F   _____

171. During a single-process color service on virgin hair, you should avoid applying haircolor to the porous ends.

T   F   _____

FILL IN THE BLANK

Complete the sentences below.

172. You may want to perform a strand test with _____ strand(s) because hair _____

and _____ can be different throughout the hair.

173. If the strand test shows that the hair is not light enough, _____ the mixture's

_____ and/or _____ the processing _____ for the lightening service.

174. If the hair strand is too light after completing the strand test, _____ the mixture's

_____ and/or _____ the processing _____ before proceeding with the

lightening service.

175. In all procedures requiring a towel to check for lightening level, ensure that the towel is

_____, not dry. Blot—do not _____—the strand. _____ could roughen

the _____, giving a _____ reading for the entire lightening testing process.

CASE STUDY

176. Your textbook describes some time factors when performing a lightener service on a client. For this exercise, pair up with a partner and work together to determine how each factor affects processing time. Then do a hair analysis on each other to determine the amount of processing time you think it would take for each aspect (short, average, longer time) found in the table below. Then, considering all the factors, guess if your partner would need a short, average, or longer time for a lightening service and note that determination at the end of the table. For a bonus, search online or in beauty magazines for a lightening product and consider its strength to determine an actual processing time. (*Hint:* Most processing times are 50 to 60 minutes.)

TIME FACTOR	HOW THIS AFFECTS PROCESSING TIME	CLASSMATE'S HAIR	SHORT, AVERAGE, OR LONGER TIME?
Melanin			
Porosity			

Tone			
Texture			
Wave and Curl Pattern			
BONUS: Product and Strength			

PARTNER'S PROCESSING TIME (short, average, longer): _____

REFLECTION

177. Now that you've practiced the procedures for various haircolor and lightener applications, as well as patch/strand tests, consider what you knew about these services before you began this section compared to what you've studied. Write a few sentences in which you reflect on and answer the following questions:

   • Can you picture yourself performing the haircolor and lightener application procedures confidently during your examination?

   • Which haircolor/lightener application steps or techniques do you excel at? Which ones are you uncertain about?

   • What surprised you the most about the haircolor/lightener application procedures after you had a chance to practice them?

   • Which procedure turned out the most successfully—for example, in terms of results matching expectations, the safety of your client/health of their hair, or impressive colors? Be specific.

   • Overall, how can you make your haircolor/lightener application flawless for the examination?

   When you're finished, meet with a classmate and discuss your responses. As you do so, look for opportunities to fill in each other's gaps and help each other master the haircolor/lightener application techniques and specifics.

SHORT ANSWER

178. What are the two main parts of the double-process color application?

   _____

   _____

   _____

179. Which beauty goal of a client will require the double-process color application?

_____

_____

_____

180. When using powdered lightener, which ingredient goes into the bowl first—powder or developer? Why?

_____

_____

_____

181. What happens if lightener dries? What can you do to prevent it from drying?

_____

_____

_____

182. What are three possible reasons to stop applying lightener?

_____

_____

_____

183. Describe the strand test that you should conduct when preparing for the toner application part of the double-process color service.

_____

_____

_____

184. After removing the toner from the hair, and rinsing and shampooing it, what type of conditioner should you use? Why?

_____

_____

_____

Indicate whether each statement below is true or false. For any false statements, explain why they are false.

185. For the regrowth application, the mixture is applied only to the new growth as long as that growth is 1 inch (2.5 centimeters) long or less.

    T   F   _____

186. If your client wants to have all-over bleached hair, they will need retouches every three to five weeks to maintain an even tone.

    T   F   _____

187. As with the complete lightener service, pre-stretching may be required for ease of application on curly and coily hair for the retouch service as well.

    T   F   _____

Highlighting Techniques

SHORT ANSWER

188. In general terms, what do highlighting techniques refer to?

    _____

    _____

    _____

189. What are three beauty goals that highlighting (or lowlighting) techniques can help your clients achieve?

    _____

    _____

    _____

190. In your own words, describe the difference between highlighting and lowlighting.

_____

_____

_____

191. What are the two most frequently used highlighting techniques?

_____

_____

_____

192. In the slicing version of the foil technique, what size should the hair sections be? What are three possible consequences of including too much hair in the sections?

_____

_____

_____

193. What two purposes are served by using foil in the foil technique?

_____

_____

_____

194. Which foil technique offers the strongest highlighting effect—slicing or weaving?

_____

_____

_____

195. Describe how a tail comb is used in the weaving foil technique.

_____

_____

_____

196. Why is it important to make sure your subsections are consistent?

_____

_____

_____

197. What is the effect of doing a back-to-back application when using the foil technique?

_____

_____

_____

198. What size should standard subsections be?

_____

_____

_____

LABELING

199. Label the types of foil sections depicted here.

    a. Slicing   c. Weaving (medium)   e. Subsections
    b. Weaving (thin)   d. Weaving (thick)

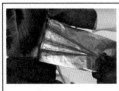 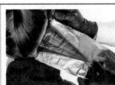 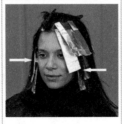 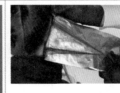 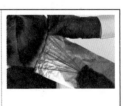

_____ _____ _____ _____ _____

200. What is another term for balayage?

_____

_____

_____

201. Is lightener painted onto wet or dry hair in the balayage technique?

_____

_____

_____

202. What are three keys to performing a successful balayage?

_____

_____

_____

203. What are pintura highlights?

_____

_____

_____

204. How is a balayage board used?

_____

_____

_____

205. What is the maximum level of lift you can expect when using the balayage technique?

_____

_____

_____

206. What are three ways you can process hair when using the balayage technique?

_____

_____

_____

207. How is the color melt technique different from balayage?

_____

_____

_____

208. In the color melt application, where is the base color (the first color) applied on the hair? Where is the second color applied on the hair?

_____

_____

_____

209. How should you blend the two colors to blur any hard lines in the color melt application?

_____

_____

_____

210. How do you use the diffusing technique to achieve a shadow root effect in the color melt procedure? How do you use it to achieve an ombre effect?

_____

_____

_____

TRUE OR FALSE

Indicate whether each statement below is true or false. For any false statements, explain why they are false.

211. Foilayage is a popular newer technique combining balayage with foiling.

T   F   _____

212. The balayage technique enclosed in foil creates a soft balayage look with minimum lift.

T   F   _____

213. Foilayage allows for maximum control in the root and mid-lengths for optimum lift and blending.

T   F   _____

214. If a client has previously tinted hair, a foilayage will be unable to achieve an even lift.

T   F   _____

SEQUENCE

215. Number the steps for performing the pintura balayage procedure, from 1 to 16. Two steps have been numbered for you.

_____ Apply a haircolor glaze/toner from scalp to ends, concentrating on areas where lightener was applied.

_____ Allow lightener to process according to strand test.

_____ Drape client for a chemical service.

_____ Work glaze into hair to ensure it is completely saturated and process per the manufacturer's directions.

_____ Prepare the lightening formula and use it immediately.

_____ Depending on heaviness of lightening desired, select a curl in the same area of the first curl or coiled section, about 1 inch (2.5 centimeters) away and repeat.

_____ Rinse hair, shampoo, condition, and style as desired.

___4___ If product buildup is evident on hair, the hair may need to be shampooed, conditioned, detangled, and dried before application.

_____ Perform hair and scalp analysis.

___10___ Continue working in the horseshoe section, repeating the same steps until the application is complete.

_____ Brush hair out, if possible.

_____ Check for even saturation throughout.

_____ Working in horseshoe-shaped sections around the head and starting at the nape, drop down sections 1 to 2 inches (2.5 to 5 centimeters) thick depending on density.

_____ Brush lightener starting from the desired distance from the scalp or up to the scalp through to the ends, ensuring there is good saturation.

_____ Rinse hair with lukewarm water immediately to prevent color from affecting untreated hair.

_____ Select a gathered curl or coiled section and hold hair taut.

216. Number the steps for starting the cap highlighting procedure, from 1 to 7.

_____ Brush the hair straight back.

_____ Add dots or circles throughout the cap where you want to pull additional hair for specific effects.

_____ Add a shine spray to the shampooed/dried hair if the hair is not slick or tangles easily.

_____ Customize the highlighting by using a thick marker to draw the part line on the cap to indicate where the client normally wears it. (This will help you avoid pulling strands on the part line where regrowth would be most noticeable.)

_____ Conduct a preliminary strand test.

_____ Apply the cap from the forehead to the back, pulling it down to ensure a snug fit that is flat to the scalp.

_____ Shampoo, lightly condition, and then dry the hair.

LABELING

217. Label each type of balayage technique depicted below.

   a. Single point   b. Dual point   c. Three point (or chevron)

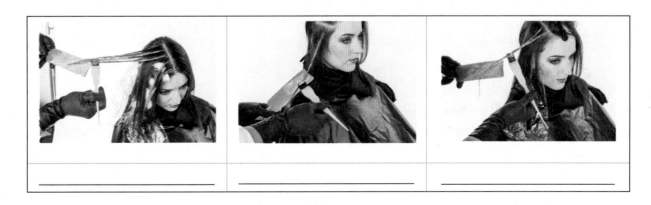

_____ _____ _____

218. Now that you've practiced the procedures for various highlighting techniques, consider what you knew about these services before you began this section compared to what you've studied. Write a few sentences in which you reflect on and answer the following questions:

- Can you picture yourself performing highlighting procedures confidently during your examination?

- Which highlighting application steps or techniques do you excel at? Which ones are you uncertain about?

- Which procedure turned out the most successfully—for example, in terms of the results matching expectations and the safety of your client/health of their hair? Be specific.

- Overall, how can you make your highlighting techniques flawless for the examination?

When you're finished, meet with a classmate and discuss your responses. As you do so, look for opportunities to fill in each other's gaps and help each other master the highlighting techniques and specifics.

Gray Hair Coverage Techniques

SHORT ANSWER

219. Why is it important to become an expert in gray coverage?

_____

_____

_____

220. What is the medical term for hair grayness or whiteness? What causes it?

_____

_____

_____

221. List four solutions for reducing or eliminating a yellow cast in gray hair.

_____

_____

_____

222. What are three other considerations, in addition to the guidelines in Tables 16-4 and 16-5 in your text, for gray hair formulation?

_____

_____

_____

LABELING

223. Label each image of natural level 5 hair with the percentage of gray depicted.

    a. 30 percent gray   c. 75 percent gray
    b. 50 percent gray   d. 100 percent gray

Roman Samborskyi/Shutterstock.com   Yaroslav Astakhov/Shutterstock.com   NinaMalyna/Shutterstock.com

_____   _____   _____   _____

TRUE OR FALSE

Indicate whether each statement below is true or false. For any false statements, explain why they are false.

224. Level 8 or lighter haircolors give complete coverage of gray hair despite their low dye concentration.

    T   F   _____

225. It can be challenging to cover gray hair because it of its low porosity.

    T   F   _____

226. Clients with both coarse hair and greater than 70 percent gray can be the most difficult to cover.

    T   F   _____

227. When covering the unpigmented hair on a salt-and-pepper head, formulate one to two levels darker than the natural level to ensure a more natural result when doing complete coverage.

T   F   _____

228. For a strand test and final formulation, you should use a manufacturer's product color chart in conjunction with Tables 16-4 and 16-5 to select a color within the proper level.

T   F   _____

229. Natural redheads and warm blondes will not have an ash tone as they gray.

T   F   _____

230. For clients who are 80 to 100 percent gray, a haircolor within the blonde range is generally less blendable and more maintenance than darker shades.

T   F   _____

231. You can counteract the resistance to color by using a higher developer volume to strengthen the color mixture or by pre-softening the hair.

T   F   _____

FILL IN THE BLANK

232. Complete the table below.

PERCENTAGE OF GRAY HAIR	SEMIPERMANENT/DEMIPERMANENT COLOR FORMULATION FOR GRAY HAIR	PERMANENT COLOR FORMULATION FOR GRAY HAIR
	Desired level	
70–90%		
	One level lighter than desired level	
		Two parts lighter level and one part desired level
		One level lighter

SHORT ANSWER

233. At what level should you formulate haircolor for the best gray coverage? What volume developer should you use?

_____

_____

_____

234. How long should you process color for gray coverage?

_____

_____

_____

235. What types of tones should you add to the formula for gray coverage? Why?

_____

_____

_____

236. What percentage of natural tones should you use in your formula if 25 percent gray is present? If 50 percent gray is present? 75 percent gray?

_____

_____

_____

237. What volume developer should you use when you prepare your haircolor formula for coverage of resistant gray hair? What level should your formula be?

_____

_____

_____

238. What size sections should you use in gray color-resistant areas?

_____

_____

_____

239. What are two different items you can apply to hair, after the application is finished, to keep resistant hairs saturated?

_____

_____

_____

Special Haircolor Challenges and Solutions

ROLE PLAY

240. Partner with a classmate to practice how you might handle a situation where a color service did not turn out as expected. Take turns playing the role of client and colorist. In this scenario, the client expected an ash blonde color, but their hair turned out darker. They have a job interview in two days and the pressure is on. The client gasps when they see the final result, and the colorist is surprised, especially given all the time and care they put into consulting with the client, examining the client's photo examples, and preparing the formulation.

As you work through the scenario (in both roles), pay attention to the tone of your voice, your body language, and the goal of the conversation. Coach each other and learn from each other. This will help you refine your approach with future clients and minimize your stress when you encounter these types of situations in the salon.

IN THE ROLE OF CLIENT	IN THE ROLE OF COLORIST
• Express your disappointment • Ask the colorist what happened (e.g., chemical mistake? communication understanding?) • Find out what can be done to fix the color • Explain the limits on your time/schedule • Indicate that you might go to another salon to correct the problem • Ask for a discount • Mention the possibility of a negative online review	• Remain calm • Determine the nature of the problem • Determine what caused the problem • Develop a solution • Always take one step at a time • Never guarantee an exact result

WORD SCRAMBLE

241. Unscramble the signs of damaged hair below.

OGRUH XRUTTEE _____ _____

VYLOER ROOPUS _____ _____

TLTEIRB NAD RYD _____ _____ _____

KRAABGEE _____

OROP LICISTEYAS _____ _____

GYPSON DNA DMETAT HWEN TWE _____ _____ _____ _____ _____

OCLOR AEFDS ILCQKUY _____ _____ _____

242. What is a common problem for clients who have color-treated red hair?

_____

_____

_____

243. How can you created warm coppery reds?

_____

_____

_____

244. What is a way to create neutral to cool reds?

_____

_____

_____

245. What are two ways to avoid orange or brassy tones when lifting brown hair?

_____

_____

_____

246. What is the best way to obtain pale blonde results?

_____

_____

_____

247. For each aspect of haircolor services specific to textured hair listed below, describe the haircolor consideration or tip associated with it.

TEXTURED HAIR FEATURES	HAIRCOLOR CONSIDERATIONS AND TIPS FOR TEXTURED HAIR
Day-to-day style	
Porosity	
Desired highlight pattern	
Stretching	
Overnight care	
Detangling	
Other chemical services	
Curl pattern	

TRUE OR FALSE

Indicate whether each statement below is true or false. For any false statements, explain why they are false.

248. To achieve natural-looking highlights in brown hair, highlighted pieces should be no more than two levels lighter than the balance of the hair.

T   F   _____

249. When lightening brown hair to blonde, there will be underlying unwanted warm tones.

T   F   _____

250. When lightening blonde hair level 7 or higher, there will be a higher concentration of pheomelanin and unwanted orange tones that will appear immediately.

T   F   _____

251. A few days at the pool or beach will have a stronger fading effect on blonde hair than on red hair.

T   F   _____

252. If highlights become too blonde or all one color, lowlights or deeper strands can be foiled into the hair to create a more natural color.

T   F   _____

253. You can use an all-over glaze to add warmth and shine to an overprocessed blonde, and choosing shades with gold tones helps keep the sparkle in pale blondes.

T   F   _____

254. Most blondes typically want to be ash blonde, which is also suitable for all skin tones.

T   F   _____

FILL IN THE BLANK

255. Complete the chart below. Some problems will have more than one solution or tip.

COMMON HAIRCOLOR PROBLEM	COMMON HAIRCOLOR SOLUTION OR TIPS
Too-light haircolor	
	Place haircolor swatches on the client's existing hair to show the difference in level and color; study the existing regrowth if there is any, and, if using a semi- or demipermanent color, select a level lighter than the targeted color
Green cast	
	Add a few highlights to give an overall appearance of lighter hair or apply haircolor remover to the areas that need lightening, then reapply the color ratios you originally used, only one to two levels lighter
Faded color	

Haircoloring Safety Precautions

DOS AND DON'TS

256. Indicate whether each safety tip or precaution for performing haircoloring services is something you should do (Do) or something that you should not do (Don't).

DO OR DON'T?	WHEN PERFORMING HAIRCOLORING SERVICES
	Apply haircolor if the patch test is negative
	Perform a strand test for elasticity, porosity, and breakage
	Perform a color service if damage is present
	Use a mild shampoo
	Allow the color to get into the client's eyes
	Perform a patch test 24 to 48 hours before each application of aniline-derivative haircolor

DO OR DON'T?	WHEN PERFORMING HAIRCOLORING SERVICES
	Use a metal bowl or whisk to mix the haircolor
	Apply haircolor if abrasions are present on the scalp
	Discard leftover haircolor
	Apply haircolor if a metallic haircolor is present
	Wear gloves when working with chemicals to protect your hands and prevent developing dermatitis
	Brush the hair before applying color
	Read and follow the manufacturer's directions
	Wash hands before and after servicing a client
	Use an alkaline or harsh shampoo
	Overlap colors during a haircolor retouch
	Perform a metallic salts test
	Use cleaned and disinfected applicator bottles, brushes, combs, and towels
	Perform the service if the strand tests positive for metallic salts
	Protect your client's clothing with proper draping
	Use an applicator bottle or bowl (glass or plastic) to mix the haircolor
	Mix haircolor before you are ready to use it

Tip: For additional safety guidelines and precautions, you may wish to visit your state's licensing website to review the specific requirements related to performing haircoloring services.

GOAL SETTING: PART 2

257. In the beginning of this chapter, you listed five things about hair color and haircoloring services that you expected to learn, along with a plan for how you expected to achieve each of the five goals you listed. You were also provided with an additional goal that all hair colorists are expected to set for themselves regarding safety procedures and chemicals.

    Now it's time to review your goals (including the safety goal) and what you learned, as well as reflect on how your plan turned out. Use the chart below to guide your reflections. (*Hint:* In the first column, copy your original five goals to make it easier to complete the rest of the chart.)

I EXPECTED TO LEARN ... ABOUT HAIR COLOR AND HAIRCOLORING SERVICES	I DID ... TO ACHIEVE THIS GOAL	MY PLAN TURNED OUT ... BECAUSE ...
I expect to learn about the chemicals, related procedures, and other precautions required to safely perform haircoloring services.		
1.		
2.		
3.		

I EXPECTED TO LEARN ... ABOUT HAIR COLOR AND HAIRCOLORING SERVICES	I DID ... TO ACHIEVE THIS GOAL	MY PLAN TURNED OUT ... BECAUSE ...
4.		
5.		

DISCOVERIES AND ACCOMPLISHMENTS

In the space below, write notes about key concepts discussed in this chapter. Share your discoveries with some of the other students in your class and ask them if your notes are helpful. You may want to revise your notes based on good ideas shared by your peers.

Discoveries:

_____

_____

_____

_____

_____

_____

List at least three things you have accomplished since you decided to enroll in school.

Accomplishments:

_____

_____

_____

_____

_____

_____

1. Identify an accurate statement related to haircoloring.

   A) Haircolor services offer creative expression and artistry for clients as well as stylists.

   B) Haircoloring is seldom a lucrative service for stylists and salons.

   C) Haircolor services seldom contribute to client loyalty.

   D) Haircolor products are typically devoid of strong chemical ingredients.

2. When the cuticle is tight and the hair is resistant to moisture, the hair has _____.

   A) high porosity   C) low porosity

   B) average porosity   D) medium porosity

3. The _____ is a measurement system that colorists utilize to determine the lightness or darkness of artificial and natural hair color.

   A) patch test   C) law of color

   B) level system   D) color system

4. Which of the following hair levels is considered the darkest according to the level system?

   A) hair level 1   C) hair level 5

   B) hair level 10   D) hair level 8

5. _____ light should be used when analyzing hair color for best results.

   A) Incandescent   C) Natural

   B) Halogen   D) Fluorescent

6. _____ colors are fundamental or pure colors that cannot be made by mixing other colors.

   A) Base   C) Primary

   B) Secondary   D) Complementary

continued

7. Demipermanent haircolor _____.

   A) is usually mixed with a high-volume developer

   B) replaces lost tonality prior to a color correction

   C) generally contains ammonia

   D) is a plant-based dye with very limited shades

8. To deposit haircolor or, when little or no lift is required, to enhance a client's natural haircolor, _____-volume hydrogen peroxide is utilized.

   A) 20

   B) 30

   C) 10

   D) 40

9. Which of the following statements is accurate about a lightener?

   A) It has a lower pH than permanent haircolors.

   B) It colorizes the natural hair pigment.

   C) It helps change the hair texture by eroding the cuticle layers and causing curl reduction.

   D) It is also known as a developer.

10. Off-scalp lighteners _____.

    A) are categorized as oil or cream lighteners

    B) create overall blonding and lightening retouches

    C) are fast-acting, strong, and formulated to lift the hair from four to seven levels

    D) have conditioning agents that allow them to be applied to the scalp with less irritation

11. Permanent, or traditional, toners are _____.

    A) great for highlighting services because they do not lift existing natural color

    B) pigmented shampoos that deposit color

    C) applied to pre-lightened hair to achieve pale blonde shades at level 9 and level 10

    D) usually mixed with a high-volume developer

continued

12. Which of the following steps needs to be followed when consulting with clients before a haircolor service?

    A) During the consultation, avoid asking questions to clients that require more than a yes or no answer.

    B) After gathering all pertinent information, avoid offering clients more than what they ask for.

    C) Refrain from asking clients to sign the salon's release statement.

    D) Refrain from promising more than you realistically can deliver.

13. Which of the following points should be kept in mind in the context of haircolor application tools and mixing haircolor?

    A) As a rule, use an applicator bottle to apply products with a thicker viscosity.

    B) Avoid measuring products using a scale to ensure formulation.

    C) When using a measuring cup to ensure formulation, rest the cup on a flat, even surface to ensure accuracy.

    D) Use an applicator brush to mix color to ensure accurate formulation and application.

14. According to the U.S. Food, Drug, and Cosmetic Act, a patch test should be performed _____ before each application of haircolor formulated with aniline derivative dyes.

    A) 24 to 48 hours   C) four to five hours

    B) eight to ten hours   D) 48 to 72 hours

15. Which of the following is a step for applying haircolor to new growth and faded ends?

    A) processing haircolor based on your analysis and the results of a strand test

    B) pulling permanent color through to the ends

    C) applying haircolor to overlap previously colored hair

    D) using a glaze to coat the hair with a permanent haircolor and extreme shine

16. Which of the following points is true regarding hair lightening processing time?

    A) The darker the natural hair color, the less melanin it has and the lesser time it takes to lighten the color.

    B) Nonporous hair of the same color level will lighten faster than porous hair.

continued

C) Stronger lighteners result in pale shades in the fastest time though they can be more damaging to the hair.

D) Fine hair has a thicker cuticle layer, resulting in a longer processing time than coarse hair.

17. Coloring some of the hair strands lighter than the natural color in order to add a variety of lighter shades and the illusion of depth is known as _____.

A) highlighting

C) fusion bonding

B) lowlighting

D) chemical hair relaxing

18. In the context of highlighting techniques, identify a tip related to the foiling technique.

A) Remember that foiling is ineffective for maximum lift.

B) When choosing your foil patterns, remember that vertical lines create width.

C) After making a straight part at the scalp, make a weaving parting by taking 1-inch hair sections.

D) Remember that a slicing parting provides the strongest effect when highlighting.

19. Which of the following guidelines should be followed when using a balayage application technique?

A) Choose this technique when only 5 levels of lift or more are desired.

B) Paint lightener directly onto clean, dry hair to provide a more natural-looking highlight.

C) Perform true balayage using the foil technique.

D) Start the technique with a heavy application of lightener on the scalp.

20. What is the medical term for hair grayness or whiteness?

A) hirsuties

C) canities

B) monilethrix

D) pityriasis

21. If the percentage of gray hair is 70–90 percent, what is the permanent color formulation for the gray hair?

A) equal parts desired and lighter level

C) desired level for all parts

B) two parts desired level and one-part lighter level

D) one level lighter for all parts

continued

22. Which of the following is a beneficial tip when haircoloring?

   A) For brunettes, lighten more than two levels above the natural color in order to avoid unwanted brassy tones.

   B) For brunettes, always use a cool red base to avoid orange or brassy tones when lifting brown hair with permanent color.

   C) For redheads, use a red-orange or red-gold base color to create neutral to cool reds.

   D) For redheads, always use a demipermanent color to refresh the shaft and ends after coloring the hair with a permanent color.

23. Identify a common haircolor solution.

   A) To correct overlightened hair caused by the formula you used or sun fade, apply a demipermanent color that is two levels lighter than the previous formula.

   B) To refresh faded color, mix a demipermanent haircolor in a different tonal family and two levels darker than the original haircolor formula.

   C) If the client's hair has mineral buildup from chlorine or well water, purify the hair with a product that is formulated to remove mineral buildup.

   D) Add a few highlights to a too-dark color to accentuate the solid dark color and give an overall appearance of darker hair.

24. Which of the following is a haircoloring safety precaution?

   A) Avoid applying haircolor if there are abrasions on the scalp.

   B) Brush the hair before applying color.

   C) Overlap during a haircolor retouch.

   D) Avoid using a mild shampoo; instead use an alkaline shampoo.

25. As a haircoloring safety precaution, cosmetologists should _____.

   A) apply haircolor when a metallic haircolor is present

   B) use a metallic applicator bottle or bowl to mix the haircolor

   C) brush the hair before applying color

   D) conduct a strand test for porosity, elasticity, and breakage

finished!

Practical Skills

Self-Evaluation Checklist

Regular self-assessment helps you to improve your technical skills and achieve success. After performing each procedure, review the procedure steps in the textbook and rate yourself as "Competent" or "Needs Work," and write in comments on how you were successful or where you can improve. Rating yourself helps you identify your strengths and weaknesses and develop your own plan for improvement.

CRITERIA	COMPETENT	NEEDS WORK	COMMENTS
PROCEDURE 16-1 PRELIMINARY PATCH TEST AND STRAND TEST			
Preparation			
Procedure			
Post-Service			
Timing			
PROCEDURE 16-2 TEMPORARY HAIRCOLOR RINSE			
Preparation			
Procedure			
Post-Service			
Timing			
PROCEDURE 16-3 DEMIPERMANENT HAIRCOLOR APPLICATION			
Preparation			
Procedure			
Post-Service			
Timing			
PROCEDURE 16-4 SINGLE-PROCESS COLOR ON VIRGIN HAIR			
Preparation			
Procedure			
Post-Service			
Timing			
PROCEDURE 16-5 PERMANENT SINGLE-PROCESS RETOUCH WITH A GLAZE			
Preparation			
Procedure			
Post-Service			
Timing			
PROCEDURE 16-6 VIRGIN LIGHTENER			
Preparation			
Procedure			
Post-Service			
Timing			
PROCEDURE 16-7 TONER APPLICATION			
Preparation			
Procedure			
Post-Service			
Timing			

Practical Skills

CRITERIA	COMPETENT	NEEDS WORK	COMMENTS
PROCEDURE 16-8 SPECIALTY HIGHLIGHTING WITH FOIL			
Preparation			
Procedure			
Post-Service			
Timing			
PROCEDURE 16-9 PINTURA HIGHLIGHTS			
Preparation			
Procedure			
Post-Service			
Timing			
PROCEDURE 16-10 COLOR MELT			
Preparation			
Procedure			
Post-Service			
Timing			
PROCEDURE 16-11 PERMANENT GRAY COVERAGE			
Preparation			
Procedure			
Post-Service			
Timing			

Ch. 17: Hair Removal

TRACK MY PROGRESS!

Use this simple tracker to record your progress as you work through the activities in each learning objective.

COMPLETED	# OF CORRECT ANSWERS	OBJECTIVE
☐	_____/3	**LO 1** - Explain how hair removal knowledge will enhance your success as a cosmetologist.
☐	_____/3	**LO 2** - Identify excessive hair growth causes.
☐	_____/13	**LO 3** - List temporary hair removal methods.
☐	_____/11	**LO 4** - Describe three permanent hair reduction methods.
☐	_____/12	**LO 5** - Outline the approach to client consultation for hair removal services.
☐	_____/4	**LO 6** - Identify hair removal contraindications.

Why Study Hair Removal?

SHORT ANSWER

1. What are the two major categories of hair removal? Which ones can be performed by cosmetologists?

_____

_____

_____

2. Other than clients seeking hair removal for fashion or image concerns, what other group tends to use hair reduction services?

_____

_____

_____

3. What are the three reasons that cosmetologists should have a thorough understanding of hair removal?

_____

_____

_____

Excessive Hair Growth

MATCHING

4. Match each statement to the corresponding type of excessive hair growth. Types will be used more than once.

   a. Hypertrichosis   b. Hirsutism

Type of Excessive Hair Growth	Description
_____	Excessive hair growth on the face, chest, underarms, and groin
_____	More common in women
_____	Excessive hair growth of terminal hair in the areas of the body that normally only grow vellus hair
_____	Genetically and ethnically inherited
_____	Can affect anyone
_____	May be caused by stimulation of male androgens at puberty, medications, illness, and stress
_____	Caused by excessive male androgens in the blood
_____	Can grow in thick patches or completely cover the face, back, or other areas of the body

5. What are three factors that can influence excessive (dense) hair growth?

_____

_____

_____

6. What is the main difference between hirsutism and hypertrichosis?

_____

_____

_____

Temporary Hair Removal

SHORT ANSWER

7. Why is there a common misconception that shaving hair makes it grow back thicker and stronger?

_____

_____

_____

8. What is an epilator? Provide an example.

_____

_____

_____

9. List the three types of temporary hair removal methods that require advanced training.

_____

_____

_____

10. Match each type of temporary hair removal method with its description. The types will be used more than once.

    a. Shaving   c. Depilatories   e. Threading
    b. Tweezing   d. Waxing   f. Sugaring

Temporary Hair Removal Method	Description
_____	Contain(s) detergents to strip the hair's sebum and adhesives to hold the chemicals to the hair shaft for the time necessary to remove the hair; during the application, the hair expands and the disulfide bonds break
_____	Razors, electric clippers, or trimmers may be used
_____	Method of entwining the hair and lifting it from the follicle
_____	Commonly used to shape eyebrows and remove undesirable hairs around the mouth and chin
_____	A common epilator
_____	Practiced in many Eastern cultures and some salons throughout the world, and is increasingly popular in the United States
_____	Similar to, but often less painful than, waxing
_____	Turns hair into a soft, jelly-like mass that can be removed from the skin
_____	Involves pulling one hair at a time out by the root
_____	The best choice for larger areas and an excellent choice for sensitive areas, such as the upper lip, inner thighs, or bikini area
_____	Common form of temporary hair removal
_____	Viewed as holistic hair removal because it is eco-friendly, in the form of a natural-ingredient paste
_____	Named for the implement that's used
_____	Available in various forms, including tubs and beads melted in a heater
_____	Can be inflammatory to skin and should not be used on sensitive skin types or on clients with waxing contraindications

11. Number the steps for performing an eyebrow waxing with soft wax, from 1 to 11, beginning after the wax has been melted in the heater for 10 to 25 minutes.

_____ Repeat steps on the other eyebrow, and then the glabella (the area between the brows).

_____ Remove the client's makeup, cleanse the area thoroughly with a mild cleanser, and dry.

_____ Brush the eyebrows with a small brush.

_____ Finish with aftercare.

_____ Test the heated wax's temperature and consistency.

_____ Apply a strip over the waxed area, leaving a free edge at the endpoint to grasp.

_____ Drape and position the client for service and then wash hands.

_____ Place the index finger and middle finger at the endpoint, holding the skin taut, and quickly pull the strip back against the hair growth, as close to the skin as possible.

_____ *Optional:* Pretreat the area to be waxed with the wax manufacturer's recommended products for soft wax.

_____ Immediately apply pressure to the waxed area with your gloved finger, holding for approximately five seconds to relieve any discomfort.

_____ Standing behind the client, glide the applicator at a 45-degree angle along the underside of the brow from the nose point to the outer edge, following the desired line for hair to be removed.

12. Indicate whether each safety tip or precaution for performing wax services is something you should do (Do) or something that you should not do (Don't).

Do or Don't? | **When Performing Wax Services**

_____ Always test the heated wax's temperature on your and your client's wrist

_____ To heat wax quickly, use a microwave or stovetop

_____ When removing hair from the same client, you can reuse the same spatula

_____ Avoid applying wax over warts, moles, abrasions, or irritated skin, even if there is hair there

_____ Use hard wax for sensitive skin, such as underarm skin

_____ Apply aloe gel and a cool compress after a waxing service

_____ Allow the wax to come in contact with the client's eyes

_____ Hold the skin loosely when removing a wax strip

_____ Use a wax pot that warms from both the bottom and the sides

FILL IN THE BLANK

13. The table below is a quick reference guide intended to show which temporary hair removal methods are appropriate for which parts of the body. Place an X where the method is appropriate for the body area.

TEMPORARY HAIR REMOVAL SERVICES						
BODY AREA	SHAVING	TWEEZING	DEPILATORY	WAXING	SUGARING	THREADING
Face/upper lips/eyebrows						
Underarms						
Arms						
Bikini line						
Back/shoulders						
Legs						
Tops of feet/toes						

TRUE OR FALSE

Indicate whether each statement is true or false. For any false statements, explain why they are false.

14. The two forms of wax, hard and soft, are both made primarily of resins and polymers but can also be made from sugars, honey, and sometimes beeswax.

   T   F   _____

15. Electric clippers or trimmers are not recommended for removing unwanted hair at the nape of the neck.

   T   F   _____

16. The eyebrow's natural arch follows the occipital bone, or the curved line of the eye socket, but hair can grow above and below the natural line.

     T   F   _____

17. Sugaring can be applied and removed in both directions (with hair growth and against hair growth), depending on the manufacturer's instructions.

     T   F   _____

18. Hard wax is somewhat thicker than soft wax and requires fabric strips for removal.

     T   F   _____

REFLECTION

19. As you expand your knowledge of the range of services that a cosmetologist can offer, think about the six types of temporary hair removal methods available and envision yourself performing them in a salon. Now rank them below, in order from the one that you find most appealing (1) to the least (6), and briefly explain your ranking for each one.

    Shaving, Tweezing, Depilatories, Waxing, Threading, Sugaring

    1. _____

    2. _____

    3. _____

    4. _____

    5. _____

    6. _____

Permanent Hair Reduction

SHORT ANSWER

20. What tool is used for electrolysis, and how is it performed?

    _____

    _____

    _____

21. What is another term for intense pulsed light (IPL)?

_____

_____

_____

22. In addition to achieving permanent hair reduction, what is an advantage of using IPL?

_____

_____

_____

23. What is a risk associated with IPL, making it a less popular technique for permanent hair reduction?

_____

_____

_____

CROSSWORD

24. Complete the crossword on different types of permanent hair reduction and temporary hair removal services.

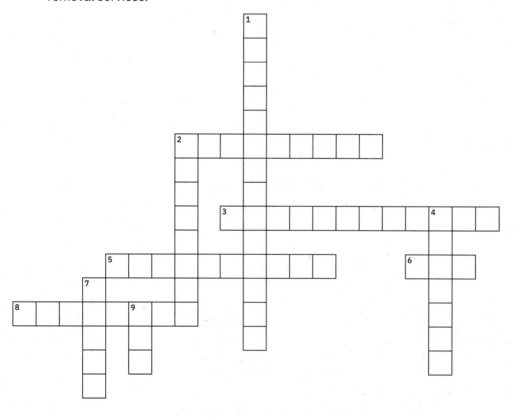

Across

2. Implement that is twisted and rolled along the skin, entwining the hair and lifting it from the follicle
3. Removal of hair by means of an electric current that destroys the growth cells of hair
5. Uses chemicals to dissolve hair at the skin's surface
6. The most common epilator that removes hair from the follicle's base
8. Uses a thick paste made of all-natural ingredients to remove hair from the follicle's base

Down

1. Technique that uses intense light to destroy the growth cells of the hair follicles
2. Pulls one hair at a time out by the root and is usually done as part of a professional makeup service
4. Both manual and electric tools used to cut the hairs at the skin
7. Reduction method in which a beam pulses on the skin, impairing hair growth
9. The abbreviation for the method that uses pulsed light to destroy the follicle's growth cells

TRUE OR FALSE

Indicate whether the statements below are true or false. For any false statements, explain why they are false.

25. Depending on state law, some cosmetologists can administer IPL in salons.

    T   F   _____

26. Laser hair removal is most effective on follicles that are in the telogen phase.

    T   F   _____

27. In certain states, certified cosmetologists or estheticians can perform laser hair removal under a physician's supervision. This method requires specialized training, which is most commonly offered by laser equipment manufacturers.

    T   F   _____

28. Light-haired clients have the best results with laser hair removal; clients whose hair is darker than the surrounding skin have less success.

    T   F   _____

29. Laws regarding IPL and laser hair removal services vary by state, so it's important to check with your regulatory agency for guidelines.

    T   F   _____

RESEARCH

30. Because state laws and regulations vary regarding who can perform certain methods of permanent hair reduction, it's important to find out what your options and limitations are as a cosmetologist. Use the Internet to search your state's laws regarding who is permitted to perform electrolysis, IPL, and laser hair removal. Find out what the licensing, certification, and other requirements are. Then check out your state's scope of practice for these services. Jot down your resources and findings here.

If you're interested in eventually performing these services, this information will be very helpful to as you continue to make choices about your studies and career path. (And even if you think, at this point, that you might not be interested in performing these services, it will be useful to have a sense of what's possible in case you change your mind or an interesting opportunity arises in the future.)

_____

_____

_____

Client Consultation

SHORT ANSWER

31. Where should the cosmetologist record the information about allergies or sensitivities that were provided on the client intake form?

_____

_____

_____

32. What is the purpose of the waxing release form?

_____

_____

_____

33. Why is it important to know the medications a client is on before performing a hair removal service?

_____

_____

_____

34. Review the client intake form (Figure 17-12) in your textbook, then follow the link below to find a copy you can print or fill out online. Take a few moments to complete the form; you can be honest about your allergies or the medications you're on, or you can make up your answers for an imaginary client. Then pair up with a classmate and take turns being client and cosmetologist. As the cosmetologist, would you perform hair removal services on your client? As the client, how would you react if you were denied the service? As the cosmetologist, be sure to explain your answer to your client about why you can or cannot do the service, answer their questions, and remain firm in your decision while being respectful. This exercise is meant to be good practice for a situation you will find yourself in with clients in a salon, so when you're done, share with your partner what you learned from each other's responses.

+ BONUS

Visit: bonus.milady.com/cos-wb/toc

TRUE OR FALSE

Indicate whether the statements below are true or false. For any false statements, explain why they are false.

35. After eyebrow, lip, or chin waxing services, brush on a 100 percent pure mineral face powder to camouflage residual redness.

    T   F   _____

36. Avoid applying an aloe vera gel or other product to the waxed area for the first 24 hours.

    T   F   _____

37. Soak in a hot tub or Jacuzzi within two hours following a body waxing service.

    T   F   _____

38. Avoid sunbathing or prolonged sun exposure for all waxed areas for at least 48 hours. Thereafter, protect the skin with a broad-spectrum, mineral-based sunscreen.

    T   F   _____

39. Use a mild exfoliating scrub or loofah, starting one week after a body waxing, to prevent ingrown hairs.

    T   F   _____

40. Why is it important to ask on the client intake form if the client requires accommodations?

_____

_____

_____

41. What are three or four questions you can ask your client during the consultation to elicit more specific answers, and therefore provide a more customized and accurate hair removal experience?

_____

_____

_____

SEQUENCE

42. Put the following steps of the post-service procedure in order, from 1 to 15. Some steps are given to you.

_____ Escort client to the reception desk, where they can purchase the recommended home care products and discuss when the next service should be.

_____ Remove all dirty laundry from the hamper and spray the hamper with disinfection spray or wipe it down with a disinfectant.

___14___ Change disinfection solution.

_____ Turn off and unplug all equipment, including wax heaters.

_____ Replenish the room with fresh spatulas, linens, utensils, and other supplies for the next day, including replacing any empty jars.

_____ Vacuum and mop the room with a disinfectant. (*Optional:* You can also spray the air in the room with a disinfectant aerosol spray).

_____ Ask the client how they feel and how their skin feels. Discuss any skin conditions and what can be done to improve them.

___5___ Record service information, observations, and product recommendations on the service record card.

_____ Thoroughly clean and disinfect all multiuse tools and supplies.

_____ Put on a fresh pair of gloves.

_____ Schedule next appointment and thank the client.

_____ Empty waste container and replace with a clean liner.

_____ Clean and disinfect all counters, the treatment chair, machines, other furniture, and both sides of the magnifying lamp.

_____ Outline proper home care and explain each home care product step by step.

_____ Discard all used single-use brushes, spatulas, utensils, and supplies.

Hair Removal Contraindications

SHORT ANSWER

43. What are your two options, as a cosmetologist, if you suspect your client has any of the contraindications for waxing services?

_____

_____

_____

44. What is one of the main purposes of the client consultation?

_____

_____

_____

45. Complete the table below.

CONTRAINDICATIONS	WHAT TO AVOID	WHY?
Heart conditions/pacemaker		
		Steroids can cause thinning of the skin, which can result in blistering or injury.
Metal bone pins or plates in the body		
Open sores, herpes simplex		
	Facial or body waxing and extraction without physician's permission	
	Known allergens, fragrances	
	Electrical or light treatments	
Exfoliating drugs (Retin-A®, Differin®)		
	Electrical treatments; any questionable treatment without physician's written permission, possible waxing sensitivities	

46. Choose two of the contraindications for receiving wax services from the list in your textbook and conduct some research on them. Use the Internet, go to the library, check medical books, and so on to learn more about each one, such as what the condition causes or medication treats (including the side effects) and how waxing services can be harmful to the client. Then use that information to write a more detailed explanation (one to two paragraphs) explaining why you think those conditions or medications might prevent a client from receiving hair removal services. Think of this as a primer so that if you must decline a waxing service, you can kindly explain why to your client. Once you've completed your paragraphs, meet with a classmate and explain your findings to each other. What did you learn from your classmate's research?

DISCOVERIES AND ACCOMPLISHMENTS

In the space below, write notes about key concepts discussed in this chapter. Share your discoveries with some of the other students in your class and ask them if your notes are helpful. You may want to revise your notes based on good ideas shared by your peers.

Discoveries:

_____

_____

_____

_____

_____

_____

_____

List at least three things you have accomplished since you decided to enroll in school.

Accomplishments:

_____

_____

_____

_____

_____

_____

_____

1. Cosmetologists should have a thorough understanding of hair removal because _____.

   A) performing procedures that are listed under any podiatry license is a primary responsibility of cosmetologists

   B) removing unwanted hair is many clients' primary concern and advising them on various types of hair removal enhances the ability of cosmetologists to satisfy their clients

   C) they are physicians specialized in a medical branch of science that involves the study of hair and its structure

   D) they are required to inform clients about the parts of the hair that will be affected by the hair removal services availed by the clients

2. Identify a reason why cosmetologists should have a thorough understanding of hair removal.

   A) Cosmetologists are required to perform procedures that are listed under any medical license.

   B) Cosmetologists are required to inform clients about all hair removal techniques in detail before performing any services on them.

   C) Offering clients hair removal services that can be scheduled while they are already in the salon is a valuable extra service.

   D) Learning about hair structure and hair removal is essential in order to tell a client that a specific hair disease or disorder is present and to suggest ways to treat it.

3. Which of the following is a condition of excessive hair growth on the face, chest, underarms, and groin in females?

   A) trichoptilosis   C) hirsutism

   B) tinea   D) canities

4. _____ is excessive terminal hair growth in body areas that normally grow only vellus hair.

   A) Monilethrix   C) Trichoptilosis

   B) Hypertrichosis   D) Pityriasis

5. Identify a temporary hair removal method.

   A) electrolysis   C) shaving

   B) photoepilation   C) laser hair removal

continued

6. Which of the following statements is true of tweezing?

   A) It does not require a client consultation.

   B) It involves twisting and rolling cotton thread along the surface of the skin, entwining the hair in the thread, and lifting it from the follicle.

   C) It is commonly used to shape eyebrows and remove undesirable hairs around the mouth and chin.

   D) It can be used to remove hair from the arms, underarms, and legs.

7. A(n) _____ is a substance, usually a caustic alkali preparation, used to temporarily remove superfluous hair by dissolving it at the skin's surface.

   A) curette   C) emollient

   B) epilator   D) depilatory

8. Which of the following is a substance that is used to remove hair by pulling them from the follicle's base?

   A) a depilatory   C) a curette

   B) an epilator   D) an emollient

9. Why should you perform a patch test on the client before a waxing service?

   A) to determine how thick the wax should be for effective results

   B) to ensure the wax does not cause rashes or redness on the client's skin

   C) to test the temperature of the wax

   D) to ensure the wax does not remove the hair protruding from any moles or abrasions

10. Identify a true statement about waxing.

    A) The time between waxings is generally eight to ten weeks.

    B) The hair should be at least 0.10-inch long for waxing to be effective.

    C) Hard wax is an excellent choice for sensitive areas, such as the upper lip, inner thighs, or bikini area.

    D) Soft wax does not require fabric strips for removal.

continued

11. Which of the following is a concern for soft wax that is *not* a concern for hard wax?

    A) the temperature of the wax

    B) the thickness of the wax

    C) the direction of removal

    D) the angle of application to the skin

12. Which of the following guidelines should you follow when using soft wax?

    A) Use soft wax only for sensitive areas such as the underarms.

    B) Take off the hair removal strip in the direction of the hair growth.

    C) Always apply the wax in the direction of the hair growth.

    D) Apply the wax in a thin layer perpendicular to the skin.

13. Identify a safety precaution that you should take when performing a waxing service.

    A) Use a wax pot that heats the wax only from the bottom.

    B) Never apply aloe gel on waxed skin.

    C) Only apply soft wax over moles or abrasions.

    D) Hold the skin taut to prevent lifting or bruising.

14. Which of the following safety precautions should you take when performing waxing?

    A) Always heat the wax in a microwave or on a stovetop.

    B) To prevent burns, always test the heated wax's temperature on the tip of your index finger.

    C) Never double dip wax.

    D) Never use hard wax on sensitive skin.

15. Identify a true statement about sugaring.

    A) It is appropriate for sensitive skin types.

    B) It is often more painful than waxing.

    C) It can only be used on hair that is shorter than 0.05 inches.

    D) It can be applied and removed in only one direction.

continued

16. Which of the following methods of hair removal can be applied and removed both in the direction of hair growth and against it?

    A) waxing

    C) banding

    B) sugaring

    D) tweezing

17. Sugaring is viewed as holistic hair removal because _____.

    A) it produces better results than soft and hard wax

    B) it is eco-friendly—the natural-ingredient paste is made of sugar, water, and lemon juice

    C) it uses sugar, which is a component of soft wax—an excellent epilator for sensitive areas

    D) it is a permanent hair removal method and, as such, aids resource conservation

18. Which of the following services use strips for removal?

    A) hard waxing and spatula-applied sugaring

    B) hard waxing and soft waxing

    C) soft waxing and spatula-applied sugaring

    D) soft waxing and hand-applied sugaring

19. Identify a temporary hair removal method that involves twisting and rolling cotton thread along the surface of the skin, entwining the hair in the thread, and lifting it from the follicle.

    A) sugaring

    C) threading

    B) waxing

    D) tweezing

20. In the context of hair reduction methods, _____ refers to hair removal using an electric current that destroys the hair's growth cells.

    A) electrolysis

    B) chemical hair relaxing

    C) lanthionization

    D) electrophoresis

continued

21. Intense pulsed light is a hair reduction method that is also known as _____.

    A) electrolysis   C) depilation

    B) photoepilation   D) sugaring

22. Intense pulsed light is not often used for hair removal because _____.

    A) it is a temporary method of hair removal

    B) it can cause burning, especially in higher Fitzpatrick scales

    C) it is illegal for cosmetologists and estheticians in all US states to administer this method in salons

    D) clinical studies have shown that intense pulsed light can provide only 10 to 15 percent hair clearance in 20 weeks

23. Identify a permanent hair reduction treatment.

    A) tweezing   C) laser hair removal

    B) sugaring   D) depilation

24. During a waxing consultation, clients will be asked to complete a _____, which discloses medications, known medical issues, skin disorders, or allergies that might affect or preclude treatment.

    A) service record card   C) release form

    B) hold harmless form   D) client intake form

25. The _____ is the client's permanent progress documentation of services received, service results, and products purchased or used.

    A) hold harmless form

    B) client analysis and

    C) service record card

    D) client intake form consultation card

finished!

Practical Skills · Self-Evaluation Checklist

Regular self-assessment helps you to improve your technical skills and achieve success. After performing each procedure, review the procedure steps in the textbook and rate yourself as "Competent" or "Needs Work," and write in comments on how you were successful or where you can improve. Rating yourself helps you identify your strengths and weaknesses and develop your own plan for improvement.

CRITERIA	COMPETENT	NEEDS WORK	COMMENTS
PROCEDURE 17-1 PRE-SERVICE PROCEDURE			
Prepare The Treatment Room			
Prepare For The Client			
Timing			
PROCEDURE 17-2 POST-SERVICE PROCEDURE			
Preparation			
Advised Client and Promoted Products			
Scheduled Next Appointment and Thanked Client			
Post-Service at the End of the Day			
Timing			
PROCEDURE 17-3 EYEBROW TWEEZING			
Preparation			
Procedure			
Post-Service			
Timing			
PROCEDURE 17-4 EYEBROW WAXING USING SOFT WAX			
Preparation			
Procedure			
Post-Service			
Timing			
PROCEDURE 17-5 LIP WAXING USING HARD WAX			
Preparation			
Procedure			
Post-Service			
Timing			
PROCEDURE 17-6 BODY WAXING USING SOFT WAX			
Preparation			
Procedure			
Post-Service			
Timing			

Ch. 18: Facials

TRACK MY PROGRESS!

Use this simple tracker to record your progress as you work through the activities in each learning objective.

COMPLETED	# OF CORRECT ANSWERS	OBJECTIVE
☐	_____/3	LO 1 - Explain why cosmetologists should have an understanding of facial treatments and skin care products.
☐	_____/7	LO 2 - Discuss the pros and cons of pursuing an esthetics career, or a dual hair and skin care career.
☐	_____/25	LO 3 - Describe at least three types of basic equipment used for esthetics services.
☐	_____/23	LO 4 - Describe the four skin types and common skin conditions that are addressed during facial treatments.
☐	_____/44	LO 5 - Explain the different categories of skin care products used in facial treatments and for home care and provide examples of each.
☐	_____/19	LO 6 - Explain the five techniques used to perform a facial massage.
☐	_____/17	LO 7 - Explain how galvanic, high-frequency, and light therapy treatments are used in facial services.
☐	_____/5	LO 8 - Explain the purpose and importance of client forms and record keeping.
☐	_____/7	LO 9 - Explain the pertinent information to gather during a client consultation and skin analysis before performing facial treatments.
☐	_____/5	LO 10 - Identify examples of contraindications that prohibit performing facial treatments.
☐	_____/22	LO 11 - Perform preservative and corrective facial treatments.

Why Study Facials?

SHORT ANSWER

1. In broad terms, what is a facial (or facial treatment)?

_____

_____

_____

2. List five reasons that it's important to study and gain a thorough understanding of facial treatments. (Hint: Think about the benefits to both you and your clients.)

_____

_____

_____

FILL IN THE BLANK

3. Complete the sentences below using words from the word bank. Each word will be used once.

   Word bank: cleaner, home, wrinkled, supple, firmer, moist, salon, smoother, healthier

   Proper skin care can make dry skin look and feel more _____ and _____; oily skin look

   _____ and _____; and aging skin look _____, _____, and less _____. Clients

   who combine _____ facial treatments with effective, individualized _____care regimens

   will see obvious results.

Esthetics Career Path

SHORT ANSWER

4. What is the biggest challenge for cosmetologists who choose to pursue both the esthetician and hair stylist career paths?

   _____

   _____

   _____

5. What is an advantage of combining the hair stylist career path with that of the esthetician?

   _____

   _____

   _____

6. What are three aspects of becoming an expert in skin care that appeal to cosmetologists?

_____

_____

_____

7. List two possible scheduling options that would help you comfortably manage a dual career as both esthetician and hair stylist.

_____

_____

_____

8. If you choose to split your day between esthetician and hairstylist services, why is it recommended that you devote mornings to skin care services instead of hairstyling appointments?

_____

_____

_____

MATCHING

9. Match each cosmetologist career path with its description. Each career path will be used more than once.

   a. Hair stylists   b. Estheticians

   Career Path   **Description**

   _____ Beauty-driven artistic perspective

   _____ Take a holistic approach to skin care treatments by focusing on the mind, body, and spirit

   _____ Classes for this career path are typically advanced and might include multiday workshops to grow knowledge, increase expertise, and network

   _____ Identify with the beauty industry

   _____ Generally wear short, manicured nails, soft-soled shoes to minimize noise, lab coats, and neutral makeup

   _____ Identify with the wellness community

_____ Expected to be outgoing and to converse in an upbeat, lively manner

_____ Thrive in a reassuring, tranquil environment, as do their clients

_____ Typically enhance their industry knowledge by learning from the beauty world around them, such as trends and techniques, and the most fashionable haircuts and haircolors of the moment

RESEARCH

10. Much of your studies so far have focused on hair services, but now as you begin to take a closer look at skin care services in this chapter, you will find it beneficial to learn more about current career opportunities for estheticians. Use the Internet to search job sites for three open esthetician positions. Then either use the table or follow the link to record your findings.

   When you've completed your research, discuss what appeals to you about the opportunities for estheticians, list a few areas where you might need to build your skills or knowledge, and describe what kind of salon you could offer your services to.

+ BONUS

Visit: bonus.milady.com/cos-wb/toc

FEATURES OF POSITION	ESTHETICIAN POSITION #1	ESTHETICIAN POSITION #2	ESTHETICIAN POSITION #3
Job/Career Site (Source)			
Title of Position			
Name of Employer			
Top Three Qualifications/Skills	1. 2. 3.	1. 2. 3.	1. 2. 3.
Prior Experience Required			
Personality Traits Suggested/ Requested			
Expected Duties			
Special Qualifications or Requirements			
Type of Clientele			
Expected Hours/Schedule			
Compensation Structure			
Training Offered? (Yes/No)			

Basic Facial Equipment

11. As you begin to learn about facial equipment, who should you consult with for its safe operation? What is another resource for specific information about an individual piece of equipment used in facial treatments?

_____

_____

_____

12. Why do precautions vary among types of facial equipment?

_____

_____

_____

13. Is use of all facial equipment by cosmetologists permitted in all states? How can you find out?

_____

_____

_____

14. What is the most important feature to consider when selecting and using facial equipment such as chairs or tables? Why?

_____

_____

_____

15. What are four main functions of magnifying lamps (mag lights), from an esthetician's perspective?

_____

_____

_____

16. Describe a magnifying lamp.

_____

_____

_____

17. How is magnification measured—that is, what does magnification measure? What does a diopter measure?

_____

_____

_____

18. How many diopters is a typical magnifying lamp that's used by estheticians? What is the magnification of such lamps?

_____

_____

_____

FILL IN THE BLANK

Complete the sentences below using the word bank. Some words will be used more than once.

Word bank: upright, massage, higher, lower, space, hydraulic, manual, raise, recline, tables, chair, platform, footprint

19. _____-end treatment _____ resemble portable _____ tables.

    _____-end equipment is attached to a _____ base and has _____ or

    electric/hydraulic controls.

20. A treatment _____ is a deluxe _____ saver because it can remain

    _____ to minimize its _____, and it will _____ only during facial

    treatments. This type of facial equipment has either manual adjustments or electric/_____

    controls that recline and _____ the _____ with the touch of a button.

21. Label each type of chair, table, and stool depicted below.

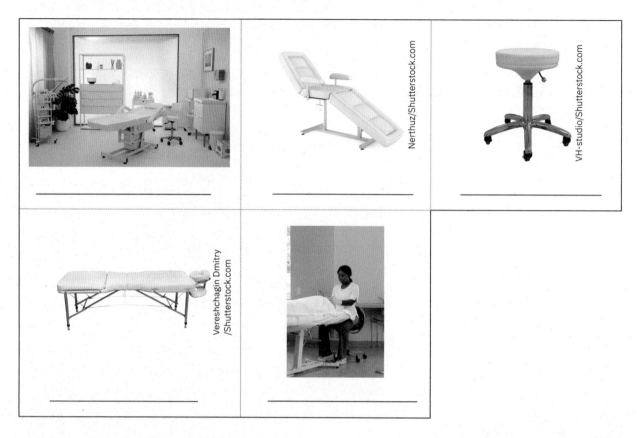

Nerthuz/Shutterstock.com

VH-studio/Shutterstock.com

Vereshchagin Dmitry/Shutterstock.com

_____   _____   _____

_____   _____

MATCHING

22. Match each type of advanced skin analysis equipment with its description. Each type will be used more than once.

a. Wood's lamp
b. Skin scope

c. Digital skin analysis system

d. Skin moisture analyzer

Type of Advanced Skin Analysis Equipment

Description

_____ Clearly defines the moisture needs of each skin zone

_____ Assesses skin using two light modes

_____ Specific fluorescent colors revealed by black light pinpoint skin conditions, pigment disorders, and the presence of certain bacteria or fungi

_____ Among many features, analyzes skin-aging issues; pinpoints presence and severity of acne and other conditions on or below the skin's surface; determines the client's skin type

_____ Uses black light to make skin fluoresce

_____ Among many features, detects and maps sun damage; determines pore size in sections; detects amount of sebum in pores; identifies hyperpigmentation and inflammation; detects bacterial and fungal infections

_____ Analyzes and calculates moisture levels in the skin in multiple zones

_____ Simulated daylight reveals visible concerns; LED-UV light identifies underlying issues

23. Match each type of skin prep equipment with its description and precautions.

a. Hot towel cabinets   b. Facial steamers   c. Ozone facial steamers

Type of Skin Prep Equipment   **Description and Precautions**

_____ Dispense a fine mist of steam and O_3

_____ Should be equipped with a UV sterilizing unit to prevent the proliferation of molds, bacteria, and viruses

_____ Can heat and produce a stream of warm steam that can be focused on the client's face or other areas of the skin

_____ Empty this type of equipment each night and manually disinfect the unit's interior and exterior

_____ In a medical setting, gas emitted by this type of equipment is used to treat wounds and speed up their healing

_____ Help dilate pores and soften clogged follicles, making them easier to extract

_____ Also called hot cabis

_____ Topical applications of this gas proven to oxygenate skin's cutaneous layer; also has germicidal and bactericidal capabilities

_____ Heat damp or dry towels

_____ Help soften the tissues, making them more accepting of moisturizers and treatment products

_____ Prolonged exposure to gas can deplete antioxidant content in skin

24. What is an extraction in the field of esthetics?

_____

_____

_____

25. In addition to preparing the skin for extractions, what are two other ways that esthetics equipment can be used to prepare the skin for treatments?

_____

_____

_____

26. List three medical conditions your clients might have that require you to either take precautions when using steam or steamed towels, or avoid using them altogether.

_____

_____

_____

FILL IN THE BLANK

Complete the sentences below using words from the word bank. Each word will be used once.

Word bank: larger, cleanse, small, disinfected, brushing, soft, face, natural, electric, cleaned, firm, facial, immersed, strength, exfoliate

27. A rotary brush, also known as a _____ brush or _____ machine, is used to

_____ and lightly _____ the skin with a rotating _____ appliance.

Brushes come in _____ sizes for the face and _____ sizes for the body, with

bristle textures ranging from _____ to _____ .

28. The softest bristles are recommended for the _____; _____ bristles are

prohibited because they cannot be _____ or _____. You should use only brush

heads that can be fully _____ in a disinfectant of appropriate _____.

29. Describe the mechanical action of an ultrasonic spatula.

   _____

   _____

   _____

30. List at least three ways an ultrasonic spatula can improve and prepare the skin for facial treatments.

   _____

   _____

   _____

31. If a client is taking keratolytic drugs such as Retin-A®, Differin®, Tazorac®, or other medications that thin or exfoliate the skin, which three types of skin prep equipment should not be used?

   _____

   _____

   _____

32. If a client has rosacea, sensitive skin, acne, or other forms of skin inflammation or redness, which two types of skin prep equipment should not be used on them?

   _____

   _____

   _____

33. What are waxing units (warmers) and how do they work?

   _____

   _____

   _____

34. Label each type of facial cleansing, exfoliation, or waxing services equipment depicted below.

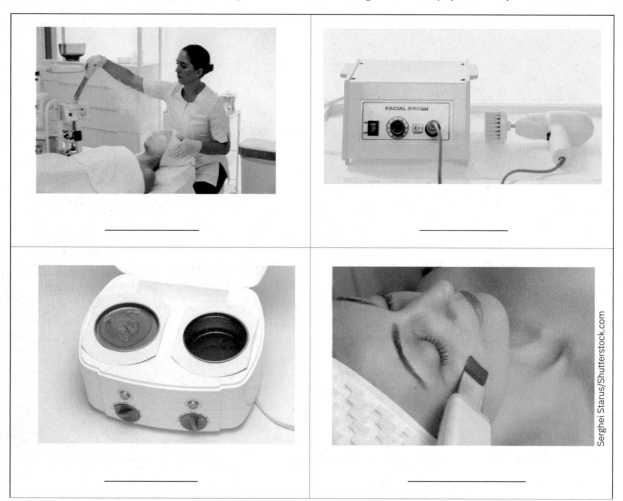

Serghei Starus/Shutterstock.com

Skin Types and Common Skin Conditions

SHORT ANSWER

35. What do skin type classifications describe?

_____

_____

_____

36. What are the four skin types? What three characteristics determine the skin types?

_____

_____

_____

SEQUENCE

37. Number the steps of the facial procedure for dry skin, from 1 to 14. Some steps have been numbered for you.

_____ Remove the scrub with moist facial sponges; moist cotton pads; or warm, moist towels.

_____ Remove the mask with moist cotton pads; moist facial sponges; or warm, moist soft towels.

___3___ Focus steam on the face and allow steaming for five minutes.

_____ Apply a cream or hydrating gel mask starting at the neck and using a soft mask brush; apply from the center outward.

_____ Before you begin, perform the Pre-Service Procedure from Chapter 17.

_____ Apply eye cream under the client's eyes.

___14___ Apply moisturizer or sunscreen designed for dry skin.

_____ If massage cream has been used, remove the cream with moist facial sponges; moist cotton pads; or warm, moist towels.

_____ Apply cold cotton eye pads and allow the mask to process for seven to ten minutes. Make sure the client is comfortable and warm.

_____ Complete steps 1–12 from the Basic Facial Procedure 18-1 in this chapter (up through cleansing and removing the cleanser).

___9___ *Optional:* Choose an electrotherapy treatment from the following:
A. Electrotherapy option 1, galvanic treatment
B. Electrotherapy option 2, high-frequency indirect current treatment
   Complete this step by applying additional moisturizing or specialty product for dry skin with slow massage movements.

_____ During or after steaming, apply a mild granular exfoliating product designed for dry skin.

_____ Apply toner for dry skin with cotton pads.

_____ Apply a moisturizing lotion, cream, or massage product designed for dry skin. Massage the skin with manipulations.

TRUE OR FALSE

Indicate whether the statements below are true or false. For any false statements, explain why they are false.

38. Normal skin is not too dry and not too oily but can have large pores in the T-zone area.

    T   F   _____

39. Every skin care professional strives to balance the skin to achieve the radiant appearance of a normal skin type.

    T   F   _____

40. The medical term for the dry skin type is alipidic skin.

    T   F   _____

41. The dry skin type is characterized by lipid overactivity and large, visible pores.

    T   F   _____

42. Dehydrated skin is unique to dry skin types.

    T   F   _____

43. Dehydrated skin is a condition, not a skin type, and is marked by a lack of sufficient moisture.

    T   F   _____

SHORT ANSWER

44. What substance do oily skin types produce too much of?

    _____

    _____

    _____

45. What are two typical indications that a client has an oily skin type?

    _____

    _____

    _____

46. What three skin conditions are most commonly associated with oily skin? Can other skin types have these conditions?

_____

_____

_____

47. What is a comedo?

_____

_____

_____

48. Describe the combination skin type.

_____

_____

_____

49. What skin types can be sensitive? What are the markers of sensitive skin?

_____

_____

_____

50. What is sensitized skin?

_____

_____

_____

51. What are five sources of ingredients used in facial treatments that estheticians should avoid when performing services for clients with sensitive or sensitized skin?

_____

_____

_____

52. What are the three primary treatment goals for estheticians who have clients with sensitive/sensitized skin?

_____

_____

_____

SEQUENCE

53. Number the steps for the facial procedure for oily skin, from 1 to 20. Several steps have been numbered for you.

_____ Unfold precut gauze across the face and apply direct high frequency using the mushroom-shaped electrode, according to the machine manufacturer's directions.

_____ Cover the client's eyes with moistened cotton pads. Focus steam on the face and allow steaming for 5 minutes.

_____ Complete steps 1–8 from the Basic Facial Procedure 18-1 in this chapter (up through makeup removal and before the cleansing steps).

_____ If skin is not extremely clogged, apply a hydration fluid or massage fluid designed for oily and combination skin, and perform massage manipulations.

_____ Apply a desincrustation lotion or gel to any area with clogged pores.

_____ Apply toner for oily skin with cotton pads.

_____ Remove with moist cotton pads; moist facial sponges; or a warm, moist soft towel.

_____ Before you begin, perform the Pre-Service Procedure from Chapter 17.

_____ Put on a fresh pair of disposable gloves prior to performing extractions.

___17___ Using a disposable mask brush or spatula, apply a clay-based mask to all oily areas, allowing it to process for about 10 minutes.

___3___ Apply cleanser designed for oily skin. Gently massage to apply and then remove with moist facial sponges; moist cotton pads; or warm, moist towels. Do not tone at this time.

___12___ *Optional:* If galvanic desincrustation was performed prior to extraction, apply positive galvanic current to the face after extractions are complete. This will help to re-establish the proper pH of the skin surface.

___7___ *Optional:* Negative galvanic current may be applied over the desincrustation lotion, depending on the manufacturer's instructions.

_____ After extraction is complete, dispose of gloves and supplies properly.

_____ Apply moisturizer or sunscreen designed for oily or combination skin.

_____ Apply an astringent lotion, a toner for oily skin, or a specialized serum designed to be used following extraction. Allow the skin to dry.

_____ Place the comedone on a tissue and proceed to other areas, but do not extract for more than 5 to 10 minutes for the entire face.

_____ Remove the mask with damp cotton pads; moist facial sponges; or a warm, moist soft towel.

_____ During or after steaming, apply a mild granular exfoliating product designed for oily or combination skin. Remove with moist facial sponges; moist cotton pads; or warm, moist towels.

_____ Cover your gloved fingertips with cotton and (using the magnifying lamp) gently press out open comedones.

FILL IN THE BLANK

54. Complete the chart below.

SKIN TYPE	SIGNS OF SKIN TYPE	CONDITIONS ASSOCIATED WITH SKIN TYPE
	Pores are very small or not visible to the naked eye; skin appears dull and flaky; feels rough, thin, and tight to the touch	
		Comedones, clogged and enlarged pores in the center of the face; flakiness on the cheeks and temples
Normal		
		Prone to blackheads (open comedones), papules, and pustules; prone to acne; can develop seborrhea (condition triggered by excess sebum)

CASE STUDY

55. Based on what you've studied about the different skin types and what you already know about your own skin, now take a look at the skin on your face.

- Use bright lighting and a magnifying mirror to examine your pores, and the color, texture, and various areas of your face.
- Write a brief assessment of what you think your skin type is—be specific and use the terms from your text to support your assessment.
- Partner with a classmate and conduct the same analysis of each other's skin.
- Write a brief assessment of your classmate's skin type and, similar to the one you wrote for yourself, be specific and use the proper terminology.

When you're finished, share your assessments with each other. How accurate were you? Where did your assessments differ? How would you present such an assessment to a client?

FILL IN THE BLANK

Complete the sentences below using words from the word bank. Each word will be used once.

> **Word bank:** hormonal, appearance, sun, hygiene, internal, extrinsic, vitamin, common, health, conditions, UV, pollution, lifestyle, acne

56. Dehydration, hyperpigmentation, sensitized skin, adult _____, _____

    aging caused by _____ exposure and the environment, and problems related to

    _____ fluctuations are the most _____ skin _____.

57. Many _____ and external factors affect the skin's condition. Diet, stress, poor

    _____ choices, hormones, aging, _____ deficiencies, _____, poor skin

    _____, and _____ exposure all play a part in our _____, which in turn

    is reflected in our skin's _____.

Facial Treatment and Care Products

SHORT ANSWER

58. Why is it important to have an in-depth knowledge of specific brands and products within each of the various skin care categories? How does this help you and your clients?

    _____

    _____

    _____

59. What are the seven categories of skin care products?

_____

_____

_____

60. What are three of the most common allergens in skin care products?

_____

_____

_____

61. Describe how to conduct a patch test for skin care product ingredients. What type of results indicate that you should not use the product?

_____

_____

_____

TRUE OR FALSE

Indicate whether the statements below are true or false. For any false statements, explain why they are false.

62. Serums and ampoules are applied over a moisturizer, sunscreen, mask, or massage cream.

    T   F   _____

63. Serums and ampoules are concentrated products that generally contain higher concentrations of ingredients that penetrate the skin and treat various skin conditions.

    T   F   _____

64. Serums are more concentrated and packaged in small sealed vials.

    T   F   _____

65. Ampoules contain a single premeasured application for targeted treatment.

    T   F   _____

66. Match each type of cleanser with its description. Each type will be used more than once.

a. Foaming cleanser   c. Cleansing lotion   e. Cleansing oil
b. Cleansing cream   d. Cleansing milk   f. Cleansing water

Type of Cleanser	Description
_____	Light emulsion suitable for normal to dry skin types
_____	Contains beneficial oils that break down makeup, dirt, excess sebum, and pollutants
_____	Lightweight foam with cream or gel consistency when massaged on damp skin; contains surfactants (detergents)
_____	Nonfoaming lotion cleanser
_____	Does not strip skin's natural oil or pH balance
_____	Suitable for very dry and mature skin
_____	Cleanses, tones, and conditions skin; formulated for all skin types
_____	Can be formulated for specific skin types and conditions
_____	Rich water-in-oil emulsion used primarily to dissolve makeup and dirt
_____	Made of microscopic oil molecules (micelles) suspended in purified water
_____	Suitable for all skin types
_____	Formulations available for normal to combination and oily skin types, and acne-prone skin
_____	Cleanses dry and sensitive skin types; removes makeup

TRUE OR FALSE

Indicate whether the statements below are true or false. For any false statements, explain why they are false.

67. The term *sunblock* refers to products that can block 100 percent of UVA and UVB radiation.

T   F   _____

68. The U.S. Food and Drug Administration (FDA) prohibits manufacturers from labeling sunscreens as waterproof or sweatproof because these claims would overstate the product's effectiveness.

    T   F   _____

69. Sun protection (sunscreen) products work by absorbing, scattering, or reflecting UV rays before they interact with the skin.

    T   F   _____

70. The majority of skin cancers are caused by genetics.

    T   F   _____

71. Sunscreen doesn't need to be used on cloudy days.

    T   F   _____

SHORT ANSWER

72. What are two functions of moisturizer products?

    _____

    _____

    _____

73. What are three factors that determine the best moisturizer to use on a client's skin?

    _____

    _____

    _____

74. What is the difference between oily skin moisturizers and dry skin moisturizers?

    _____

    _____

    _____

75. Which ingredient that is often included in day moisturizers is not included in a night cream? What is its purpose?

_____

_____

_____

76. What are day moisturizers usually formulated with? What is their general purpose?

_____

_____

_____

DOS AND DON'TS

77. For each statement about aromatherapy and essential oils, indicate whether it is something you should do (Do) or something you should not do (Don't).

Do or Don't?	When Considering the Use of Aromatherapy and Essential Oils
_____	Use essential oils for aromatherapy (the therapeutic use of plant aromas) for balancing, invigorating, or relaxing purposes
_____	Apply essential oils on sensitive skin
_____	Check your state board regulations to determine if essential oils and aromatherapy services fall within your scope of licensure before using them
_____	Use large quantities of essential oils
_____	Use essential oils preblended with carrier oils such as grapeseed extract or sweet almond oil
_____	Use pure, undiluted essential oils on the skin
_____	Use organic essential oils as opposed to synthetic or artificial oils
_____	Use essential oils and aromatherapy without advanced education

78. What is the difference between nonsetting masks and setting masks?

_____

_____

_____

79. What are six possible functions of masks?

_____

_____

_____

80. If a client is allergic to the iodine in seaweed or shellfish (a contraindication), which type of mask should you avoid using on them?

_____

_____

_____

81. What are three possible uses for gauze when applying a mask to a client?

_____

_____

_____

82. What are desincrustation products?

_____

_____

_____

83. What do desincrustation products do? When are they used?

_____

_____

_____

84. Match each type of mask with its description. Each type will be used more than once.

   a. Alginate   d. Gel   g. Sheet
   b. Clay-based   e. Modelage
   c. Cream   f. Paraffin wax

Type of Mask	Description
_____	Can be used for sensitive or dehydrated skin
_____	Mask material first heated up, checked for temperature, and applied to the face, as opposed to being self-heating
_____	Most often seaweed based; comes in a powder form and is mixed with warm water
_____	Similar to paraffin wax masks, treatment serums or creams applied to the face first, followed by the mask application for enhanced product penetration
_____	Oil-absorbing cleansing masks with an exfoliating and astringent effect on oily and combination skin, making large pores temporarily appear smaller
_____	Collagen-infused versions of this mask are very popular, as they are plumping, calming, and hydrating; also diminish the appearance of wrinkles
_____	Used for the same purpose as modelage masks
_____	Have a conditioning effect on dry and/or dehydrated skin; remain moist and pliable
_____	Available as a single packaged moist or freeze-dried sheet
_____	Freeze-dried version of this type of mask similar to a piece of paper and infused with performance ingredients; moistened after it's pressed onto the skin and remains wet until removal
_____	Often contain oils and emollients, as well as humectants (also known as hydrators or water-binding agents—ingredients that attract water)
_____	Often contain hydrators and soothing ingredients to help plump surface cells with moisture, making the skin look more supple and hydrated
_____	Form a seal that encourages the skin's absorption of the serum or treatment cream underneath

_____ The prepackaged moist version of this type of mask applied directly on the skin until removal

_____ Self-heating masks that harden as they dry on the skin

_____ Might have additional beneficial ingredients such as antibacterials like sulfur, which are helpful for acne-prone skin

_____ Doesn't dry hard, but does firm up

_____ After mixing, quickly applied to the face and then allowed to dry to a rubberized texture

SHORT ANSWER

85. What does the process of exfoliation accomplish? What is the overall result of exfoliation?

_____

_____

_____

86. What are the two main categories of exfoliants?

_____

_____

_____

87. List six of the eight benefits of exfoliation.

_____

_____

_____

88. A fellow esthetician tells you that they recently performed microdermabrasion on a client. Based on what you know about microdermabrasion, what can you guess about the client? Why?

_____

_____

_____

89. Complete the sentences below using the words from the word bank. Each word will be used once.

    Word bank: jojoba, brushes, aluminum, buildup, crystals, physically, scrubs, spatulas

    Mechanical exfoliation is a method used to _____ remove dead cell _____.

    Some of the methods include using facial _____ and ultrasonic _____;

    facial _____ made with rice bran, almond meal, _____ beads, and/or other

    ingredients; and scrubs containing _____ oxide or sodium bicarbonate _____.

MATCHING

90. Match each type of microdermabrasion method with its description. Each type will be used at least once.

    a. Crystal   b. Crystal-free   c. Hydrodermabrasion

    Type of Microdermabrasion Method

    Description

    _____ Promotes healthier, more balanced skin

    _____ Therapeutic procedure that combines liquid exfoliation with serum penetration

    _____ Does not require the clean-up or expense of crystals

    _____ Uses a closed vacuum system to spray crystals onto the skin and then vacuum up the dead skin cells and the crystals in one action

    _____ Also known as wet microdermabrasion

    _____ Popular because it consists of a diamond-tip applicator that polishes away the skin's upper layers

91. Which types of mechanical exfoliation devices should not be used on clients taking blood thinning medication to avoid damaging the skin?

_____

_____

_____

92. When consulting with a client, they mention they have heard good things about rotary brushes and want them included in their facial. What are seven contraindications you should discuss with your client before you consider including these brushes in a facial treatment?

_____

_____

_____

93. What are two ways that you might end up overexfoliating the skin? What is a consequence of overexfoliating?

_____

_____

_____

94. How do hydroxy acids work to remove dead skin cells on the skin's surface?

_____

_____

_____

95. Are treatments involving hydroxy acids considered to be basic or advanced facial services?

_____

_____

_____

96. What are two possible effects of a single hydroxy acid facial treatment? What are three possible results of a series of such treatments?

_____

_____

_____

97. What are two types of enzyme exfoliants? What are their main ingredients?

_____

_____

_____

98. How do enzyme exfoliants work?

_____

_____

_____

MATCHING

99. Match each type of hydroxy acid with its description. Each type will be used more than once.

a. Alpha hydroxy acids (AHAs)
b. Glycolic hydroxy acid
c. Lactic acid
d. Beta hydroxy acids (BHAs)
e. Polyhydroxy acids (PHAs)

Type of Hydroxy Acid	Description
_____	A type of AHA; not recommended for sensitive skin, but recommended for dry skin and photo (sun) damage because it draws moisture and prevents moisture loss
_____	Most common types are gluconolactone, galactose, and lactobionic acids
_____	Does not penetrate as deeply as glycolic acid and is gentler than glycolic acid; recommended for sensitive skin types because it causes less inflammation
_____	Best suited for oilier, acne-prone skin
_____	Part of a group of acids that smooth, tighten, firm, and brighten the skin

_____ Used to treat hyperpigmentation and aids in general skin brightening

_____ Considered second-generation AHAs

_____ Most used as standalone treatments, or in specific combinations with each other, to achieve targeted results

_____ Group of hydroxy acids, with salicylic acid being the top performer for skin care treatments

_____ Recommended for normal to dry skin

_____ Oil soluble (dissolves sebum); breaks apart pore debris where _Propionibacterium (P.) acnes_ bacteria thrive; lightens sun spots and age spots

_____ Smallest hydroxy acid molecule; penetrates deepest and most quickly

_____ Molecules cannot penetrate as deeply as AHAs or BHAs; work exclusively on the surface

_____ Less irritating and reduce the risk of skin photosensitivity caused by overexposure to UV rays; recommended for sensitive skin

_____ Less likely to trigger inflammatory hyperpigmentation than alpha hydroxy acids; can mildly dry the skin

RESEARCH

100. Use the Internet or beauty supply catalogues, or visit a drug store or beauty supply shop, to find two examples of each skin care product category. Focus your research on products appropriate for a client with a specific skin type. Follow the link here or use a separate sheet of paper to record your findings. The chart below is an example of the information you should gather.

Skin type (choose one): normal, oily, dry, combination

Other skin characteristics or factors (choose one or two): mature, sensitive, allergic, acne-prone, taking medications

What was most challenging about your research? What was most enlightening?

+ BONUS

Visit: bonus.milady.com/cos-wb/toc

SKIN CARE PRODUCT	SOURCE	NAME/ BRAND	PRICE	MAIN/ACTIVE INGREDIENTS	FRAGRANCE	ADVERTISED RESULTS
Cleanser A						
Moisturizer A						
Serum and ampoule A						
Mask A						
Desincrustation product A						
Exfoliant A						
Sun protection A						

MATCHING

101. Match each type of enzyme treatment with its description.

    a. Enzyme masks   b. Gommages

Type of Enzyme Treatment   **Description**

_____ Do not dry on the skin

_____ Form a crust as they dry on the skin; crust then rolled off the skin

_____ Made of powder mixed with warm water to form a paste or gel, or premixed with the same consistencies

_____ Cream- or paste-type enzyme masks

_____ Considered a hybrid treatment because it is both a mechanical and chemical exfoliant

_____ Recommended for most skin types, but be sure to check the client for any citrus allergies before using this type

_____ Make the skin look healthier and more polished

_____ Also known as roll-off masks and usually contain papain

Basic Techniques Used in Facial Massage

FILL IN THE BLANK

102. Complete the sentences below using the words from the word bank. Each word will be used once.

    Word bank: disease, inflammation, surgery, intake, enhancements, soothing, contraindicate, laser, chemical, purifying, acne, medical

    Consult the client's _____ form to note and discuss any _____ condition

    that may _____ a facial massage. These include recent facial _____

    or _____ treatment, facial paralysis, recent cosmetic _____ (fillers) or

    _____ exfoliation, or any skin _____ affecting the facial skin. Do not massage

    areas with _____ breakouts. Replace massage with a _____ or _____

    skin treatment if the breakout is widespread or general _____ is present.

SHORT ANSWER

103. In general terms, what is massage?

    _____

    _____

    _____

104. What are the three overall expected benefits of massage?

    _____

    _____

    _____

105. What type of knowledge and practice are required for you to master massage techniques?

    _____

    _____

    _____

106. List four ways that you can enhance your hands and wrists to provide a high-quality massage for each client.

_____

_____

_____

LABELING

107. Label the motor points for the face and neck depicted below.

Word bank: brachial plexus (Erb's point), cervical nerve (2 times) facial nerve (buccal branch), facial nerve (main trunk), facial nerve (mandibular branch), facial nerve (temporal branch), occipital nerve, plexus nerve, posterior auricular nerve, trapezius nerve

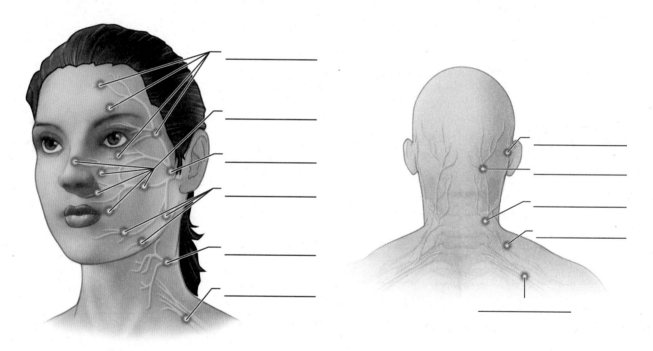

SHORT ANSWER

108. Describe what a motor point is, including what happens if pressure is applied to it.

_____

_____

_____

109. What is a benefit of manipulating the proper motor points?

_____

_____

_____

110. What are the four immediate benefits of massage first visible on the skin?

_____

_____

_____

FILL IN THE BLANK

Complete the sentences below using the words from the word bank. Some words will be used more than once.

Word bank: sagging, skeleton, origin, resiliency, wrong, farthest, closest, muscle, fixed, moveable, insertion, movement

111. In a massage treatment, the direction of _____ is always from the muscle's _____

toward the muscle's _____. Massaging a muscle in the _____ direction could result in

loss of _____ and _____ skin and muscles.

112. The _____ is the portion of the muscle at the more _____ attachment (where it

is attached to another _____ or to a movable bone or joint) and _____ to/from

the skeleton. The _____ is the portion of the muscle at the _____ attachment (an

immovable section of the _____) and _____ to/from the skeleton.

TRUE OR FALSE

Indicate whether the statements below are true or false. For any false statements, explain why they are false.

113. For facial massage, relaxation is achieved through light but firm slow rhythmic movements, or very slow light hand vibrations over the motor points for a short time.

T   F   _____

114. After you have asked whether your touch should be more or less firm, be sure to keep the conversation with your client light and casual during the massage to keep the client relaxed.

T   F   _____

115. When performing a facial massage on a client, your routine must be started on the forehead.

T   F   _____

116. Massage pressure, type, and duration will vary according to skin type.

T   F   _____

117. For clients with facial hair, use the same up and down massage techniques you would use on clients without facial hair, as they can be especially relaxing in the beard area.

T   F   _____

FILL IN THE BLANK

118. Complete the chart below.

Massage Modality	Description of Movement
_____	Kneading movement performed by lifting, squeezing, and pressing the tissue with a light, firm pressure
_____	Fingertips strike the skin in rapid succession or fast tapping movements.
Effleurage	_____
_____	A rapid shaking movement in which the balls of the fingertips are pressed firmly on the application point.
Friction	_____

SEQUENCE

119. Number the steps of the basic facial procedure, from 1 to 14.

_____ Properly drape the client and wash your hands.

_____ Apply a mask for approximately 10 minutes.

_____ Analyze the skin with a magnifying lamp.

_____ Recommend initial home care products.

_____ Perform exfoliation. Remove exfoliant and tone skin.

_____ Steam or apply a hot, moist towel to face.

_____ Apply toner.

_____ Apply a moisturizing and sunscreen for daytime.

_____ Massage.

_____ Book the client's next visit.

_____ Remove the mask.

_____ Perform a full facial cleansing to remove makeup.

_____ Apply serums, as well as eye and lip treatments.

_____ Perform extractions.

120. Label each of the techniques of the facial massage routine in the space provided. The first step is provided for you. Write the steps for the facial routine and use the correct terms for the massage techniques, such as petrissage, effleurage, vibration, tapotement, and friction.

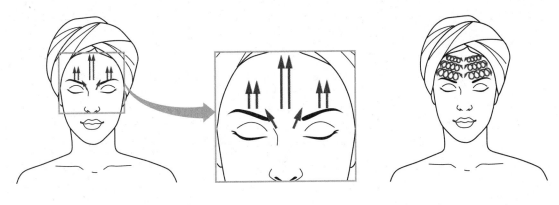

Effleurage strokes on the forehead _____

_____

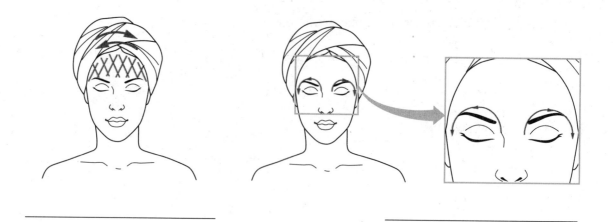

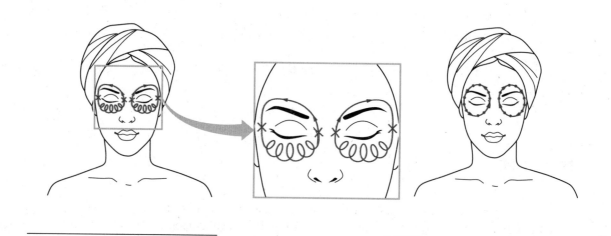

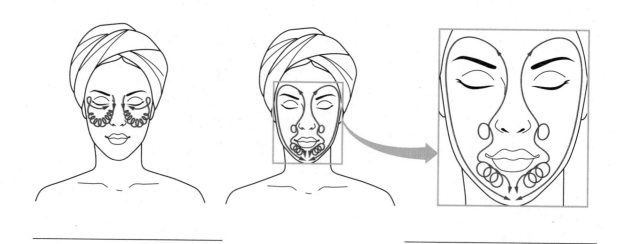

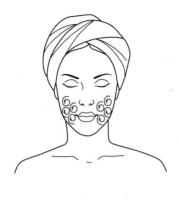

_____

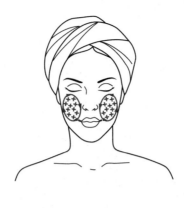

_____

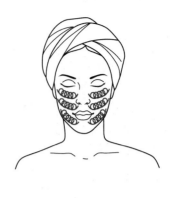

_____

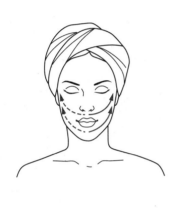

_____

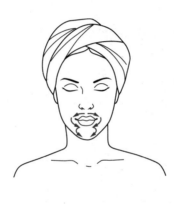

_____

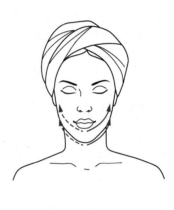

_____

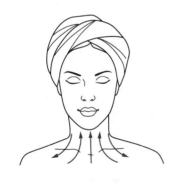

_____

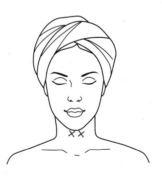

_____

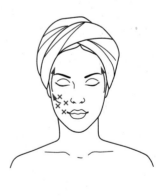

_____

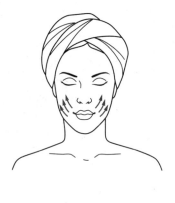
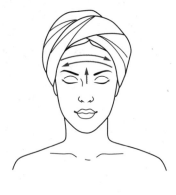
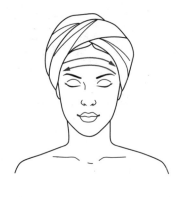

_____

Electrotherapy and Light Therapy

SHORT ANSWER

121. Define electrotherapy.

_____

_____

_____

122. What are two of the more challenging skin conditions that electric devices are especially effective for treating?

_____

_____

_____

123. What are the three types of electrotherapy?

_____

_____

_____

124. Which electrical machines are approved for use by estheticians in your state? (Check your state regulatory agency to determine this.)

_____

_____

_____

FILL IN THE BLANK

125. Complete the sentences below using words from the word bank. Each word will be used once.

    Word bank: fear, current, jewelry, heart, seizure, galvanic, electrotherapy, metal, piercing, open

    Never administer _____ on clients with the following conditions: (1) _____ conditions, pacemakers, _____ implants, or braces; (2) epilepsy or _____ disorders; (3) _____ or broken skin; (4) _____ or apprehension of electrical _____; or (5) pregnancy. In addition, the client must remove _____ and _____ before you can use electrical devices such as the _____ machine.

SHORT ANSWER

126. What are two facial treatment goals that can be achieved by using galvanic current?

_____

_____

_____

127. What specific category of skin care products is most commonly prepared for use in iontophoresis?

_____

_____

_____

128. Is any special training required to perform iontophoresis?

_____

_____

_____

129. What type of activity in the human body is most similar to the very low level of electric current used in the microcurrent treatment?

_____

_____

_____

130. On which side of the body should you always place an electrode? Why?

_____

_____

_____

FILL IN THE BLANK

131. Complete the following chart with the three forms of electrotherapy:

MODALITIES	PURPOSE	BENEFIT
Galvanic current		
Microcurrent		
High-Frequency Current		

SEQUENCE

132. Number the steps for using galvanic current to accomplish desincrustation, from 1 to 6.

_____ The positive electrode (in this case, the inactive electrode) is held by the client in their right hand or attached to a pad that is placed in contact with the client's right shoulder.

_____ Refer to the product manufacturer's recommendations and usage specifications to ensure that you understand the directions for your machine.

_____ Extract sebum deposits with gentle pressure.

_____ Cover the entire positive electrode that makes contact with the client with a piece of dampened cotton around the electrode.

_____ Confirm that your client has no contraindications for the use of galvanic current. If there are none, proceed with desincrustation.

_____ Apply the active electrode—in the case of desincrustation, the negative electrode—to the oily areas of the face for three to five minutes.

MATCHING

133. Match each type/color of light with the description of its purpose in facial treatments. Each type/color will be used at least once.

a. Infrared
b. Light-emitting diode (LED)
c. Red light
d. Yellow light
e. Green light

Type/Color of Light	Description of Light's Purpose
_____	Used to minimize redness, warm lower-level tissues, stimulate blood flow, and improve skin smoothness
_____	Traditionally used to heat the skin and increase blood flow; also used for hair and scalp treatments
_____	Popular light therapy type involving concentrated light that flashes very rapidly
_____	Calms and soothes; lessens hyperpigmentation
_____	Can be used for relaxation, warming up muscles, detoxifying the body, and reducing pain
_____	Reduces inflammation and improves lymphatic flow
_____	Treats aging and redness
_____	When set to blue, applied to improve acne-prone skin

134.

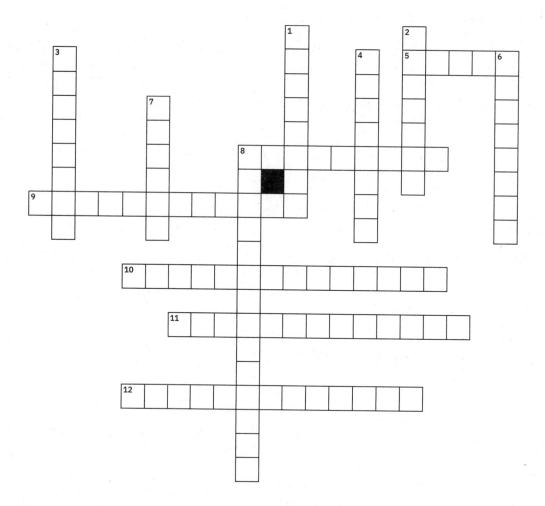

Across

5. A positive electrode
8. The applicator for directing the electrical current to the client's skin
9. Also known as wave therapy; uses a very low level of electrical current best known for toning the skin
10. The process of softening and emulsifying hardened sebum stuck in the follicles
11. The process of using galvanic current to enable water-soluble products that contain ions to penetrate the skin
12. A kind of current discovered by Tesla that is used after extraction or during treatments for acne-prone skin due to its germicidal effect

Down

1. The name for a high-frequency treatment that involves the client holding the electrode during treatment
2. A negative electrode
3. A type of current that uses two electrodes
4. The most common electrode used in high-frequency treatments
6. A condition that causes seizures; a contraindication for electrotherapy
7. The name for a high-frequency current applied on the skin
8. The use of electrical currents to treat the skin

135. When using any light therapy equipment to treat your client, how do you protect their eyes?

_____

_____

_____

136. Although they are safe for most clients, people with what specific medical condition should avoid LED treatments?

_____

_____

_____

137. If a client has a questionable health condition but is requesting LED treatment, what should you do?

_____

_____

_____

138. In addition to following the manufacturer's directions for operating light therapy machines (including LED and infrared devices), what is required to safely and effectively perform advanced light therapy services for your skin care clients?

_____

_____

_____

Client Forms and Record Keeping

SHORT ANSWER

139. What should you do with the client forms once they have been completed?

_____

_____

_____

140. Why is it useful to specify the client's birth date on their service record form?

_____

_____

_____

141. On the client service record, why might you note specific products and the date the client purchased them?

_____

_____

_____

142. What is a contraindication? Why is it important to find out early on in your consultation if your client has one or more?

_____

_____

_____

FILL IN THE BLANK

143. Complete the chart below.

	CLIENT INTAKE FORM	SERVICE RECORD FORM	CONSENT FORM
Other Terms for the Form			
Purpose			

	CLIENT INTAKE FORM	SERVICE RECORD FORM	CONSENT FORM
Type of Information Collected/ Recorded			
Who Completes			
When to Complete			

Conduct a Client Consultation

SHORT ANSWER

144. What two important opportunities does the client consultation offer you, as the esthetician, before the service and after the service?

_____

_____

_____

145. What does a skin analysis determine about a client?

_____

_____

_____

146. Partner with a classmate, preferably someone you have not partnered with before, to practice conducting a client consultation for skin care services.

- Use the chart below to ask your partner the typical skin care consultation questions.

- Before you begin, set a timer for 15 minutes for each consultation.

- When asking the questions (and answering them), be as natural, authentic, and conversational as possible.

- For each question, note your partner's answer in the chart. Listening carefully will be key.

- When your 15 minutes are up:

  - Review the chart to see how far you made it through the list, if you skipped any questions, and whether you changed the order in which you asked them

  - Go through each question and repeat your partner's answers back to them to see if you accurately captured what they told you

- Finally, discuss the following with each other:

  - How well you think you did overall

  - How you could have either sped up or slowed down the consultation

  - What you would do differently next time

ESTHETICIAN: CONSULTATION QUESTIONS	CLIENT'S RESPONSE
What is the reason for your visit? (What brought the client in? Is it for a treatment or just relaxation?)	
Tell me what you like about your skin. Tell me what you would change about your skin.	
What are your skin care goals? Are you preparing for a special event? When is it?	
What is your home skin care routine? (How many products does the client use at home? What are the ingredients, and how often are they used?)	
Have you had treatments before? (Is this the client's first treatment of this type?)	
Do you have allergies to products or scents?	

ESTHETICIAN: CONSULTATION QUESTIONS	CLIENT'S RESPONSE
Is this a normal state for your skin? (Is it normally clearer? Is it usually less irritated?)	
How does your skin feel during different times of the day? (What is the degree of oiliness or dryness?)	
Do you wear sunscreen? What is the SPF value?	
Tell me about your diet. Do you eat a healthy diet?	
How much water do you drink daily?	
How stressful is your lifestyle? Are you under a lot of stress right now?	
Before we begin your treatment, would you please sign our client consent form?	

TRUE OR FALSE

Indicate whether the statements below are true or false. For any false statements, explain why they are false.

147. Every new client should receive a thorough post-service consultation regarding proper home care for their skin conditions, including recommendations for services and products that will benefit the client.

    T   F   _____

148. To allow enough time to thoroughly give home care recommendations to new clients, add an additional hour to your service.

    T   F   _____

149. Home care is a minor factor in a successful skin care program.

    T   F   _____

150. A skin care program consists of a long-range plan involving home care, facial treatments, and client education.

    T   F   _____

Contraindications for Facial Treatments

151. Which two treatments should you avoid (unless you have their physician's permission) if a client indicates they are taking blood thinners and NSAIDs (nonsteroidal anti-inflammatory drugs, e.g., ibuprofen)? Why?

_____

_____

_____

152. General caution is advised for clients who have which medical condition (mainly because they heal slowly and are likely experiencing neuropathy, meaning they may not feel pain in affected areas)?

_____

_____

_____

153. What are four examples of exfoliating drugs that would contraindicate performing all waxing on the area where the client has been using the drug for a week or more? What other facial services should you avoid if the client said they were taking these drugs?

_____

_____

_____

154. Which drug, if taken in the last six months by the client, would contraindicate all waxing anywhere on the body or the use of any peeling agent or drying agent, including alpha hydroxy acids (AHAs), scrubs, microdermabrasion, and brushing machines? Why?

_____

_____

_____

155. Complete the chart below.

CONTRAINDICATIONS	WHAT TO AVOID	WHY?
	Electrical treatments	Electricity can possibly affect rhythms and pacemakers
Pregnancy		Unknown; general safety precaution
Open sores, herpes simplex (cold sores)	All treatments until clear with doctor	
Recent facial surgery or laser treatment		Client should refer to medical provider for safety reasons
	Electrical treatments	Electricity can possibly affect metal
Use of oral steroids such as prednisone	• Any stimulating or exfoliating treatment • Waxing	
	Electrical or light-based treatments that pulsate	Could trigger seizure reaction
Sensitive, redness-prone skin		Can aggravate redness

Perform Facial Procedures

156. Describe what is included in five-minute makeup. Why would you offer this to a client?

_____

_____

_____

157. Recall the guidelines that should be followed for performing a professional facial service that your clients will love. Now list seven ways that you might end up leaving a client dissatisfied after your facial service—think of them as "Don'ts."

_____

_____

_____

FILL IN THE BLANK

Complete the sentences below using words from the word bank. Some words may be used more than once.

Word bank: massage, oiliness, tone, corrects, glands, preservative, aging, texture, circulation, conditions, nerves, comedones, improved, corrective, regular, correctly, acne

158. The two categories of facial treatments are _____ and _____. The

_____ facials maintain facial skin health by cleansing _____, increasing

_____, relaxing the _____, and activating the skin _____ and

metabolism through _____.

159. The other category of facials _____ certain facial skin _____, such as dryness,

_____, _____, _____ lines, and minor _____ conditions.

160. When clients receive professional facials on a _____ basis, their skin _____,

_____, and appearance are noticeably _____.

161. For each aspect related to providing a professional facial service listed below, write the guideline(s) that you should follow to ensure that clients are satisfied and continue seeking your services.

ASPECTS OF PROFESSIONAL FACIAL SERVICES	GUIDELINES FOR PERFORMING PROFESSIONAL FACIAL SERVICES
Organization	
Hand temperature	
Trusted, knowledgeable professional	
Atmosphere/work style	

ASPECTS OF PROFESSIONAL FACIAL SERVICES	GUIDELINES FOR PERFORMING PROFESSIONAL FACIAL SERVICES
Fingernail quality	
Voice/tone	
Cleanliness	

REFLECTION

162. Now that you've practiced the procedures for the basic facial and the facial massage, consider what you knew about these services before you began this section compared to what you've studied. Write a few sentences in which you reflect on and answer the following questions:

- Can you picture yourself performing the basic facial and a facial massage confidently for a client?

- Which facial and facial massage steps or techniques do you excel at? Which ones are you uncertain about?

- Overall, how can you make your facial and facial massage services flawless for your clients?

When you're finished, meet with a classmate and discuss your responses. As you do so, look for opportunities to fill in each other's gaps and help each other master the facial and facial massage techniques and specifics.

DOS AND DON'TS

163. For each statement about special considerations for facial hair and skin care treatments below, indicate whether it is something that you should do (Do) or something that you should not do (Don't).

Do or Don't?   **When Giving Facials to Clients Who Have Facial Hair**

_____ Go against the pattern of any facial hair (beard, goatee, etc.)

_____ Use calming and healing products during the service if your client recently shaved

_____ Incorporate grooming services such as trimming or waxing eyebrows if your client appears to have a need

_____ Use sponges or towels on areas with excess facial hair

_____ Use cotton when giving facials to clients who have beard hair

_____ Flow with the hair growth

Indicate whether the statements below are true or false. For any false statements, explain why they are false.

164. Acne bacteria are anaerobic, which means they can easily survive in the presence of oxygen.

    T   F   _____

165. It is rare for estheticians to see adult acne.

    T   F   _____

166. Acne is a disorder in which the hair follicles become clogged with solidified sebum and dead cell buildup, which prevents oxygen from getting to the bottom of the follicle where acne bacteria live, ultimately causing an infection of the follicle with redness and inflammation.

    T   F   _____

167. If you are ever unsure about treating a client with acne, refer them to a dermatologist.

    T   F   _____

168. Because skin with acne contains infectious matter, you must wear protective gloves and use disposable materials such as cotton cleansing pads when working with clients with acne.

    T   F   _____

LABELING

169. Label each image below with the correct acne-related term.

    a. Open comedones   b. Papules   c. Pustules

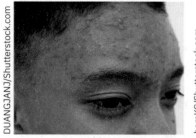
DUANGJAN3/Shutterstock.com

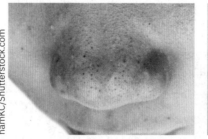
hamKC/Shutterstock.com

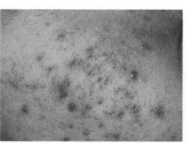
thawatchai_bandit/Shutterstock.com

_____   _____   _____

170. What are three important ways that cosmetologists can help their clients who have acne?

_____

_____

_____

TRUE OR FALSE

Indicate whether the statements below are true or false. For any false statements, explain why they are false.

171. Cultural differences in diet, hygiene, and traditions have no bearing on aging, acne, or barrier skin concerns.

   T   F   _____

172. No matter what a client's skin type or ethnic background, everyone needs an individualized skin care consultation and treatment plan to maintain healthy skin.

   T   F   _____

173. When it comes to skin treatments, everyone's level of skin reactivity is the same.

   T   F   _____

174. Individuals with darker skin may experience adverse reactions such as hyper- or hypopigmentation and keloid scarring due to aggressive treatments.

   T   F   _____

175. Individuals with darker skin types are generally more sensitive, while individuals with light skin have larger melanin deposits in the stratum corneum (SC), which gives more protection from the sun.

   T   F   _____

176. Sun protection is not necessary for all skin types.

   T   F   _____

177. Number the following steps in the proper sequence for the acne procedure, from 1 to 12.

_____ Steam and apply serum.

_____ Wash hands and put on gloves.

_____ Apply a clay-based mask for deep cleansing. Remove the mask.

_____ Apply moisturizer.

_____ Analyze the skin.

_____ Apply astringent/toner.

_____ Perform galvanic or high-frequency treatment.

_____ Perform extractions.

_____ Proceed with desincrustation, then remove product.

_____ Perform deep cleansing.

_____ Apply a soothing mask. Remove with wet cotton.

_____ Finish with the post-treatment consultation.

DISCOVERIES AND ACCOMPLISHMENTS

In the space below, write notes about key concepts discussed in this chapter. Share your discoveries with some of the other students in your class and ask them if your notes are helpful. You may want to revise your notes based on good ideas shared by your peers.

Discoveries:

_____

_____

_____

_____

_____

_____

_____

List at least three things you have accomplished since you decided to enroll in school.

Accomplishments:

_____

_____

_____

_____

_____

_____

_____

1. Cosmetologists should have a thorough understanding of facial treatments and skin care products because _____.

    A) they are required to inform clients in detail about the parts of the skin that will be affected by a facial treatment

    B) having knowledge of the basics of skin care products and skin analysis allows them to give advice to clients when they ask for it

    C) they are licensed to diagnose, prescribe, treat, or work on unhealthy skin and perform any service required in the process

    D) skin services are listed under a podiatry license and performing procedures that are listed under any podiatry license is a primary responsibility of estheticians

2. Identify a difference between estheticians and hair stylists.

    A) Estheticians seldom attend classes and typically learn their skills from the world around them, whereas hair stylists typically take advanced classes to learn their skills.

    B) Unlike estheticians, hair stylists often take a holistic approach to skin care treatments by focusing on the mind, body, and spirit.

    C) Estheticians usually identify with the wellness community, whereas hair stylists identify with the beauty industry.

    D) Unlike hair stylists, estheticians are expected to be sociable and to converse in an upbeat, lively manner.

3. Magnifying lamps are used for _____.

    A) cleansing and exfoliation   C) comedone extractions

    B) removing excess sebum   D) dilating the pores on the skin's surface

4. Which of the following is a benefit of using a facial steamer?

    A) It is used to cleanse and lightly exfoliate the skin.

    B) It stimulates circulation and removes excess sebum.

    C) It helps constrict pores and harden clogged follicles, making them easier to extract.

    D) It helps soften the tissues, making them more accepting of moisturizers and treatment products.

continued

5. Identify a true statement about alipidic skin.

   A) It has large pores.

   B) It appears thick and rough.

   C) It does not produce enough sebum.

   D) It has a waxy or yellowish appearance.

6. Which of the following is a skin condition commonly associated with oily skin?

   A) alopecia

   B) accentuated fine lines and wrinkles

   C) skin dehydration

   D) open and closed comedones

7. Which of the following statements is true of combination skin?

   A) It has a waxy or greasy appearance.

   B) Pores become bigger toward the edges of the face.

   C) No skin conditions are associated with a combination skin type.

   D) It has a wider distribution of large pores in the T-zone.

8. Which of the following is a rich water-in-oil emulsion used mainly to dissolve makeup and dirt and is suitable for very dry and mature skin?

   A) cleansing lotion

   B) foaming cleanser

   C) cleansing cream

   D) cleansing water

9. Which of the following statements is true of ampoules?

   A) They are diluted products that usually contain lower concentrations of ingredients that penetrate the skin and treat various skin conditions.

   B) They are packaged in small, sealed vials containing a single premeasured application for targeted treatment.

   C) They are applied over a mask, sunscreen, massage cream, or moisturizer.

   D) They are typically packaged in a dropper bottle or pump container.

continued

10. Which of the following is a benefit of proper exfoliation of the skin?

    A) It eliminates fine lines and wrinkles.

    B) It slows down the shedding of dead skin cells.

    C) It reduces moisture content in the skin.

    D) It decreases clogged pores and oiliness of the skin.

11. In the context of basic massage techniques, _____ is a light, continuous stroking movement applied in a slow, rhythmic manner with the fingers or the palms.

    A) percussion   C) effleurage

    B) petrissage   D) vibration

12. In the context of massage techniques, which of the following is an invigorating rubbing movement in which you apply pressure on the skin while your fingers or palms move over the underlying structures?

    A) vibration   C) effleurage

    B) petrissage   D) friction

13. Identify the massage technique that involves the fingertips striking the skin in rapid succession or fast tapping movements.

    A) tapotement   C) vibration

    B) effleurage   D) petrissage

14. Galvanic current is used when _____.

    A) the objective of the treatment is to assist in delivering targeted products to the skin or prepare the skin for extractions

    B) a client has open wounds or inflamed pustular acne

    C) the objective of the treatment is to stimulate blood flow and oxygenate the skin

    D) a client has metal implants, a pacemaker, braces, or any heart condition

continued

15. Which of the following statements is true of high-frequency treatments?

    A) They can be applied using iontophoresis and desincrustation.

    B) They can be used to stimulate blood flow and oxygenate the skin.

    C) They use two electrodes.

    D) They can be applied only before extraction because they have a germicidal effect.

16. In the context of light therapy, which of the following colors of light should be used to treat acne-prone skin?

    A) blue light   C) yellow light

    B) green light   D) red light

17. The purpose of _____ is to determine whether the client has any contraindications that might prohibit certain skin treatments.

    A) a client chart   C) the consent form

    B) the service record form   D) the client intake form

18. Which of the following is a customary written agreement between the cosmetologist and the client for applying pre- or postoperative treatment following the medical provider's directions or for applying a simple routine treatment?

    A) the consent form   C) the service record form

    B) the client intake form   D) the health history form

19. Which of the following should you most likely do as a skin care professional?

    A) Perform skin analysis before starting a facial treatment.

    B) Avoid selling products under all circumstances.

    C) Designate a loud, chirpy area for facial treatments.

    D) Complete the client intake form after the completion of a service.

20. Which of the following is a common skin care consultation question?

    A) What is your monthly income?

    B) How does your skin feel during different times of the day?

continued

C) Do you have any children?

D) Are you okay with the use of a curette on your skin?

21. If a client has used oral steroids such as prednisone, you should most likely _____.

A) avoid all treatments until the doctor has cleared them

C) avoid waxing

B) use an exfoliating treatment

D) give a stimulating massage

22. If a client is pregnant, has a history of seizures or epilepsy, has metal bone pins or plates in the body, or has a pacemaker, you should most likely avoid _____.

A) stimulating massages

C) waxing anywhere on the body

B) electrical treatments

D) using scented products

23. If a client has sensitive, redness-prone skin, you should most likely _____.

A) give a stimulating massage

C) avoid cold packs and use heat

B) use mechanical treatments

D) avoid harsh scrubs

24. Which of the following guidelines should you follow when considering skin care treatments and facial hair?

A) Always move opposite the pattern of any facial hair.

B) Select calming and healing products during the service if the skin has abrasions.

C) Use cotton pads instead of towels or sponges on areas with excess facial hair.

D) Never combine waxing with other grooming services such as trimming eyebrows.

25. Which of the following guidelines should you follow when working with clients who have acne?

A) Avoid using ozone steamers on such clients as ozone lacks bactericidal and germicidal capabilities.

B) Only perform preservative facial treatments and not corrective facial treatments on such clients.

C) Use disposable materials such as cotton cleansing pads when working with clients with acne.

D) Wear nondisposable latex gloves during acne treatment procedures.

finished!

Practical Skills Self-Evaluation Checklist

Regular self-assessment helps you to improve your technical skills and achieve success. After performing each procedure, review the procedure steps in the textbook and rate yourself as "Competent" or "Needs Work," and write in comments on how you were successful or where you can improve. Rating yourself helps you identify your strengths and weaknesses and develop your own plan for improvement.

CRITERIA	COMPETENT	NEEDS WORK	COMMENTS
PROCEDURE 18-1 BASIC FACIAL			
Preparation			
Procedure			
Post-Service			
Timing			
PROCEDURE 18-2 FACIAL MASSAGE			
Preparation			
Procedure			
Timing			
PROCEDURE 18-3 FACIAL FOR DRY SKIN			
Preparation			
Procedure			
Post-Service			
Timing			
PROCEDURE 18-4 FACIAL FOR OILY SKIN WITH OPEN COMEDONES			
Preparation			
Procedure			
Post-Service			
Timing			
PROCEDURE 18-5 FACIAL FOR ACNE-PRONE SKIN			
Preparation			
Procedure			
Post-Service			
Timing			

Ch. 19: Makeup

Why Study Makeup?

SHORT ANSWER

1. What are two important concepts to understand for successful makeup application, in addition to the guidelines presented in this chapter?

   _____

   _____

   _____

2. What two perspectives do cosmetologists need to balance, style-wise, to excel in makeup application?

_____

_____

_____

3. List four reasons that cosmetologists should develop a thorough understanding of makeup.

_____

_____

_____

Color Theory for Makeup

FILL IN THE BLANK

4. Complete the sentences below using the words from the word bank. Some words will be used more than once.

    Word bank: red, orange, yellow, green, blue, wheel, makeup, blue-green, contrasting, contrast, theory, complementary, red-yellow, middle

    Color _____ is the foundation of a successful _____ application. The color

    _____ is a guide that will help you learn about pairing _____ or _____

    colors. Divide a color wheel in half through the _____ of the _____ and

    _____ wedges. The wheel's _____ side represents warm colors. The

    _____ side represents cool colors. The dividing line shows that _____ and

    _____ can be both warm and cool. For example, _____-based red is warm,

    while _____-based red is cool. _____-based green is warm, but

    _____-based green is cool. Colors directly across from each other on the color wheel

    offer the most _____ and are therefore considered complementary.

5. Fill in the color wheel below with the proper colors to show the primary, secondary, and tertiary colors. Draw lines to indicate the warm and cool sides of the wheel. Finally, indicate the complementary colors.

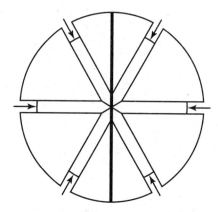

TRUE OR FALSE

Indicate whether the statements below are true or false. For any false statements, explain why they are false.

6. Neutral colors are colors that contrast with all other colors.

   T   F   _____

7. Neutral colors cannot have a warm or cool base.

   T   F   _____

8. Your client's skin type is the most important factor when choosing the color palette for their makeup.

   T   F   _____

9. Examples of a cool neutral are orange-brown and bronze-gold; examples of a warm neutral are charcoal-gray and blue-gray.

   T   F   _____

10. Eyeshadows in complementary colors will emphasize the eyes and make the colors pop, while monochromatic colors that match the eye color will have less of an impact.

    T   F   _____

11. Because orange contains yellow and red, eyeshadows with any of these colors will make blue eyes look bluer.

    T   F   _____

12. The complementary color for green eyes is red, which means you should always use pure red tones.

    T   F   _____

SHORT ANSWER

13. What are the four color-related factors of your client's physical features that you should consider when choosing their makeup color palette? List the types of colors or tones associated with each one.

    _____

    _____

    _____

14. What does skin tone refer to?

    _____

    _____

    _____

15. What are the traditional skin tone categories, according to cosmetics companies?

    _____

    _____

    _____

16. Your ability to properly identify the depth of your client's skin tone will affect your choice of which type of cosmetic for your client?

_____

_____

_____

FILL IN THE BLANK

Complete the sentences below.

17. Undertone refers to the _____ beneath the skin's _____ layer. Undertone is generally classified into three categories:

    • _____ colors—equal mix of _____ and _____ undertones

    • _____ colors—pink, red, or bluish undertones

    • _____ colors—yellow, peachy, or golden undertones

Undertone, more so than _____ tone, is responsible for the overall _____ of your

client's complexion and determines if their skin is seen as _____, _____, or neutral.

Performing a color _____ test using various shades is the most effective way to select a proper

_____ color.

CREATE

18. While your text mentions the color match test, there are many ways to determine the skin's undertones. For this exercise, work with a partner to create your own test for determining skin undertones. Research various beauty, skin, and cosmetics websites or blogs to review the types of tests they offer and the questions they ask. Use search terms such as "skin undertones," "selecting the proper foundation," "how do I determine my skin undertone," and so on. Compile questions and screenshots of color tables or charts and use the information you find to create a short (three- to six-question) quiz.

Next, partner with another group and take each other's quizzes. How accurate do you think the results of your quizzes are? What color foundation would you recommend for each other? Does it differ from a foundation color that you may have typically used in the past?

19. Label each color palette depicted below to indicate which eye color it best complements.

     a. Blue eyes   b. Brown eyes   c. Green eyes

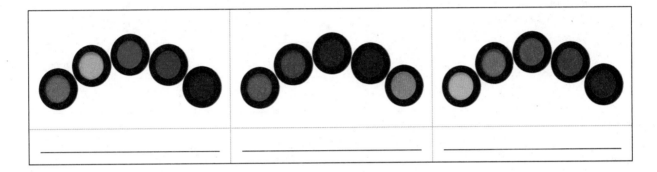

20. Although eye color is often divided into three categories (brown, blue, and green), multiple variations exist. Find images in magazines or celebrity Instagram posts, or pair up with a few different classmates and look closely at their eyes. Describe the variations that you noticed among those main categories. Be specific and accurate in the terms you use for the different colors. Partner with a classmate to review and discuss each other's terms. Do your partner's terms sound like colors you observed? How may the lighting—sunlight, fluorescent lighting, professional photos, and so on—affect eye colors?

Brown	
Blue	
Green	

21. What color category should you coordinate the cheek and lip makeup with?

_____

_____

_____

22. Provide an example of the lip and cheek color (warm, cool, or neutral) that you might choose for a client who has light brown-golden eyes and wears rosy peach eyeshadows.

_____

_____

_____

23. When selecting eyeshadow, what else should you consider aside from eye color? Why?

_____

_____

_____

24. If you have a client with blue eyes and cool blue-black hair, would you use a warm or cool color of eyeshadow?

_____

_____

_____

MATCHING

25. Match each warm or cool tone to the corresponding hair color in the table below. Each tone will be used once.

   a. Red-violet, violet
   b. Copper, red

   c. Yellow, orange
   d. Violet, blue

   e. Gold, copper, orange, red
   f. Ash, silver

HAIR COLOR	WARM HAIR COLOR TONE		COOL HAIR COLOR TONE	
Blonde		_____		White-blonde, ash
Red		_____		_____
Brown		Yellow, gold, orange		Ash
Dark brown/ black		_____		_____
Gray or white		[Not applicable]		_____

Makeup Is for Everyone

SHORT ANSWER

26. Are salon makeup services gender or age specific?

_____

_____

_____

27. Provide an example of two different purposes—for a minimal and a fuller application—that makeup for everyday wear might serve.

_____

_____

_____

28. List four ways you can incorporate camouflaging techniques using everyday makeup.

_____

_____

_____

29. What are four products that typically provide a full coverage look for everyday makeup application?

_____

_____

_____

30. What are three ways you can enhance the basic full coverage look with everyday makeup?

_____

_____

_____

REFLECTION

31. Write a few sentences in response to each question below. Allow yourself some time to think carefully about the range of clients you will encounter in the role of a professional makeup artist.

- What does the term "makeup for everyday" mean to you—personally and in general?

- How does the concept of "makeup for every day" relate to the notion that makeup is for everyone?

- List one or two specific examples of how embracing those concepts (makeup is for every day and everyone) can help build your clientele and enhance your professional approach to makeup application.

32. For each statement about how to work with mature skin when applying makeup, indicate whether it is something you should do (Do) or something that you should not do (Don't).

Do or Don't?   **When Applying Makeup for Clients with Mature Skin**

_____ Blend in muted eyeshadow colors with pops of light shimmer for clients with mature skin

_____ Hold the skin firmly when applying makeup

_____ Use glitter or frosted colors if your client has wrinkles, age spots, or skin tags

_____ Prepare the skin before applying makeup

_____ Leave hard lines in the makeup application

_____ Minimize the appearance of wrinkles with a hydrating serum

_____ Use products that help conceal sun damage

_____ Use heavy powders

_____ Use a lightweight powder formula sparingly

33. Number the steps for performing makeup applications on clients who have textured skin, from 1 to 7.

_____ Use a matte (nonshiny, dull) blush color to avoid accenting the uneven texture.

_____ Determine if the client's skin texture is due to enlarged pores, scars, active acne, or excessive sun damage.

_____ Temper your client's expectations in advance by letting them know that makeup cannot eliminate uneven skin texture.

_____ Once you have determined the source of your client's skin texture, take some time to educate them about skin care.

_____ Select a long-wear foundation that contains a setting agent that will create a more even canvas.

_____ After completing the makeup application, offer the client your products and services that address their skin condition.

_____ Properly prepare the skin for makeup application. For example, if the skin is acneic, consider using an oil-absorbing product before applying the foundation.

Facial Makeup

34. What are three examples of skin imperfections that foundation can hide?

   _____

   _____

   _____

35. List four formulations for foundation. How do you choose the best formulation of the foundation for your client?

   _____

   _____

   _____

36. What is the role of primer in relation to foundation?

   _____

   _____

   _____

37. Describe how primer and foundation are applied.

   _____

   _____

   _____

Indicate whether the statements below are true or false. For any false statements, explain why they are false.

38. Ensure that the ingredients in a liquid foundation product are noncomedogenic, meaning they do not contain ingredients that will clog the follicles and aggravate acne-prone skin.

   T   F   _____

39. Some liquid foundations are marketed as oil free and are not intended for oilier skin types.

   T   F   _____

40. Cream foundations provide heavier coverage and are usually intended for hyperpigmented or mature skin types.

   T   F   _____

41. *Mineral makeup* most commonly refers to the highly pigmented powder, not liquid, formulations for foundation.

   T   F   _____

42. Mineral makeup formulations are popular for clients with acne, rosacea, allergies, and/or sensitive skin because, when applied properly, they feel weightless on the skin.

   T   F   _____

RESEARCH

43. Use the Internet, review beauty catalogues, or visit a beauty supply store to identify and research three different foundations: a cream, liquid, and powder. Use the table below to record your findings. Which foundation brand or type could you imagine yourself using most often on clients?

FEATURES	CREAM FOUNDATION	LIQUID FOUNDATION	POWDER FOUNDATION
Source (Store/Website)			
Name/Brand			
Form (Liquid, Cream, Mineral)			
Color			
Oil or Water Based			
Noncomedogenic?			
Sunscreen Included			
Cost/Size			

SHORT ANSWER

44. What are concealers used to hide?

_____

_____

_____

45. Provide three examples of how concealers are packaged.

_____

_____

_____

46. What is the formulation of concealer if light coverage is desired? What is the formulation for greater coverage?

_____

_____

_____

47. What cosmeceutical ingredient would you look for in a concealer if you wanted to control blemishes? If you wanted to build collagen?

_____

_____

_____

FILL IN THE BLANK

48. Complete the sentences below using the words from the word bank. Each word will be used once.

   Word bank: lavender, green, cancel, opposite, dark, correcting, discoloration, hyperpigmentation, theory, sallow, wheel, lift, neutralizing

   The formulation for color-_____ concealers is based on the color

   _____, which states that when colors _____ each other on the

   color _____ are layered, they _____ each other out. In other

   words, they are formulated in various _____ shades. So, _____

   concealer helps hide redness associated with ruddy skin. Concealer formulated with a

   _____ pigment reduces a _____ (dull yellow) skin appearance.

   An orange-to-peach concealer cancels out _____. For deep skin tones,

   orange, peach, or red can also help _____ the complexion or neutralize

   _____ spots or under eye _____.

RESEARCH

49. Use the Internet, review beauty catalogues, or visit a beauty supply store to identify and research three different concealers, such as ones to control blemishes or build collagen, ones with light coverage or oil-based creams, or those with different packaging. Use the table below to record your findings. Which concealer brand or type could you imagine yourself using most often on clients?

FEATURES	CONCEALER #1	CONCEALER #2	CONCEALER #3
Source (Store/Website)			
Name/Brand			
Packaging (e.g., Stick, Jar)			
Color/Color Correction			
Silicone or Oil Based			
Cosmeceuticals (if any)			
Cost/Size			

SHORT ANSWER

50. What is face powder used for in makeup application?

_____

_____

_____

51. What is the difference between translucent and color-correcting face powders?

_____

_____

_____

52. Which face powder is best for touch-ups on oily skin throughout the day?

_____

_____

_____

53. Which ingredient in face powder is considered best for use by clients who might be on camera? Why?

_____

_____

_____

54. Match each type of eye makeup with its description. Each type will be used three times.

    a. Eyeshadow   b. Eyeliner   c. Eyebrow color

Type of Eye Makeup	Description
_____	Available in every color, from warm to cool, neutral to bright, and light to dark
_____	Can darken the eyebrows, alter their shape, or fill in sparse areas
_____	Pencil version of this type of eye makeup is available in both soft and hard forms for use on the upper and lower eyelids
_____	Adds color and shape to the eyebrows
_____	Defines the eyes and makes the lash line appear fuller
_____	Chemistry of the pencil version is similar to that of eyeliner pencils; chemistry of the powder version is similar to that of eyeshadows
_____	Available in pencil, liquid, pressed (cake), gel, and felt-tip pen forms
_____	Comes in various finishes, including metallic, matte, frost, and shimmer
_____	Available in cream, as well as pressed and loose powder forms

TRUE OR FALSE

Indicate whether the statements below are true or false. For any false statements, explain why they are false.

55. Lip color is available in many forms, including creams, glosses, pencils, gels, and sticks.

    T   F   _____

56. Lakes are water soluble and will not mix with oils; dyes are insoluble, can be mixed with oils, and may be more color stable.

    T   F   _____

57. Lip liner is generally applied before lip color to define the lip's shape and keep color from bleeding.

T   F   _____

58. You must follow proper infection control procedures by sharpening the lip pencil before each client and cleaning it after each use. Also clean and disinfect your sharpener every day.

T   F   _____

59. Lip conditioner is used as a lip moisturizer when starting the makeup application so that it can soak in and moisturize before you start to apply the liner, while lip gloss can give a shiny, moisturized look to the lips.

T   F   _____

60. A primer, foundation, or plumper can be applied after the lip color.

T   F   _____

RESEARCH

61. Use the Internet, review beauty catalogues, or visit a beauty supply store to identify and research three types of eye makeup: eyeshadow, eyeliner, and eyebrow color. Use the table below to record your findings. Keep this as a record for when you are putting together your makeup kit for the salon.

FEATURES	EYESHADOW	EYELINER	EYEBROW COLOR
Source (Store/Website)			
Name/Brand			
Form (e.g., Powder, Cream, Pencil)			
Range/Examples of Colors Available			
Applicator Included?			
Cost/Size			

62. What are the two types of cheek color? What effects can you achieve with each form?

   _____

   _____

   _____

63. Which forms of cheek color are layered over and then directly blended into the foundation?

   _____

   _____

   _____

64. How do makeup artists lend a sheer, natural-looking glow with cheek colors?

   _____

   _____

   _____

65. What are three types of mascara? What is the most common type?

   _____

   _____

   _____

66. A client comes in asking for a way to increase their eyelash thickness without adding the color of mascara. What product would you recommend to them?

   _____

   _____

   _____

67. Use the Internet, review beauty catalogues, or visit a beauty supply store to identify and research three different lip colors and lip products. Use the table below to record your findings. Keep this as a record for when you are putting together your makeup kit for the salon.

FEATURES	LIP COLOR #1	LIP COLOR #2	LIP COLOR #3
Source (Store/Website)			
Name/Brand			
Type (e.g., Lipstick, Lip Liner, Lip Gloss or Conditioner)			
Range/Examples of Colors Available			
Ingredients			
How Long Is It Promised to Last?			
Cost/Size			

MATCHING

68. Match each type of other cosmetics with its description. Each type of cosmetic will be used at least twice.

a. Eye makeup removers   b. Grease paint   c. Cake makeup

Types of Other Cosmetics

Description

_____ Can be either water based or oil based; water-based versions of this cosmetic comprise a solution with added solvents

_____ Also known as pancake makeup

_____ Primarily used for theatrical purposes because it does not shift during performances

_____ Oil-based versions of this cosmetic generally used to remove heavy, dramatic makeup and break down the latex glue used to apply false eyelashes

_____ Heavy cream foundation that provides heavy coverage

_____ Special preparations for removing eye makeup, including water-resistant products

_____ Applied to the face with a moistened cosmetic sponge

_____ Heavy makeup

_____ Cosmetics most commonly used to cover scars and uneven pigmentation

_____ Great for correcting little errors during the makeup application process

Makeup Brushes, Tools, and Implements

FILL IN THE BLANK

69. Complete the missing information in the chart below.

PART OF THE MAKEUP BRUSH	DESCRIPTION
	Comes in various lengths and can be made of wood, acrylic, plastic, or metal
	Bristles of the makeup brush
	Metal part that holds the brush intact and supports the bristles' strength, ideally with double crimping or a ring around it

70. Complete the missing information in the chart below.

TYPE OF MAKEUP BRUSH OR TOOL	DESCRIPTION AND USE	IMAGE OF STANDARD BRUSH OR TOOL
Eyeshadow brush		
	Tapered soft bristles; used to blend makeup all over the face in broad sweeps; hard-to-reach areas like corners of the nose, hairline; around the eyes and mouth	

TYPE OF MAKEUP BRUSH OR TOOL	DESCRIPTION AND USE	IMAGE OF STANDARD BRUSH OR TOOL
	Firm, thin bristles; used to apply powder to the eyebrows or eyeliner at the lash line	
Lip brush		
Concealer brush		
	Short brush with dense bristles for powder or blush; mainly used in a circular motion to apply and blend powders	
Eyeliner brush		
Powder brush		
	Smaller, more tapered version of the powder brush; excellent for applying powder cheek color	

SHORT ANSWER

71. What are the two types of materials that makeup brushes can be made of?

_____

_____

_____

72. What are the three parts of a makeup brush?

_____

_____

_____

73. What can you do to ensure that the high-quality makeup brushes you invest in will last for years?

_____

_____

_____

74. List two or three regulations for cleaning makeup brushes specified by your state's regulatory agency.

_____

_____

_____

75. Which direction should you point your brush when cleaning and disinfecting it? Why?

_____

_____

_____

76. Which two materials used in makeup brushes cannot be disinfected? Why?

_____

_____

_____

77. What should you do after using a single-use implement? Why?

_____

_____

_____

78. What are two benefits of using single-use implements?

_____

_____

_____

SEQUENCE

79. Number the steps for cleaning and disinfecting makeup brushes, from 1 to 8.

_____ Cleanse them with a commercial cleaning solution.

_____ Store brushes in a clean, covered container.

_____ Rinse brushes thoroughly after cleansing.

_____ Rinse brushes thoroughly after disinfecting.

_____ Gently cleanse brushes with an antibacterial detergent.

_____ Reshape the wet bristles.

_____ Disinfect the brushes for the required length of time.

_____ Lay brushes flat on a clean towel until dry.

DOS AND DON'TS

80. For each statement related to safety guidelines for working with makeup brushes, indicate whether it is something you should do (Do) or something that you should not do (Don't).

Do or Don't?	Safety Guidelines when Working with Makeup Brushes
_____	Use brushes that have natural bristles on multiple clients
_____	Pick up a portion of the product from a clean palette when applying makeup
_____	Keep disposable brushes after use
_____	Sell brushes with wooden handles and/or natural bristles to clients for personal use
_____	Use brushes with wooden handles on clients
_____	Clean and disinfect synthetic brushes
_____	Use disposable brushes

81. Identify each makeup tool pictured below and fill in its description and use.

MAKEUP TOOL	NAME	DESCRIPTION AND USE

82. What are three advantages or benefits of using airbrush makeup?

_____

_____

_____

83. What is the main objective when using airbrush makeup?

_____

_____

_____

84. What are some types of makeup that more experienced makeup artists apply with airbrush tools?

_____

_____

_____

MATCHING

85. Match each single-use implement with its description.

Single-Use Implements	Description
_____	May be made of velour and are used to apply and blend powder, powder foundation, and powder blush
_____	May be used to minimize the risk of infection; check with your instructor, state, and regulatory agency for proper guidance
_____	Disposable applicators for hygienically applying lip color
_____	Disposable applicators for applying mascara
_____	Used to apply shadow and lip color and blend eyeliner; may be used damp to intensify eyeshadow color
_____	May be used with toner or makeup removers
_____	Available in various sizes and shapes, including wedges and circles, and work well to apply and blend foundation, cream or powder blush, pressed powder, and concealer
_____	May be used to apply shadow, blend eyeliner, apply lip balm, and correct application mistakes; allow for focused and detailed work
_____	Have a wide, flat base; used to dispense makeup from containers

Complementing Face Shapes and Features

SHORT ANSWER

86. What are two overall qualities of your client's face that you, as a makeup artist, should try to create with makeup techniques?

_____

_____

_____

87. How are the techniques and goals of makeup application similar to those of artists?

_____

_____

_____

88. To evaluate the degree of symmetry in a client's face, what are the three horizontal sections that you should visually divide it into? Briefly describe each section.

_____

_____

_____

89. What are three examples of a client's facial components you should examine once you've visually divided their face into the horizontal thirds, in order to determine the symmetry of their face?

_____

_____

_____

90. Which three makeup products can be used to perform highlighting and contouring?

_____

_____

_____

91. Complete the sentences below using words from the word bank. Each word will be used once.

     Word bank: lighter, darker, light, highlight, shadow, noticeable, emphasizes, prominent, contour

     The basic rule when using facial cosmetics is that drawing _____ to an area

     _____ features, while creating a _____ minimizes them. A _____ is

     produced when a product _____ than the client's skin tone is placed on the high planes of

     the face. A _____ is formed when a product _____ than the client's skin tone is

     used to create shadows over _____ features to make them less _____.

92. Listed below are a variety of objectives that your clients may have regarding their facial shapes and
    features. They typically want to use makeup to enhance or de-emphasize certain facial features.
    For each objective, do the following (one example is provided for you):

    1. Use colors and shading to indicate how you would bring balance and harmony with your
       makeup skills to each face below, based on the client's face shape.

    2. Write a brief description of what your drawing shows.

CLIENT'S OBJECTIVE FOR ENHANCING AND DE-EMPHASIZING FACIAL FEATURES	YOUR DRAWING OF CLIENT'S FACIAL SHAPE WITH MAKEUP TO ACHIEVE CLIENT'S OBJECTIVE	YOUR DESCRIPTION
Example: Add width to overall face		1. Applied a darker foundation along the hairline and under the cheekbones to create the illusion of wider cheekbones 2. Blended a light foundation shade over the outer edge of the cheekbones to bring out the sides of the face
Reduce width from jaw area		

CLIENT'S OBJECTIVE FOR ENHANCING AND DE-EMPHASIZING FACIAL FEATURES	YOUR DRAWING OF CLIENT'S FACIAL SHAPE WITH MAKEUP TO ACHIEVE CLIENT'S OBJECTIVE	YOUR DESCRIPTION
Emphasize receding chin		
Reduce prominent forehead		
Reduce width from overall face		
Create illusion of a longer nose length		
Reduce width from lower portion of face		

CLIENT'S OBJECTIVE FOR ENHANCING AND DE-EMPHASIZING FACIAL FEATURES	YOUR DRAWING OF CLIENT'S FACIAL SHAPE WITH MAKEUP TO ACHIEVE CLIENT'S OBJECTIVE	YOUR DESCRIPTION
Add height to forehead		
Reduce width from forehead area		
Minimize width of cheekbone		
Reduce nose width		

FILL IN THE BLANK

Complete the sentences below.

93. Blend eyeshadow color outward to elongate _____.

94. To lift _____ eyes, place a dot of highlighter directly under the brow arch with a thin line of

_____ slightly thickened at the outside edge.

95. To soften and define the _____ of the eyelid, create a dense line then blend.

96. To add width to close-set eyes, use a _____ color at the inner corners and blend a

_____ shade out to the edge.

97. To minimize the distance between wide-set eyes, apply _____ along the lash line

extending toward the _____ then soften by blending with an eyeshadow.

98. _____ eyelashes can open, elongate, and create balance to the face.

SHORT ANSWER

99. What effect do unkept brows have on the eyes?

_____

_____

_____

100. What is the effect of overtweezed brows?

_____

_____

_____

101. When determining the three lines to create a well-balanced eyebrow shape, where should the
client look?

_____

_____

_____

102. Now that you've studied techniques for helping clients achieve objectives such as bringing balance to their eye shape, it's time for you to practice these techniques on yourself. For this activity, you will practice different techniques on your own eyes to see for yourself what the various effects are. Follow the steps below.

1. Take a photo of your own eyes (or work with a partner to make it easier).

2. Describe what you think your eye shape and eye features are. _____

3. Describe one aspect about your eyes that you might want to change with makeup. _____

4. Apply makeup to make the change you described in step 3.

5. Take a photo of the finished look (or work with a partner to do so).

6. Describe the techniques you used in step 4 to achieve the finished look. _____

7. Remove the eye makeup.

Next, use three different techniques to create three different looks for your eyes. For each of the three applications, be sure to take a photo of the finished look (or have a partner do so) and completely remove the eye makeup after each application. Finally, record the following information about your three applications in the table.

DESCRIBE	EYE MAKEUP APPLICATION #1	EYE MAKEUP APPLICATION #2	EYE MAKEUP APPLICATION #3
Types of eye makeup used (e.g., liners, pencils, shadows, concealers, mascara)			
Color palette of makeup			
Placement of the types of eye makeup (e.g., outer edge of eye, lid, lashes, near nose)			
Effects (e.g., widened eyes, made eyes smaller, rounder, narrower)			
Whether you liked the effects and why			
Your discoveries about the techniques, and color and makeup choices			

103. Draw the lines used to determine brow placement and shape on the images below and order them from 1 to 4. Label each line that you've drawn with the appropriate step.

1. Alternative method for determining the arch's highest part

2. Determine the arch's highest part

3. Determine where the eyebrow should end

4. Determine the start of the brow

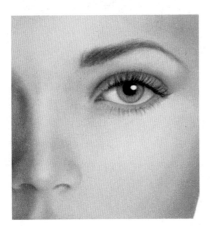 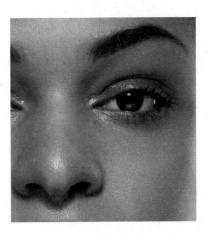

MATCHING

104. Match each eyebrow objective with the recommended technique for achieving it.

a. Raise the brow
b. Lower the brow

c. Reduce the width between the eyes

d. Increase the width between the brows

Eyebrow Objective	Recommended Technique to Achieve Objective
_____	Extend the eyebrow lines slightly outward beyond the outer corners of the eyes
_____	Fill in the lower part of the brow with an eyebrow pencil or shadow; outline the area with concealer to define the eyebrow
_____	Extend the eyebrow lines inward toward the inside corners of the eyes but be careful not to give your client a frowning look
_____	Fill in the top part of the brow with a pencil or powder and accent the brow bone

105. On the diagram below, use colored pencils to illustrate how lipstick can be applied to create the illusion of more balanced and proportioned lips.

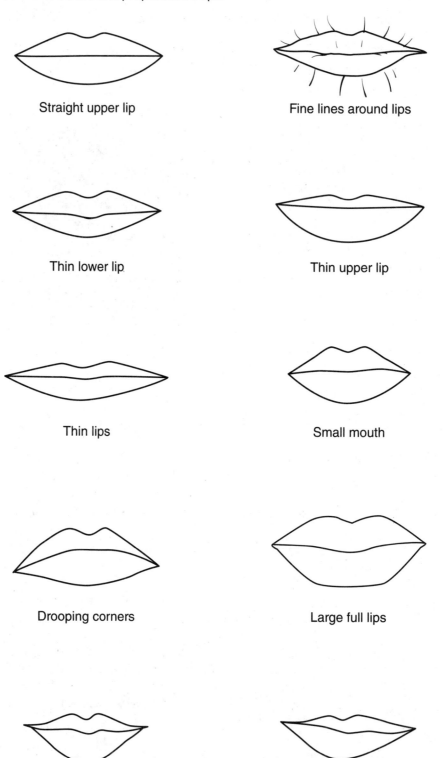

Straight upper lip

Fine lines around lips

Thin lower lip

Thin upper lip

Thin lips

Small mouth

Drooping corners

Large full lips

Cupid's Bow

Uneven lips

106. Match each skin tone with its description and the technique for balancing it. Each skin tone will be used more than once.

a. Ruddy   b. Sallow   c. Hyperpigmented

Skin Tone	Description and Technique for Balancing
_____	Skin that is uneven, or has blemishes or melasma
_____	Avoid red or pink blush
_____	Apply a pink-based foundation, concealer, or primer on the affected areas and blend carefully into the jaw and neck; set with translucent powder
_____	Skin with a yellowish hue
_____	Skin with a reddish hue that may be sensitive, wind-burned, or affected by rosacea
_____	Cancel out brown macules with an orange-color corrector then follow with foundation; set with powder
_____	Apply a green concealer or primer to the affected areas and blend carefully; you may then apply a light foundation layer with a warm yellow tone to balance the complexion; set it with translucent powder
_____	Avoid yellow-based colors for eyes, cheeks, and lips

SHORT ANSWER

107. What are three types of skin issues that camouflage makeup can conceal?

_____

_____

_____

108. What are two possible methods of applying camouflage makeup? Which method is considered advanced and requires much practice to master?

_____

_____

_____

Makeup Consultation and Application

109. What two things should you do when your client responds to your consultation questions?

_____

_____

_____

110. After completing the makeup service, what kind of form should you fill out and review with your client? Who keeps the form?

_____

_____

_____

111. What is the purpose of the form that you complete after the makeup service is completed?

_____

_____

_____

112. List the top five questions you plan to ask during the client consultation for makeup services. Then compare it with the list in your text. Does your list match? If not, what is missing or different on your list?

_____

_____

_____

Indicate whether the statements below are true or false. For any false statements, explain why they are false.

113. When lighting your client's face, use the dark shadows caused by overhead lighting as a guide for where to contour and highlight their features.

    T   F   _____

114. Adequate and flattering lighting is essential for both the consultation and the application portions of the makeup process.

    T   F   _____

115. Artificial light is the best choice when applying makeup but use daylight if necessary.

    T   F   _____

116. If you must choose between fluorescent and incandescent, incandescent light is more flattering.

    T   F   _____

117. LED panels accentuate the face's highlights and contours, while ring lights offer even, balanced light.

    T   F   _____

118. Setting the lights so that they are a balance of fluorescent light (cool industrial light) and incandescent light (warm bulb light) is conducive to makeup application.

    T   F   _____

SHORT ANSWER

119. What is the main purpose of bracing during makeup application?

    _____

    _____

    _____

120. When working around the face, how do you position your dominant hand or fingers on the client's face? Which hand do you use to manipulate the applicator, brush, or pencil?

_____

_____

_____

121. Does your state require you to demonstrate bracing techniques during your practical exam?

_____

_____

_____

SEQUENCE

122. Number the steps for choosing and applying foundation, from 1 to 7.

_____ Use a cotton swab to apply a small amount of three different skin-matching shades to the jawline, hairline, or collar bone.

_____ If you see obvious lines of demarcation (where the foundation begins and ends), gently blend those line until they are no longer visible.

_____ Place the foundation on a palette to avoid contaminating the container.

_____ To choose the correct foundation—one that is closest to the client's natural skin tone—seat the client in a well-lit area.

_____ Use a sponge, your fingertips, or a brush to blend the foundation downward using short strokes.

_____ Start at the area requiring the greatest amount of coverage, such as the center of the face, over hyperpigmented cheeks, or along the hairline.

_____ After choosing the correct color—the color that disappears is the right choice—use a spatula to remove the makeup from its container.

FILL IN THE BLANK

Complete the sentences below.

123. Under the eyes, apply concealer with a _____ and focus on concealing

_____ areas and discoloration. Be sure to use a concealer that is only

_____ shade(s) _____ than the client's skin tone.

124. Applying concealer in a _____ from nose to the temple will lift the _____ for a more dramatic look.

125. A _____ fiber concealer brush produces the most natural result.

126. When hiding a blemish, avoid applying a color _____ than your client's skin tone, as this will draw attention to the concealed area.

SHORT ANSWER

127. Why is it suggested that you select one area of the face as your focal point when applying makeup?

_____

_____

_____

128. What is the resulting effect if the foundation color is too light? What is the effect if it is too dark?

_____

_____

_____

129. What three tools or single-use items can you use to apply loose powder?

_____

_____

_____

130. What are some signs that your powder application was less than ideal?

_____

_____

_____

131. Why should you avoid using pressed powder in compacts (usually accompanied by a powder puff applicator) in the salon?

_____

_____

_____

132. How should you prepare the eyebrow pencil for use in application?

_____

_____

_____

133. Describe the application technique that is used with both eyebrow pencils and eyebrow powders. What is the difference between the techniques?

_____

_____

_____

134. Which eyebrow makeup is often paired with eyebrow wax?

_____

_____

_____

135. Where do you apply powder eyeshadow?

_____

_____

_____

136. How and where do you apply cream eyeshadow?

_____

_____

_____

137. Match each type of eyeshadow color with its description.

    a. Highlight color   c. Contour color
    b. Base color   d. Transition color

Type of Eyeshadow Color	Description
_____	Darker than the client's skin tone
_____	Generally a medium shade close to the client's skin tone
_____	Used to diffuse the contour color
_____	Usually applied across the lid, up to the crease to make the eyes appear larger
_____	Accents specific areas, such as the brow bone or the inner corners to add width between the eyes
_____	Applied to minimize unwanted fullness/puffiness or elongate the eye
_____	Blended into the area between the crease and brow bone
_____	Lighter than the client's skin tone and may have a matte or iridescent finish

SHORT ANSWER

138. What should you do once you've applied cream eyeshadow if it's not waterproof?

    _____

    _____

    _____

139. Should you attempt to coat all the hairs of the eyelashes with mascara? Can you use mascara on both top and bottom lashes?

    _____

    _____

    _____

140. If planning to curl the lashes, when should you do so? Why?

_____

_____

_____

141. What type of wand should you use for mascara application? How many mascara wands should you use on a client?

_____

_____

_____

FILL IN THE BLANK

Complete the sentences below using the words from the word bank. Each word will be used once.

Word bank: angle, dramatic, inner, lash, lid, outer, powder, sharpen, sharpener, short, tissue, wet, wipe

142. To minimize the chance of cross-contamination, _____ the eyeliner pencil and

_____ it clean before each use, and also clean the _____ before each use.

143. With the client's eyes closed, hold the _____ taut and apply liner along the

_____ line from the _____ corner to the _____ corner with

_____ strokes and gentle pressure.

144. You can also use _____ shadow as eyeliner; simply place a small amount onto a

_____ and apply to the eyes with a clean _____ brush. For a more

_____ look, _____ the brush before the application.

145. Number the steps for applying lip color, from 1 to 11.

_____ Connect the center peaks with rounded strokes, following the natural lip line with the pencil.

_____ Select a lip pencil that coordinates well with the chosen lipstick; the liner color should match the shade of either the natural lip or the lipstick.

_____ Apply the lip color with a clean brush; begin by applying color at the outer corners of each side of the top lip and work toward the middle.

_____ Outline the lower lip by moving from the outer corners of either side to the center of the lip.

_____ Connect the center peaks (the Cupid's bow) using rounded strokes.

_____ After lining the lips, remove the lip color with a spatula.

_____ Ask the client to relax their lips and part them slightly; then ask them to smile slightly so that you can fill in the corners.

_____ Rest your ring finger on the client's chin to steady your hand as you prepare to apply the lip color.

_____ Beginning at the outer corner of the upper lip and working toward the middle, trace the natural lip line with the pencil.

_____ Then, using the same technique, fill in the bottom lip with lip color.

_____ Repeat on the opposite side of the upper lip.

TRUE OR FALSE

Indicate whether the statements below are true or false. For any false statements, explain why they are false.

146. Use a clean blush brush to apply color to the cheeks before foundation and face powder are applied.

T   F   _____

147. Sweeping blush just below the cheekbones results in a more chiseled, sophisticated look.

T   F   _____

148. A more vertical application of blush will tend to widen the face, whereas a more horizontal application will make it look narrower.

    T   F   _____

149. Apply cream blush before powder so that it blends into the foundation and looks soft and natural.

    T   F   _____

150. Never apply blush in a solid circle on the apple of the cheek, beyond the corner of the eye, or blended inward between the cheekbone and the nose.

    T   F   _____

151. For a fresh look, apply color to the apples of the cheeks, blending outward towards the temples, and right into the hairline.

    T   F   _____

152. Cream and gel blush result in a sheer finish that simulates naturally flushed cheeks.

    T   F   _____

FILL IN THE BLANK

153. For each topic related to performing makeup services, write the safety guideline for maintaining infection controls.

TOPICS RELATED TO MAKEUP SERVICES	SAFETY GUIDELINES FOR MAINTAINING INFECTION CONTROLS
Eye pencils, per eye	
Lip color tubes or containers	
Powder makeup materials	
Multi-use utensils, chairs, and counters	
Clients with suspected eye or other infections on the face	
Eye pencils, per client	
Possibly contaminated products	
Your hands	

154. Now that you've practiced the procedures for the basic professional makeup application, consider what you knew about these services before you began this section compared to what you've studied. (And if you haven't practiced these techniques yet, be sure to partner with a classmate, willing friend, or relative and, under your instructor's supervision, practice.) Write a few sentences in which you reflect on and answer the following questions:

   • Can you picture yourself confidently performing the basic professional makeup application techniques for a client?

   • Which makeup techniques do you excel at? Which ones are you uncertain about?

   • Are you comfortable with the array of products, colors, and tools available?

   • Do you feel that you can perform makeup application services safely for you and your clients?

   • Overall, how can you make your professional makeup services flawless for your clients?

   When you're finished, meet with a classmate and discuss your responses. As you do so, look for opportunities to fill in each other's gaps and help each other master the makeup application techniques and specifics.

Eyelash Enhancements

SHORT ANSWER

155. What are three ways that artificial lashes can benefit your clients?

   _____

   _____

   _____

156. What are the three types of materials that eyelashes can be made from?

   _____

   _____

   _____

157. Can clients wear their contact lenses when receiving artificial lash services?

   _____

   _____

   _____

158. Describe how to position and light your client for the lash services.

_____

_____

_____

159. If the lash services are being performed as part of a makeup application, at what point do you perform the lash services? Where does the mascara application fit into the process?

_____

_____

_____

160. Match each type of lashes with its description.

    a. Strip lashes   b. Individual lashes

Type of Lashes   **Description**

_____ Eyelash hairs on a strip applied with adhesive to the natural lash line

_____ Type of lashes that create a full, natural-looking lash line; the result generally lasts longer than the other type

_____ Also known as band lashes

_____ Can be clustered or flared; clustered versions also referred to as tabs

_____ Separate artificial eyelashes applied one at a time on top of the client's lashes

_____ Can trim the outside edge of this type of lash if it's too long to fit the curve of the upper eyelid

_____ Term *eye tabbing* sometimes used to describe the process of applying groups of this type along the lash line

_____ Before application, need to be bent (with your fingers) into a horseshoe shape to make them more flexible so they fit the contour of the eyelid

_____ Not to be confused with synthetic eyelash extensions that last six to eight weeks

161. Label the types of artificial lashes depicted below.

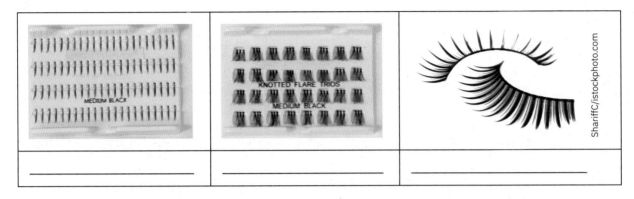

162. Describe the two types of allergy patch tests that you can perform on clients who might be allergic to eyelash adhesive.

_____

_____

_____

163. How long do you need to wait for the allergy patch test results on the adhesive?

_____

_____

_____

164. Number the steps for removing artificial eyelashes, from 1 to 5.

_____ Hold the eye pads or cloth over the eyes for a few seconds to soften the adhesive.

_____ Use wet cotton pads or swabs to remove any makeup and adhesive remaining on the eyelid.

_____ Starting from the outer corner, remove the lashes carefully to avoid pulling out the client's own lashes.

_____ Saturate eye pads with an oil-based eye makeup remover formulated to remove waterproof mascara. Or saturate a facecloth or cotton pad with warm water and a gentle cleanser.

_____ While removing strip lashes, pull them off parallel to the skin, not straight out.

SHORT ANSWER

165. List the tools and equipment needed to perform lash extension services.

_____

_____

_____

166. What are lash extensions made of? How are they applied?

_____

_____

_____

167. How long does the process of applying lash extensions take? How long will the bond last?

_____

_____

_____

168. Why are fills (or touch-ups) needed for lash extensions?

_____

_____

_____

169. What kind of setting in the salon is recommended for performing lash extension services?

_____

_____

_____

170. Briefly describe eyelash perming.

_____

_____

_____

171. Does your state allow you to perform lash perming services?

_____

_____

_____

Complete the sentences below using the words from the word bank. Not all words will be used.

Word bank: add-on, brow, client, cosmetologist, days, effective, excess, expensive, mascara, penciling, physician, precisely, quick, quickly, regulatory agency, skin, sparse, weeks

172. Rather than _____ in brows or wearing _____ every day, tinting darkens

the brows and lashes for a few _____. In addition to the convenience for the

_____, tinting eyelashes and eyebrows is a _____ procedure that is a

great _____ service from the perspective of the _____. However, consider

that if hair is _____, tinting may not show up enough to be _____ .

173. When tinting the eyebrows, keep the tint off of the _____. The application must

_____ define the _____ shape. Color takes very _____,

so any _____ tint must be removed immediately. Finally, always check with your

_____ before performing any lash or brow tinting services.

174. Now that you've practiced the procedures for applying artificial eyelashes, consider what you knew about these services before you began this section compared to what you've studied. Write a few sentences in which you reflect on and answer the following questions:

   • Can you picture yourself confidently applying artificial lashes for a client?

   • Which parts of the lash application procedure do you feel comfortable with? What aspects are you uncertain about?

   • Do you feel that you can perform lash application services safely for your clients?

   • Overall, how can you make your lash application technique flawless for your clients?

   When you're finished, meet with a classmate and discuss your responses. As you do so, look for opportunities to fill in each other's gaps and help each other master the lash application techniques and specifics.

DISCOVERIES AND ACCOMPLISHMENTS

In the space below, write notes about key concepts discussed in this chapter. Share your discoveries with some of the other students in your class and ask them if your notes are helpful. You may want to revise your notes based on good ideas shared by your peers.

Discoveries:

_____

_____

_____

_____

_____

_____

_____

List at least three things you have accomplished since you decided to enroll in school.

Accomplishments:

_____

_____

_____

_____

_____

_____

_____

1. Which of the following is a reason why cosmetologists should have a comprehensive understanding of makeup?

   A) because makeup services are listed under a medical license and performing procedures that are listed under any medical license is a primary responsibility of cosmetologists

   B) because it will help them diagnose, prescribe medications for, and provide treatment for irregular skin conditions, illnesses, or diseases

   C) because contouring, highlighting, and other face shape-enhancing techniques will help them emphasize the best features of their clients

   D) because cosmetologists are physicians specialized in a medical branch of science that involves the study of the skin and its nature, structure, and functions

2. Which of the following statements is true of cool colors?

   A) They range from yellow and gold through oranges and red-oranges, most reds, and even some yellow-greens.

   B) They represent natural, soft colors that complement any skin tone.

   C) They are dominated by blues, greens, violets, and blue-reds.

   D) They do not contrast with any other color.

3. In makeup, _____ represent natural, soft colors that complement any skin tone, eye color, or hair color.

   A) warm colors   C) cool colors

   B) complementary colors   D) neutral colors

4. In the context of factors affecting makeup color selection, the term _____ refers to the color of the skin's surface, and it can be affected by heredity, food habits, and sun exposure, so it may vary at different times of the year.

   A) undertone   C) transition color

   B) base color   D) skin tone

5. In the context of complementary color choices, _____ are neutral, and therefore, any color can be applied to highlight them.

   A) brown eyes   C) blue eyes

   B) green eyes   D) purple eyes

continued

6. Identify a true statement about everyday makeup.

   A) It excludes camouflaging techniques to cover dark circles, rosacea, acne, in-grown facial hair, and hyperpigmentation.

   B) It is exclusively for wealthy clients.

   C) It usually requires a full coverage look including a tinted moisturizer, lip balm, eyebrow gel, and a little setting powder.

   D) It is exclusively for women.

7. Which of the following guidelines should you follow when applying makeup on mature skin?

   A) Use heavy powders instead of a light-weight formula.

   B) Hold the skin loosely when applying makeup.

   C) Use glitter or frosted colors to conceal age spots and skin tags typical of mature skin.

   D) Nourish the skin with a hydrating serum to reduce the appearance of wrinkles.

8. When applying makeup on textured skin, you should use a _____ blush color to avoid enhancing the uneven texture.

   A) shiny   C) glossy

   B) bright   D) matte

9. In the context of facial makeup, identify a function of foundation.

   A) It is primarily used to fill in uneven skin surfaces.

   B) It is used to cleanse, hydrate, detoxify, and nourish the skin.

   C) It can conceal acne, hyperpigmentation, and birthmarks.

   D) It is used to add color to the cheeks.

10. It is recommended that people with oily skin use products that are _____, which means that they do not include ingredients that will block the follicles and worsen acne-prone skin.

    A) alipidic   C) noncomedogenic

    B) comedogenic   D) inflammatory

continued

11. Which of the following is usually applied before lip color to define the lip's shape and keep color from bleeding?

A) lipstick

C) lip gloss

B) rouge

D) lip liner

12. Which of the following steps should you take to clean and disinfect makeup brushes?

A) Always place the brush into still or running water with the ferrule pointing upward.

B) Reshape the wet bristles of the brush after cleansing and disinfecting them.

C) Disinfect all brushes with wooden handles after each use.

D) Clean synthetic brushes only with water as they cannot be disinfected.

13. Which of the following statements is true of a spoolie?

A) It is used to lift and curl the upper eyelashes.

B) It is used to brush brows into place.

C) It is used to apply powder on the eyebrows.

D) It is used to apply liquid liner on the lash line.

14. Which of the following is a single-use makeup implement that may be used to apply lip balm, blend eyeliner, apply shadow, and correct application mistakes?

A) cotton swabs

C) sponges

B) spoolies

D) powder puffs

15. The basic rule when using facial cosmetics is that _____.

A) redefining every facial feature of your client can make the client look naturally beautiful

B) a highlight is produced when a product darker than the client's skin tone is placed on the high planes of the face

C) the face can be divided into five equal horizontal sections

D) drawing light to an area emphasizes features, while creating a shadow minimizes them

continued

16. Identify a reshaping technique to reduce width from the overall face.

A) Apply and blend a darker foundation shade from the center of the forehead down the center of the face to the tip of the chin.

B) Apply and blend a light foundation shade over the outer edges of the cheekbones to bring out the sides of the face.

C) Apply and blend a lighter foundation over the chin and neck.

D) Apply and blend a darker foundation shade on the outer edges of the temples, cheekbones, and jawline.

17. Identify a reshaping technique to enlarge small lips and mouth.

A) Use a medium-color liner to draw a soft curve inside the peaks of the Cupid's bow.

B) Draw a thin line just inside the natural lip line and use soft, flat lipstick colors.

C) Outline upper and lower lips with a soft color to create proportion and fill in with flattering color.

D) Outline both the upper and lower lips and fill in the lips with soft or shimmery colors.

18. In the context of balancing skin tones, for ruddy skin (skin with a reddish hue that may be sensitive, wind-burned, or affected by rosacea), you should apply a _____ concealer or primer on the affected areas and blend carefully.

A) green   C) pink

B) orange   D) blue

19. During a makeup consultation with a client, you should _____.

A) gather important information about the client, including skin condition and sensitivities

B) prepare the tools that will be required for the makeup application process

C) determine whether the client will be able to pay for the makeup service

D) check if the client is fine with the use of a curette

20. Which of the following statements is true of lighting in the context of makeup application?

A) Artificial lighting is the best choice for makeup application.

B) Ring lights enhance the contours and highlights of the face.

continued

C) Overhead lighting should create a pattern of light and dark shadows on the face.

D) Fluorescent light is more flattering than incandescent light.

21. Which of the following guidelines should you follow during blush application?

A) A vertical application of blush will make the face look wider, whereas a horizontal application of blush will tend to make the face look narrower.

B) Blush should blend into the hairline.

C) Apply cream blush before powder so it blends into the foundation.

D) Always apply blush in a solid circle on the apple of the cheek, beyond the corner of the eye, or blended outward between the cheekbone and the nose.

22. Identify a guideline that you should follow to avoid the spread of infection during makeup application.

A) Perform a makeup service on a client with a suspected eye infection only after performing a thorough medical exam.

B) Wash your hands properly before any service.

C) Never sharpen the eye pencil once you start applying eye makeup on a client.

D) Apply gloss or lipstick directly to the lips from the tube or container.

23. In the context of types of lashes, _____ are eyelash hairs on a strip applied with adhesive to the natural lash line.

A) flared lashes   C) individual lashes

B) clustered lashes   D) band lashes

24. Which of the following terms is sometimes used to describe the process of applying groups of individual eyelashes along the lash line?

A) eye tabbing   C) eyelash tinting

B) eyelash perming   D) eye curling

25. The process of chemically curling the lashes is known as _____.

A) eye curling   C) eye tabbing

B) eyelash perming   D) eyelash tinting

finished!

Practical Skills

Self-Evaluation Checklist

Regular self-assessment helps you to improve your technical skills and achieve success. After performing each procedure, review the procedure steps in the textbook and rate yourself as "Competent" or "Needs Work," and write in comments on how you were successful or where you can improve. Rating yourself helps you identify your strengths and weaknesses and develop your own plan for improvement.

CRITERIA	COMPETENT	NEEDS WORK	COMMENTS
PROCEDURE 19-1 BASIC PROFESSIONAL MAKEUP APPLICATION			
Preparation			
Procedure			
Post-Service			
Timing			
PROCEDURE 19-2 FALSE EYELASH APPLICATION			
Preparation			
Procedure			
Post-Service			
Timing			

ch. 20: Manicuring

Why Study Manicuring?

SHORT ANSWER

1. Describe the general procedures that are involved in a manicure.

_____

_____

_____

2. What are the possible consequences for performing certain manicure services outside of the scope of practice (SOP) for your state?

_____

_____

_____

3. In your own words, explain why cosmetologists must have a thorough understanding of manicuring.

_____

_____

_____

Manicure Station Equipment

TRUE OR FALSE

Indicate whether each statement is true or false. For any false statements, explain why they are false.

4. Fans and open windows are excellent substitutes for proper ventilation systems.

   T   F   _____

5. Only table lamps with 40- to 60-watt incandescent bulbs should be used in the salon.

   T   F   _____

6. Disinfection containers should be able to fit several service sets of implements, completely immersed.

   T   F   _____

7. If a trash receptacle with a foot-operated, self-closing lid is not available, it is acceptable to tape or clip a plastic bag to the manicure table for collecting used materials during your manicure.

   T   F   _____

8. The autoclave must remain at the optimal heat, pressure, and steam levels for at least 60 minutes to kill all harmful microorganisms and their spores.

   T   F   _____

9. Match each piece of required manicure station equipment with its description. Each piece of equipment will be used once.

a. Manicure table
b. Client arm cushion
c. Adjustable lamp
d. Cosmetologist's chair
e. Finger bowls

f. Disinfection containers
g. Autoclave
h. Gauze and cotton wipe container
i. Trash container

j. Ventilation system
k. Client's chair

Manicure Station Equipment

Description

_____ Should be made of plastic, metal, glass, or ceramic for proper disinfecting after each client's use

_____ Must be made of materials that can be disinfected; covered with a fresh, clean towel for each client

_____ Must have a lid to protect the contents from dust and contaminants

_____ Usually includes a drawer and a shelf for storing disinfected implements and professional products

_____ Required by the OSHA Hazard Communication Standard where chemical services are performed

_____ Most equipped with a lifting tray or basket that allows the implements to be removed from the solution

_____ Should be selected for ergonomics, comfort, durability, stain resistance, and cleaning ease

_____ Should have a foot-operated, self-closing lid and be located next to your manicure station

_____ Should have no or low arms on the sides so it can be moved closer to the table

_____ This equipment should be researched carefully to ensure it will not cause premature curing of nail enhancement products

_____ A machine that is required by some states to sterilize all multiuse metal implements

10. How is the finger bowl used in a nail service?

_____

_____

_____

11. How often does the Centers for Disease Control (CDC) recommend conducting spore tests on an autoclave?

_____

_____

_____

12. Describe how downdraft ventilation machines work and explain the role of the two-stage carbon filter.

_____

_____

_____

Optional Manicure Station Equipment

SHORT ANSWER

13. List the six types of optional equipment that can be used as part of your manicure services.

_____

_____

_____

14. What are three benefits of the various optional equipment used in manicuring services?

_____

_____

_____

TRUE OR FALSE

Indicate whether each statement is true or false. For any false statements, explain why they are false.

15. Electric nail polish dryers usually have a heater and a fan to speed up drying time.

    T   F   _____

16. Terry cloth mitts may be used during a service that uses a penetrating conditioning treatment.

    T   F   _____

17. Paraffin treatments are extra services or are included in upscale spa services to help enhance moisture in the skin.

    T   F   _____

18. Ultraviolet (UV) and LED curing lamps cure or harden products and are especially effective on gel polishes and traditional hard gel products.

    T   F   _____

19. Terry cloth mitts, typically used over paraffin to hold in heat, are disposable.

    T   F   _____

RESEARCH

20. Select two pieces of optional manicuring equipment that interest you, and visit a beauty supply store (or use the Internet) to conduct research on types, costs, brands, and functions that you wish to know more about. List your details here, then state whether you will consider investing in these types of optional equipment for your practice and why.

_____

_____

_____

Multiuse Manicuring Implements

MATCHING

21. Match each implement to its description or function. Some implements may be used more than once.

   a. Metal pusher
   b. Nail clipper

   c. Nail nipper
   d. Tweezers

Multiuse Implement	Description or Function
_____	Can remove implements from disinfectant solution
_____	Shortens the free edge of the nail quickly
_____	Gently scrapes tissue from the natural nail plate
_____	Can save filing time during the service if the client's nails are too long
_____	Used to trim dead skin away from nails
_____	Should be held at a 20- to 30-degree angle from the nail plate
_____	Can lift small bits of debris from nail plate
_____	Should be held with thumb on one handle and three fingers around the other, and index finger on box joint
_____	Has a spoon-shaped end

SHORT ANSWER

22. Describe what a microtrauma is and explain what can cause them.

   _____

   _____

   _____

23. Multiuse equipment that is made of what type of metal should be avoided?

_____

_____

_____

24. What are four uses for nylon nail brushes?

_____

_____

_____

25. Identify each multiuse implement below.

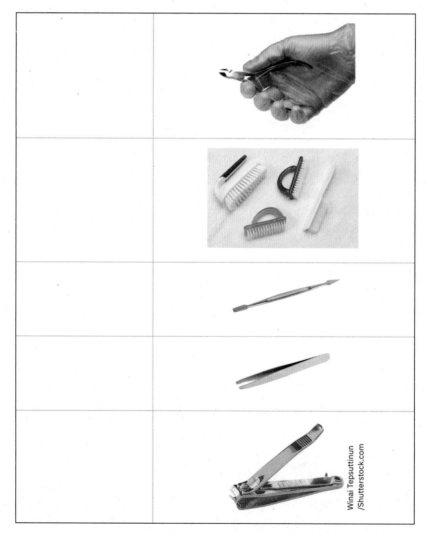

Winai Tepsuttinun
/Shutterstock.com

Single-Use Manicuring Implements

26. Describe how single-use implements are used.

_____

_____

_____

27. What are the five types of single-use implements used in nail care?

_____

_____

_____

MATCHING

28. Match each type of grit abrasive with its description. All types will be used more than once.

    a. Coarse grit   b. Medium grit   c. Fine grit

**Type of Grit
Abrasive**   **Description**

_____ Less than 100 grit

_____ Used to smooth and refine surfaces

_____ Refines, buffs, and removes very fine scratches

_____ 240 and higher grit

_____ 150 to 180 grit

_____ Mainly used for shaping and refining or removing the bulk of enhancements

_____ 150-grit version of this type shortens and shapes natural nails

Indicate whether the statements below are true or false. For any false statements, explain why they are false.

29. When creating a high shine, it's recommended that you begin with the highest grit abrasive surface, move to the next lower grit, and then finish with the shining surface.

    T   F   _____

30. Most two- and three-way buffers are single-use only and are discarded after each use.

    T   F   _____

31. Two-way buffers are generally used on natural nails or in the first steps of the two-color application of monomer liquid and polymer powder nails, such as French manicures, or nails worn without polish.

    T   F   _____

MATCHING

32. Match the following single-use implements with their descriptions. Each type will be used twice.

    a. Plastic or metal spatulas and product
        applicators

    b. Wooden pushers

    c. Product application brushes

    **Single-Use
    Implement**   **Description**

    _____ Can be used to apply nail products by completely wrapping the end
                               with a small piece of cotton and dipping it into the product

    _____ Can be used to remove products from their respective containers to
                               prevent product contamination

    _____ Do not need to be cleaned and disinfected between uses when using
                               products such as alcohol, nail polish, monomers and polymers, or
                               dehydrators and bleaches

    _____ If the same implement of this type is used to remove dissimilar
                               products, it can alter the product's chemistry

    _____ Used to apply masks, nail oils, or nail treatments to clients' nails

    _____ Used to remove cuticle tissue from the nail plate, clean under the
                               nail's free edge, and apply products

Nail Service Materials

33. Which type of glove does OSHA recommend for protection against chemicals? Which two types of gloves do not protect against chemicals?

_____

_____

_____

34. If a client receives two services together, such as a manicure and a pedicure, can the nail technician wear the same set of gloves for both services?

_____

_____

_____

35. What three things found in a salon setting should a dust mask be specifically designed for?

_____

_____

_____

36. Dust masks with which rating are highly effective at preventing dust inhalation overexposure?

_____

_____

_____

37. Why is it important for fiber or cotton pads to have a plastic backing?

_____

_____

_____

38. What kind of towel should you use to wipe up spills from the manicure table?

_____

_____

_____

Professional Nail Products Used During a Manicure

SHORT ANSWER

39. List the eleven categories of professional nail products.

_____

_____

_____

MATCHING

40. Specify which descriptions apply to which products used during a manicure. More than one of these types of nail product might fit a description.

a. Nail cream   c. Nail oil   e. Soap
b. Nail lotion   d. Cuticle removers

Type of Nail Product(s)   **Description**

_____ Barrier products because they contain ingredients that seal the surface of the skin around the nail and hold the subdermal moisture in the skin

_____ Removes more than 90 percent of pathogenic (disease-producing) microbes from the hands when used properly

_____ Absorbed into the nail plate to increase flexibility and into the surrounding skin to soften and moisturize

_____ Soften dry skin around the nail plate and increase the natural nail's flexibility

_____ Should be applied only to the nail plate

_____ Top nail product to sell to manicure and pedicure clients

_____ Excessive exposure can cause hangnails

_____ The liquid version of this product is best at preventing the growth of bacteria

41. Match each type of nail product with its description.

a. Polish
b. Top coat

c. Nail polish dryer
d. Polish Remover

e. Gel polish
f. Base coat

Nail Product   **Description**

_____ Similar to polishes, contains solvents designed to evaporate and increase the colored coating's adhesion

_____ Contains ingredients that create hard, shiny, or matte films after the solvents evaporate

_____ Requires UV light to dry and cure

_____ Other names for this: enamel, lacquer, and varnish

_____ Comes in acetone and nonacetone versions

_____ Product applied over the top coat

_____ Is more chip resistant than traditional nail lacquers

_____ Reduces smudging on regular manicures

_____ The stronger version of this product can dissolve or weaken nail enhancements

SHORT ANSWER

42. What are three types of nail hardeners? Give one fact about each of them.

_____

_____

_____

43. At what point in the manicure can a nail hardener be applied?

_____

_____

_____

44. What can be used with paraffin treatments or warming mitts to enhance penetration?

_____

_____

_____

45. Besides hardening the surface of a nail, what other benefit can a nail hardener provide if used properly?

_____

_____

_____

46. What are some reasons to apply hand creams and lotions in a manicure service?

_____

_____

_____

DOUBLE PUZZLE

47. Unscramble the words using the clues provided and write them in the squares. You'll see a number underneath some of the squares. Find the numbered square below and write that letter into that square to reveal the secret message!

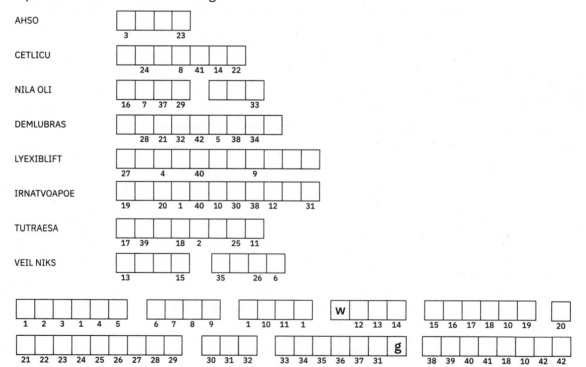

AHSO

CETLICU

NILA OLI

DEMLUBRAS

LYEXIBLIFT

IRNATVOAPOE

TUTRAESA

VEIL NIKS

Manicure Consultation

Indicate whether the statements below are true or false. For statements that are false, explain why they are false.

48. The nail technician should get to know the client and understand the client's expectations, goals, and needs for the nail service.

    T   F   _____

49. Always check the client's skin and nails to make sure they are healthy before beginning any service.

    T   F   _____

50. If a client appears to have diseased or disordered skin or nails, you should state the potential diagnosis and continue with the service.

    T   F   _____

51. It is important to consider the client's work and hobbies when determining the best service.

    T   F   _____

SHORT ANSWER

52. In addition to the questions and observations you make during the client consultation, what are three things that you can communicate to your client to help them maintain the look of their manicure afterward?

    _____

    _____

    _____

53. Which nail shape is most appropriate for clients who work with their hands, such as nurses, office workers, and landscapers?

_____

_____

_____

54. Who is the oval shape nail most appropriate for?

_____

_____

_____

55. Which nail shape is more likely worn as an enhancement than on the natural nail?

_____

_____

_____

56. Complete the table below on considerations necessary for clients with certain medical conditions.

Medical Condition	Considerations
Diabetes	_____
_____	Change massage pressure
Pregnancy	_____
_____	Suggest a dark color polish to hide bruising
Irregular split or brittle nails (onychorrhexis)	_____

57. This exercise requires six different sets of nail tips. First, label the images below with the correct name. Then use cutting and filing to create a set of tips with each of the five basic nail shapes. For the sixth set of tips, design your own nail shape and give it a name (e.g., two stiletto spikes per nail, called the vampire).

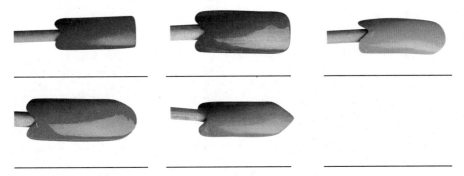

_____   _____   _____

_____   _____   _____

The Basic Manicure

Complete the sentences below.

58. You should always start with the _____ hand, _____ finger when starting a new step in the

    manicure procedure. Doing so will help you create a _____ (or routine) as you practice, which

    increases your _____ and helps you _____ steps.

59. Your basic manicure procedure should take between _____ and _____ minutes, including
    polishing.

60. List the three main parts of the manicure procedure.

    _____

    _____

    _____

61. Why is it helpful to follow a three-part procedure for manicures?

_____

_____

_____

62. When in the three-part procedure should a client was their hands?

_____

_____

_____

63. Can you offer hand sanitizer to a client rather than asking them to use soap and water to wash their hands? Why or why not?

_____

_____

_____

MATCHING

64. Listed below are some of the steps that take place during the pre-service, service, and post-service parts of the basic manicure. Match each part of the service with the steps that are in that part. The parts will be used more than once.

   a. Pre-service   b. Service   c. Post-service

   **Part of the
   Three-Part
   Procedure   Step**

   _____ Record service information, products used, observations, and retail
   recommendations on client service form or input via computer record

   _____ Remove old polish until all traces of polish are gone; check for nail
   abnormalities that could have been hidden by the polish

   _____ Apply massage lotion or oil and perform massage.

   _____ Clean and disinfect manicure table and drawer with EPA-approved disinfectant,
   according to product directions.

_____ Remove products and tools, dispose of used materials, and clean and disinfect your work area.

_____ Remove any loosely hanging dead skin tags with sharp nippers.

_____ Discuss consultation card information and determine course of action for the service.

_____ Suggest retail products that help maintain the client's service; explain why they are important and how to use them.

_____ Set out tools and implements.

_____ Apply nail oil to each nail plate, using cotton-tipped wooden pusher, cotton swab, or eyedropper.

_____ Thank client for their business and mention you look forward to their next visit.

_____ Escort client to hand washing area. Hand client a fresh nail brush and ask them to wash their hands.

SEQUENCE

65. Number the steps of a basic manicure that you would do after performing your pre-service procedures and before your post-service, from 1 to 18, from beginning to end. Some numbers have been provided for you.

___15___ Remove any rough spots on the free edges.

_____ Bleach the nails (optional).

_____ Soften eponychium and cuticle.

_____ Massage.

_____ Apply cuticle remover.

_____ Polish the nails.

_____ File and shape the nails based on client consultation.

_____ Clean under the free edge.

_____ Clean nail surfaces.

_____ Remove polish and inspect the client's nails.

_____ Remove all traces of lotion and oil from the nail plate after the massage and before polishing.

_____13_____ Smooth the nail surface.

_____ Use sharp nippers.

_____ Dry hands with a towel.

_____ Use a wooden or metal pusher.

_____ Remove debris and cuticle remover.

_____ Repeat steps 5 to 10 (as numbered for this activity) on the right hand.

_____ Apply nail oil.

Nail Polish Application

SHORT ANSWER

66. In addition to allowing clients to choose their own color to ensure their satisfaction, what are two ways that you can help your client choose a polish color?

_____

_____

_____

67. How many coats of polish are needed for a successful manicure?

_____

_____

_____

FILL IN THE BLANK

68. Complete the following sentences about polish application.

Fill in the blanks with words or phrases to complete the statements about the proper technique for the application of nail polish.

Apply a thin coat of _____ to cover the entire nail plate of all nails.

When applying nail polish, remove the brush from the bottle and _____ the side

of the brush _____ on the inside of the lip of the bottle to remove excess polish.

You should have a _____ on the end of the other side of the brush large enough

to apply _____ to the entire nail plate without having to re-dip the brush. Hold

the brush at approximately a _____ angle.

Place the tip of the brush on the nail _____ away from the cuticle area in

the _____ of the nail. Slightly _____ the brush onto the

_____, producing a slight _____, ensuring the polish and

brush do not touch the _____.

_____ the brush toward the free edge of the nail, down the center.

Move to each side of the nail and _____ in even strokes toward

the _____.

After finishing the first coat of each nail, move the brush back and forth on the

_____, barely touching, to apply color to it. Use the same technique for every

nail while applying the first coat of color.

This application technique can be used for all _____, base coats, and _____ coats and is

known as the _____-stroke method. It allows polish coverage over the _____nail plate,

making the nails look smooth, evenly polished, and _____.

SEQUENCE

69. Number the steps of the procedure for nail polish application, from 1 to 9, beginning to end. One
    number has been provided.

    _____ Apply second coat to first hand.

    _____ Apply fast drying product. If using polish-drying product or fast dry top coat, apply
    according to manufacturer's instructions.

_____ Apply first coat of polish on first hand.

_____ Coat the sides. Move to each side of the nail and pull in even strokes toward nail tip.

_____ Dry the nails; the client may sit at a separate table with hands under nail dryer or sit comfortably away from your table.

____1____ Ask your client to put on any jewelry and outerwear that may have been removed; make their car keys accessible; and, if possible, have them pay for services at this time or have payment ready to hand to the receptionist.

_____ Cap the free edge (tip sealing).

_____ Apply base coat.

_____ Apply top coat for glossy, finished look and to prevent chipping; also coat the nail's free edge.

Hand and Arm Massage

TRUE OR FALSE

Indicate whether the following statements about massage are true or false. If a statement is false, explain why.

70. The nail technician should always have one hand on the client's arm during massage.

    T   F   _____

71. All states permit massage services by a nail technician.

    T   F   _____

72. It is important to understand any health conditions that a client may have that contraindicate massage.

    T   F   _____

73. If a client has a medical condition, a good rule of thumb to follow is "When in doubt, do not massage."

    T   F   _____

74. Match each massage technique listed in the word bank with its description.

    Word bank: effleurage, friction, pétrissage, tapotement, vibration

Massage Technique	Description
_____	Rapid tapping or striking of hands against skin
_____	Succession of strokes; hands glide over an area with varying degrees of pressure/contact
_____	Hands placed around the arm, fingers in opposite directions, then gentle twisting in opposite directions
_____	Kneading, lifting, squeezing, pressing the tissue
_____	Continuous trembling/shaking applied by hand without leaving contact with the skin

SHORT ANSWER

75. List two medical conditions that are either contraindicated for a hand or arm massage or require special precautions.

    _____

    _____

    _____

76. After performing a massage, what should you do to thoroughly cleanse the client's nail plate?

    _____

    _____

    _____

Spa and Basic Manicures Compared

77. What is the general difference between a spa manicure and a basic manicure?

    _____

    _____

    _____

78. List five features and techniques associated with spa manicures that are designed for relaxation.

    _____

    _____

    _____

79. Spa manicures that are results-oriented, also known as treatment manicures, often have names that closely represent their purpose. List one example and describe it.

    _____

    _____

    _____

CREATE

80. Imagine you've just started renting a manicure station at a large full-service salon. The owner would like to begin offering upscale themed manicure services and has requested that you develop three different types. Be creative—brainstorm holidays, special occasions, sporting events, seasons, age groups, trends in current events, and so on—and design three different themed manicure services that you would like to offer.

    Write the titles of your themes here, give a brief description, and then provide details about the special treatments and techniques that support the themes you created. Then, using a computer or paper and markers, develop a flyer for them that might appear on social media; use photos, colors, graphic art, and whatever else you think will catch the eye.

Complete the sentences below.

81. Waterless manicures, also known as _____ manicures, eliminate soaking the nails in

_____.

82. You can perform _____ manicures (basic, spa, scrub, etc.) using dry manicure techniques.

83. _____ is the therapeutic use of essential _____ that are _____ or applied

to the skin. They are used in _____, pedicures, and _____ to induce relaxation or

invigoration for the client.

Paraffin Wax Treatments with Manicures

SHORT ANSWER

84. Briefly describe what paraffin is and what it does for a client's skin.

_____

_____

_____

85. What are two benefits experienced by clients who have a paraffin treatment?

_____

_____

_____

Indicate whether the following statements about paraffin treatments are true or false. For any false statements, explain why they are false.

86. Clients with impaired circulation are okay to receive paraffin treatments.

    T   F   _____

87. Do not perform paraffin wax treatments on a client with open wounds, cuts, rashes, or burns.

    T   F   _____

88. Be careful when applying paraffin wax to senior citizens or chronically ill clients, as they may be more sensitive to heat.

    T   F   _____

89. The nail technician should perform a heat tolerance test by applying a small patch of wax onto the client's skin before moving forward with the whole treatment if this is the first time they have the service.

    T   F   _____

SHORT ANSWER

90. List the five types of paraffin application methods.

    _____

    _____

    _____

91. Of the five methods of paraffin application, which one is most appealing to you? Explain why you would choose that one—both as a cosmetologist and as a client.

    _____

    _____

    _____

92. Describe how to remove paraffin from your client's hands after the treatment has been completed.

_____

_____

_____

Services for Clients with Disabilities

TRUE OR FALSE

Indicate whether the following statements are true or false. For questions that are false, explain why they are false.

93. Salons are bound by the Health Insurance Portability and Accountability Act of 1996 (HIPAA) to keep client information confidential.

   T   F   _____

94. A client with neuropathy or another neurological complication may require special care in nail services.

   T   F   _____

95. Keeping client information confidential is the most ethical practice.

   T   F   _____

SHORT ANSWER

96. Describe how you should interact with a client and their caregiver.

_____

_____

_____

97. Above all, how should you treat clients with disabilities in the salon setting?

_____

_____

_____

98. What does ADA stand for? How can that resource help you ensure the comfort of your clients who may require special considerations?

_____

_____

_____

FILL IN THE BLANK

99. Below is a chart that lists areas related to the salon environment in which you can make special considerations and small adjustments for your clients. Describe the adjustments that can be made.

Area for Adjustment	Description
Table clearance	_____
Pedicure	_____
Aisles and walkways	_____
Speed/timing	_____

MATCHING

100. Match each client's needs to the corresponding accommodation.

a. cancer
b. neuropathy
c. older clients
d. arthritis
e. heart conditions

f. autoimmune disease
g. visual impairment
h. active chemotherapy
i. neurological complications

j. attention deficit hyperactivity disorder (ADHD)
k. diabetes
l. mobility devices (wheelchair, cane)

Client's Needs   **Accommodation**

_____ Stay at least 0.025 inch (0.07 centimeter) away from eponychium and sidewalls; do not use acetone; use ridge filler to disguise uneven nail plate color

_____ Have a mobile manicuring table available

_____ Watch for brittle nails; offer light massage; avoid sharp implements

_____ Escort in salon at all times; be prepared to accommodate a service animal; throughout the service, say what you are doing and maintain physical contact, such as a hand on the arm, to help your client relax and feel more comfortable

_____ Offer a stable chair with arms and without wheels, as client may have balance issues

_____ Be sensitive to dry skin; offer light massage

_____ Offer light massage so that the client's heart rate does not elevate

_____ Use light massage; be aware of mobility and balance challenges

_____ Maintain eye contact, explain the procedure in a soothing voice, and minimize environmental distractions if possible

_____ Be aware of client sensitivity to touch and lack of flexibility; offer light massage

_____ Watch for brittle nails and a corrugated nail plate; offer a private service area if possible if client expresses concern because of loss of hair, weight, mobility, and so forth

_____ Be especially mindful when using sharp implements, hot water, paraffin baths, and UV lights; have patience and take time to perform the services

RESEARCH

101. All cosmetologists should have an understanding of how to best serve clients who may require special considerations. Conduct some research to find out about products available to help perform services on older clients or clients with physical or mental health conditions. What products are available to better accommodate clients in the salon? What products would make the clients' experience more relaxing or enjoyable? You may want to check websites like the ADA or an organization that focuses on a specific medical condition or ability (e.g., Autism Speaks or Muscular Dystrophy Association). Research products for at least five client needs, from either the terms above or from ones you are aware of in your own life, and use the table below or follow the link to a PDF. What products would be valuable for you to purchase for your own salon?

+ BONUS

Visit: bonus.milady.com/cos-wb/toc

CLIENT NEED	PRODUCT	BENEFIT TO CLIENT

Upgrading Your Manicure with Nail Art

LABELING

102. Label each image with the type of nail art that it shows.

    a. Embellishments   c. French manicure   e. Color blocking
    b. Marbleizing   d. Color fade   f. Nail stamping

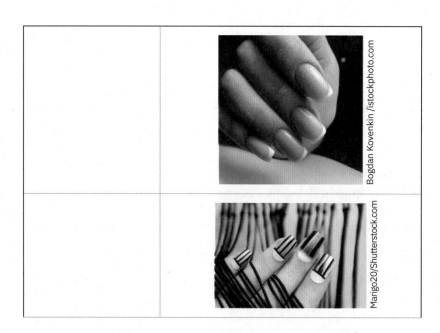

Bogdan Kovenkin /istockphoto.com

Marigo20/Shutterstock.com

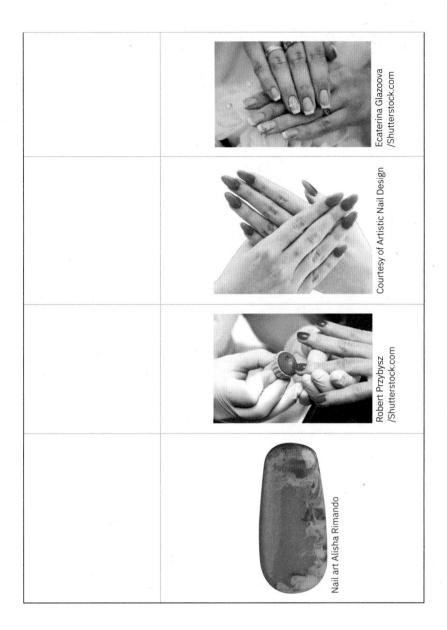

Ecaterina Glazoova /Shutterstock.com

Courtesy of Artistic Nail Design

Robert Przybysz /Shutterstock.com

Nail art Alisha Rimando

CREATE

103. Now it's your turn to create beautiful nail art! Sketch a design or shape that would work well as a stencil on nails. Design a set of stencils that could be applied to all 10 nails. Once you've sketched your stencils, find the material(s) that you want to make them from (paper, lace, fabric, etc.). Create the actual stencils, determine what your color scheme will be, and plan the sequence in which you would like to apply the stencil to the nails. Then apply them to your nails or a classmate's. Share your results with your classmates. You'll likely be very inspired by the variety!

DISCOVERIES AND ACCOMPLISHMENTS

In the space below, write notes about key concepts discussed in this chapter. Share your discoveries with some of the other students in your class and ask them if your notes are helpful. You may want to revise your notes based on good ideas shared by your peers.

Discoveries:

_____

_____

_____

_____

_____

_____

_____

List at least three things you have accomplished since you decided to enroll in school.

Accomplishments:

_____

_____

_____

_____

_____

_____

_____

1. Cosmetologists should understand that _____.

   A) they are fully liable if a client injury occurs while performing an illegal service

   B) clients prefer maintaining their own nails rather than having a professional perform this task for them

   C) improving the appearance of certain nail conditions that are medical disorders is their responsibility

   D) they are licensed to diagnose unhealthy nails

2. Which of the following guidelines should be followed when choosing manicure station equipment?

   A) An adjustable work lamp should use a 12- to 14-watt incandescent or fluorescent bulb.

   B) A client's chair should have high arms on the sides.

   C) A manicuring table should be made of a hard, impenetrable surface and remain free of clutter.

   D) A cosmetologist's drawer should contain used materials.

3. In the context of the Occupational Safety and Health Administration (OSHA), to ensure safe working conditions in a salon, cosmetologists should _____.

   A) use a local source capture ventilation system

   B) install fans and open windows as substitutes for proper ventilation

   C) use ventilated tables with filters vented to the inside rather than to the outside of the salon

   D) avoid installing portable downdraft vent machines that use a powerful fan

4. Which of the following statements is accurate about multiuse implements?

   A) Multiuse implements are often made of metal.

   B) Multiuse implements are also known as disposable implements.

   C) Multiuse implements are used once on a client and then discarded, preferably while the client is present.

   D) Multiuse implements that are nickel-plated are more expensive than those made of stainless steel.

5. Wooden pushers are typically used _____.

   A) when the nails require more shortening than the depth of routine filing

   B) when implements need to be removed from disinfectant solutions

   C) to create a beautiful shine on natural nails and some artificial enhancements

   D) to clean under the nail's free edge, remove cuticle tissue from the nail plate, and apply products

continued

6. Since the skin can absorb chemicals, the Occupational Safety and Health Administration (OSHA) recommends _____ gloves as they protect the skin from chemicals.

   A) latex

   B) nitrile

   C) cloth

   D) vinyl

7. Nail creams are barrier products because they _____.

   A) have longer-lasting effects than nail oils and lotions

   B) absorb into the nail plate to increase flexibility and into the surrounding skin to soften and moisturize

   C) contain ingredients that seal the surface of the skin around the nail and hold subdermal moisture in the skin

   D) penetrate the nail plate or skin, unlike nail oils and lotions

8. Which of the following statements is true of a base coat?

   A) It creates a colorless layer on natural nails and nail enhancements that promotes polish adhesion.

   B) It is applied over colored polish to prevent chipping and add shine or a matte finish.

   C) It allows nail polishes to create discoloration on the natural nail plate.

   D) It contains ingredients that create hard, shiny, or matte films after the nail polish solvents evaporate.

9. Identify a true statement about the squoval nail shape.

   A) It is sturdy if the nail extends only slightly past the fingertip.

   B) It is completely straight across the free edge with no rounding at the outside edges.

   C) It is slightly tapered and extends a bit past the fingertip.

   D) It is tapered and longer than usual, making it suitable for thin hands with long fingers and narrow nail beds.

10. A conservative nail shape that is considered attractive on most hands is the _____.

    A) squoval nail

    B) square nail

    C) oval nail

    D) pointed nail

11. A basic manicure, including polishing, should take _____ minutes to complete.

    A) 15 to 30

    B) 30 to 45

    C) 10 to 20

    D) 45 to 90

continued

12. When starting a new step in a basic manicure procedure, always start with the _____.

    A) pinky finger of the right hand

    B) index finger of the left hand

    C) index finger of the right hand

    D) pinky finger of the left hand

13. Identify an accurate statement about the pre-service procedure.

    A) It is an organized, step-by-step plan for accomplishing the requested service, such as a manicure and pedicure.

    B) It is an organized, step-by-step plan for cleaning and disinfecting your tools, implements, and materials.

    C) It includes caring for your client after completing the procedure.

    D) It details helping your client through the scheduling and payment process.

14. Which of the following is a guideline to file and shape nails based on client consultation?

    A) Ensure that you use low-grit abrasive to shape natural nails.

    B) Begin with the little finger on the left hand.

    C) Use a sawing back-and-forth motion while filing natural nails.

    D) Avoid removing the old nail polish.

15. The post-service procedure is an organized, step-by-step plan for _____.

    A) greeting and escorting your client to your service area

    B) accomplishing the requested service, such as a manicure and nail tips and wraps

    C) caring for your client after completing the procedure

    D) cleaning and disinfecting your tools, implements, and materials

16. Which of the following options shows the correct sequence of steps to successfully apply nail polish?

    A) Apply the base coat, followed by two coats of polish color and one top coat application to give a protective seal.

    B) Apply the base coat, followed by one coat of polish color and one top coat application to give a protective seal.

    C) Apply the top coat, followed by two coats of polish color and one base coat application to give a protective seal.

    D) Apply the top coat, followed by one coat of polish color and one base coat application to give a protective seal.

continued

17. Identify a guideline to apply nail polish.

    A) Apply thick coats for maximum smoothness and minimum drying time.

    B) Apply multiple product layers to improve appearance and polish longevity and durability.

    C) Start the application by placing the brush at the free edge of the nail.

    D) First, apply the top coat, followed by one coat of polish color and one base coat application.

18. For professional results, practice the three-stroke method to apply nail polish. This method involves _____.

    A) applying one light polish stroke down the middle and one on each side of the nail

    B) applying three thick coats for maximum smoothness and minimum drying time

    C) placing the brush at the free edge of the nail first and pushing down toward the cuticle area

    D) getting polish on the underside of the nail in order to cover the entire nail

19. Which of the following movements that are part of a massage is defined as a succession of strokes in which the hands glide over an area of the body with varying degrees of pressure or contact?

    A) petrissage   C) effleurage

    B) tapotement   D) vibration

20. In the context of the movements that are part of a massage, petrissage is a _____.

    A) movement that involves lifting, squeezing, and pressing the tissue

    B) succession of strokes in which the hands glide over an area of the body with varying degrees of pressure or contact

    C) continuous trembling or shaking movement applied by the hand without breaking contact with the skin

    D) rapid tapping or striking motion of the hands against the skin

21. Which of the following is a guideline that needs to be followed with respect to a hand and arm massage?

    A) Do not be conservative when deciding whether to perform the massage on someone with a medical condition.

    B) Do not use vigorous or strong massage techniques on clients with arthritis.

    C) Perform the massage right after polish application.

    D) Before performing the massage, ensure to lean toward your client.

continued

22. Which of the following is an accurate statement about spa manicures?

    A) Spa manicures involve the procedures of exfoliation and massage.

    B) The service times of spa manicures are usually shorter than those of basic manicures.

    C) Most spa manicures include a less detailed massage than do basic manicures.

    D) Spa manicures seldom involve advanced specialty techniques and skin treatments.

23. In the context of manicures, which of the following is a paraffin wax safety guideline?

    A) Do not use paraffin if skin irritations such as cuts, burns, rashes, eczema, or warts are present.

    B) Use paraffin treatments on clients with impaired circulation.

    C) Remelt and reuse paraffin whenever possible.

    D) Do not perform a test for heat tolerance on all clients.

24. If a client has an autoimmune disease, a nail technician performing a manicure should _____.

    A) watch for brittle nails

    B) avoid using penetrating oils

    C) use sharp implements

    D) avoid offering a light massage

25. A swirled effect created by combining two or more colors while wet and then mixing them on the nail with a stylus is called _____.

    A) marbleizing

    C) color blocking

    B) stamping

    D) color fading

finished!

Practical Skills
Self-Evaluation Checklist

Regular self-assessment helps you to improve your technical skills and achieve success. After performing each procedure, review the procedure steps in the textbook and rate yourself as "Competent" or "Needs Work," and write in comments on how you were successful or where you can improve. Rating yourself helps you identify your strengths and weaknesses and develop your own plan for improvement.

CRITERIA	COMPETENT	NEEDS WORK	COMMENTS
PROCEDURE 20-1 PRE-SERVICE PROCEDURE			
Preparation/ Infection Control			
Basic Table Setup			
Greeted The Client			
Washed Hands and Put on Gloves			
Timing			
PROCEDURE 20-2 PERFORMING A BASIC MANICURE			
Preparation			
Procedure			
Post-Service			
Timing			
PROCEDURE 20-3 POST-SERVICE PROCEDURE			
Advised Clients and Promoted Products			
Scheduled Next Appointment and Thanked Client			
Prepared Work Area and Implements for Next Client			
Timing			
PROCEDURE 20-4 POLISH THE NAILS			
Preparation			
Procedure			
Post-Service			
Timing			
PROCEDURE 20-5 HAND AND ARM MASSAGE			
Preparation			
Procedure			
Post-Service			
Timing			

Ch. 21: Pedicuring

Why Study Pedicuring?

SHORT ANSWER

1. Define pedicure and list three to five examples of the services included in a pedicure.

_____

_____

_____

2. Although manicures and pedicures are similar, what specific knowledge is required to perform pedicures?

_____

_____

_____

Pedicuring Equipment

FILL IN THE BLANK

3. Complete the sentences below by filling in the blanks.

_____ is the term used to indicate all the permanent tools used for pedicure services

that are not implements. Some examples include the pedicure _____ and footrest,

the pedicure _____ to hold implements and materials, and a footbath, all of which

are necessary at a pedicure station. _____ equipment varies but could include foot

_____ (electric or terrycloth), a paraffin _____, or hot _____.

MULTIPLE CHOICE

4. An ideal pedicure station includes a(n) _____ stool for the cosmetologist to promote healthy posture and a comfortable chair with an armrest and footrest for the client.

A) stain-resistant

C) high

B) brightly colored

D) ergonomic

5. What is the purpose of a footrest, whether it's built in or separate from the cosmetologist's stool?

A) provides a place for the cosmetologist to put their feet to maintain a healthy posture while performing a pedicure

B) provides a place for the client to put their feet to maintain a healthy posture while receiving a pedicure

C) used by the client while their toenails dry after the pedicure is complete

D) makes it easier for the cosmetologist to reach the client's feet

6. Which of the following do most pedicure carts *not* have?

A) built-in disinfection of implements   C) a hard, flat service

B) drawers and shelves   D) rollers

7. Which of the following pieces of pedicure equipment is considered optional at a pedicure station?

A) paraffin bath   C) pedicure cart

B) pedicure footrest   D) pedicure footbath

8. Which of the following is *not* a benefit typically associated with a paraffin treatment?

A) deep, moist heat   C) reduction of pain and inflammation

B) removal of excess hair   D) improved circulation to arthritic joints

9. _____ clients have skin that may be thinner and more sensitive to heat, so it's recommended that cosmetologists perform a pre-service paraffin patch test for them.

A) Teenage   C) Older

B) Pregnant   D) New

LABELING

10. Place the following examples of pedicure foot baths into order, from simplest (1) to most sophisticated (4).

_____ Portable foot basin with built-in whirlpool action

_____ Portable foot bath

_____ Throne-design chair

_____ Basin soak bath

11. If your salon supplied its cosmetologists with both electric foot mitts and terry cloth mitts, which one would you prefer to offer your clients? Explain your choice.

_____

_____

_____

12. List three precautions to consider for clients interested in paraffin bath services.

_____

_____

_____

13. List two precaution for preparing hot stone treatments.

_____

_____

_____

Pedicuring Implements

LABELING

14. Label the implements depicted below and indicate whether they are multiuse (M) or single use (S). For options that could be both, check your state guidelines to find out which is legal in your state.

LABEL THE IMPLEMENT	M OR S?	IMPLEMENTS
		mnimage/Shutterstock.com

LABEL THE IMPLEMENT	M OR S?	IMPLEMENTS
		Creatikon Studio /istockphoto.com

15. Given the requirements for maintaining a safe and clean workplace for both clients and cosmetologists, do some research on "green" salons' practices to reduce waste, recycle, or refuse materials. Visit a few local salons, their websites, or the Internet more generally to find out how nail salons are balancing the current push to recycle with the need for safety. What are some challenges for salons—for example, is it expensive? Is it complicated? Did you find any creative solutions to balancing environmental concerns with salon safety? What types of actions and procedures are most popular? On a separate sheet of paper, write a short paragraph, five to seven sentences, about your findings.

MULTIPLE CHOICE

16. Some foot paddles feature disposable and replaceable abrasive surfaces (grit). How should these be cared for between uses?

    A) clean and disinfect the handles of these files before reuse

    B) soak the abrasive surface of the paddle in disinfectant before reuse

    C) avoid implements with disposable parts

    D) carefully cover the abrasive surface with a new surface

17. A nail rasp is considered a time-saving implement and a prevention tool. What is it intended to prevent?

    A) ingrown toenails   C) calluses

    B) fungus   D) brittle nails

18. If a cosmetologist notices that a client has an ingrown toenail, the cosmetologist should _____.

    A) refer the client to a podiatrist   C) soak the area in a disinfecting solution

    B) refer the client to a dermatologist   D) check to see if the other toenails are also ingrown

19. Where is the best place to use a nail rasp?

    A) on top of the nail

    B) just past the hyponychium area of the side of the nail's free edge

    C) at the base of the nail, near the cuticle

    D) under the nail, angling the point at the nail's center

20. Which government organization mandates that technicians wear gloves—and recommends nitrile gloves—while performing pedicures or working with chemicals?

A) OSHA

C) Health and Human Services

B) DEA

D) CDC

21. How many pedicures can you perform using the same pair of gloves?

A) one

C) all that are scheduled in a single day

B) two

D) as many as you can perform in a 4-hour period

FILL IN THE BLANK

22. Complete the paragraph below using words from the word bank to fill in the blanks.

Word Bank: straight, nippers, remove, fingernails, shortening, clippers, curved, shorten

Toenail _____ are specifically designed for _____ toenails and are larger than

what is used for _____. They have _____ or _____ jaws with wider

space between the jaws, allowing them to cut thicker nails. Toenail _____ are similar to

the ones for fingernails but have a larger hinge box and longer and thicker jaws, which allows

them to _____ the nail, whereas fingernail versions of this tool are generally used to

_____ dead skin.

23. Complete these sentences using the word bank. Not all words will be used.

Word bank: edges, state, metal, single, coarse, reuse, medium, fine, discard, legal, shaping, guidelines, multi

For toenails, a _____-grit pedicure file works best for _____, and a _____

-grit pedicure file works best for finishing and sealing the _____. If an abrasive file

cannot survive proper cleaning and disinfection procedures, consider it _____-use and

_____ it or give it to the client for home use.

Before you decide to use a _____ file on a client, you should determine (1) whether they

are _____ in your _____ and (2) if they must be cleaned and disinfected or sterilized

after each use, depending on your state's _____.

24. List three precautions to take when using a curette.

_____

_____

_____

ROLE PLAY

25. Partner with a classmate to practice a scenario in which you discuss treatments for calluses. Take turns playing the role of client and cosmetologist. Scenario: A client comes into your salon with thick calluses on their feet from being on their feet all day. The calluses have started to hurt, and the client wants them to be cut off. As a cosmetologist, explain to your client (1) what is causing their calluses, (2) what could happen if you cut them off, (3) how a cosmetologist can and should treat them, and (4) and any at-home treatments between visits. Use the space below for any notes.

Unique Pedicure Materials

FILL IN THE BLANK

26. Read through the paragraph below and fill in the blanks using the word bank. Not all the words will be used.

    Word bank: rope, polishing, new, single-use, multiuse, toe separators, sanitized, rubber, fabric

    _____ help keep the toes apart while the technician is _____ the toenails.

    They can be made from a variety of materials, ranging from a foam _____ one-piece

    unit to even a _____ woven between the toes. They are considered a _____

    implement because a _____ set must be used with each client.

27. The disposable slippers provided for clients who have not worn open-toed shoes and want to avoid smudging their newly applied toenail polish are typically made of _____.

A) rubber or cotton

C) paper or foam

B) paper or plastic

D) rubber or plastic

Professional Pedicure Products

28. What products are used in pedicures that are not used in manicures?

_____

_____

_____

29. Why is it important to use a high-quality product in the foot soak part of a pedicure?

_____

_____

_____

30. Exfoliating scrubs contain an abrasive ingredient as the exfoliating agent. List three to five abrasives that are typically found in exfoliating scrubs.

_____

_____

_____

31. What are three popular ingredients in foot care masks?

_____

_____

_____

32. List at least three functions served by applying a mask to the foot.

_____

_____

_____

MULTIPLE CHOICE

33. Which type of product is put into the water in a pedicure bath to soften the skin on the feet?

A) foot soaks

C) scrubs

B) essential oils

D) masks

34. What is one reason to use a professionally formulated foot soak in a foot bath?

A) cleanse and deodorize feet at the beginning of a pedicure

B) disinfect the water

C) identify the thickest part of a client's foot

D) exfoliate dead skin cells

35. Foot soaks may also include _____.

A) moisturizers and oils

C) disinfectants

B) mild abrasives

D) all-purpose vinegar

36. Exfoliating scrubs are _____ that are massaged on the foot and leg to remove dry, flaky skin and smooth calluses.

A) gritty lotions

C) mint-scented sprays

B) thick creams

D) mild disinfectants

TRUE OR FALSE

Indicate whether the statements below are true or false. For any false statements, explain why they are false.

37. Foot lotions and creams used in standard salons are formulated in such a way that they are not available as home care products.

T   F   _____

38. Treatment-level lotions and creams are sometimes used by cosmetologists who work in podiatry or medical offices to improve medical conditions of the feet such as xerosis, an abnormal skin dryness.

   T   F   _____

39. A callus softener is a special implement used by the nail technician that shaves off the top layers of the callus.

   T   F   _____

40. Some callus softeners can be potentially hazardous if they splash onto the skin or into the eyes, so personal protective items such as safety glasses or gloves should be worn when the softeners are used or poured.

   T   F   _____

41. The time between pedicure appointments, unlike manicure appointments, is generally two months because of toenails' slower growth.

   T   F   _____

MULTIPLE CHOICE

42. Callus softener products are applied _____.

   A) directly to the callus

   B) by mixing with water in a pedicure bath

   C) by spraying on the entire foot with a mister

   D) by mixing with a softening lotion

43. Which of the following is the only chemical the Food and Drug Administration (FDA) has approved to be marketed as a callus "remover"?

   A) urea   C) potassium hydroxide

   B) salicylic acid   D) hydrogen peroxide

44. The word bank includes the three ingredients commonly found in callus softeners. Match each ingredient with its description, features, and characteristics listed below. (*Hint:* The ingredients from the word bank will be used more than once.)

Word bank: urea, salicylic acid, potassium hydroxide

Callus Softener Ingredients	Description, Features, and Characteristics
_____	An inorganic compound that degrades the protein in callus cells
_____	An organic acid originally derived from willow tree bark
_____	An organic compound originally derived from mammalian urine
_____	Intensely moisturizes and hydrates tough, thick calluses
_____	Has anti-inflammatory properties and can break down fats and lipids
_____	Quickly softens even the toughest callus
_____	Currently produced from carbon dioxide and ammonia
_____	Small amounts are often included in cuticle removers
_____	Also used to treat plantar warts and acne

CASE STUDY

46. You are opening your own nail salon and are currently in the process of choosing which product lines to carry. Select two product lines (e.g., Aveda and Pantene) and compare them according to the guidelines listed below. Jot down notes about your findings and then state which product line you would select for your nail salon and explain why you would choose it.

- Check the quality of the company's educational support and its commitment to the cosmetologists using its products.

- Find other cosmetologists who use the products and discuss the quality of the company's customer service and its shipping competence, and listen closely to their experiences. (Note: For the purposes of this exercise, consider published quotes/testimonials/reviews from experts. However, when you are preparing to actually invest in a product, be sure to consult personally with other cosmetologists.)

Client Consultation

SHORT ANSWER

47. What is the purpose of the client consultation?

_____

_____

_____

48. What role does the intake form play in the client consultation?

_____

_____

_____

SEQUENCE

49. Number the following steps of the client consultation, from 1 to 5, beginning to end.

_____ Maintain client records.

_____ Determine service.

_____ Evaluate nails and skin.

_____ Acknowledge medical conditions.

_____ Identify diseases or disorders.

CREATE

50. Develop a checklist that you can use to efficiently evaluate your client's nails and skin.

_____

_____

_____

51. When consulting with your client, which of the following is outside your scope of practice and should never be done?

    A) asking your client about discoloration or thickening of the nails

    B) noticing markings or other disorders on the nails

    C) discussing dryness, calluses, red spots, or any markings on the client's feet and legs

    D) diagnosing a disease or disorder

52. During a consultation with a new client, you notice that both their big toenails are yellowish and very thick. What should you do?

    A) ask your client about them

    C) exclude those nails from treatment

    B) say nothing to avoid offending the client

    D) ask the salon owner in private whether you can cancel the pedicure

53. You, as the cosmetologist, should record all information from the consultation on _____.

    A) the client's intake form

    C) the salon's website

    B) the client's service card

    D) your client log

ROLE PLAY

54. Develop a checklist for acknowledging and discussing medical conditions with your client during the consultation. Then pair up with a classmate and compare your lists. Discuss your choices and work together to decide what should be added or removed from your checklists when acknowledging and discussing sensitive information with your client.

55. What is the purpose of the discussion when you're identifying diseases and disorders during the client consultation?

_____

_____

_____

56. What does contraindicated mean?

_____

_____

_____

CREATE

57. As a cosmetologist, you will build a client base. It will be important to maintain service records for your clients. Think about what types of information you would like to include in their records. Find a template online and customize it or design your own form with fields for the information you want to record. Feel free to use borders, colors, images, check boxes, and so on. Make sure that it looks professional, is easy to read, and organizes the information in a logical way. Listed below are some types of information that you may wish to include in your client service record:

- Contact information: name, nickname, cell phone number, e-mail address.

- Preferred method of contact (e.g., phone, text, e-mail, voicemail)

- Birthday

- Services/updates they want to know about (e.g., sales, discounts, holiday hours)

- List of services performed and dates of service

- Colors/products they have previously chosen or preferred

- Medical history/conditions with space to update

Pedicure Services

58. What are some benefits of short pedicure services?

_____

_____

_____

59. What is meant by the term *series pedicure*? What is done during a series pedicure? Provide an example.

_____

_____

_____

60. List two examples that demonstrate how a basic pedicure could be upgraded to a spa pedicure.

_____

_____

_____

61. List at least three ways to upgrade a pedicure.

_____

_____

_____

62. What are three factors that affect the additional costs of an upgrade to a pedicure?

_____

_____

_____

63. Match the following with the type of pedicure that best serves the client.

    a. Spa pedicure
    b. Pedicure series

    c. Basic pedicure
    d. Short service

    _____ Thick calluses

    _____ Third-week appointment in a five-week series

    _____ Nail art

    _____ Four-week appointment in a six-week series

    _____ Lower leg massage and foot mask

    _____ Scaly feet not caused by a fungus

    _____ Exfoliation of dead skin cells on the feet

    _____ Polish change

    _____ To maintain healthy feet and nails

CREATE

64. You have been offered the opportunity to set up a pedicure station within a large full-service salon. The salon owner would like to review your pedicure service menu before sharing it with the salon's clientele. Prepare a realistic menu that lists the services you intend to provide, including prices, add-ons/upgrades, short services, and series options. Consider listing packages (e.g., combination manicure/pedicures), holiday offers, punch card options (e.g., "buy four, get one free"), referral bonuses, and so on. Once you've outlined your services menu, use a template from a software program (or carefully sketch it out on a separate sheet of paper) to create a one-page decorative flyer showcasing your menu. Incorporate a readable font, organize your information logically, make sure everything is spelled correctly, and use an appealing color palette. Show it to a friend, fellow student, or family member and request their feedback before finalizing it.

Pedicure Massage Benefits

Complete the following sentences.

65. According to client salon surveys, _____ is the most enjoyed aspect of any nail

    service. And the most enjoyable type is a rhythmic, slow _____ with the fingers and

    _____. Throughout this service, it's important to maintain _____ with the client,

    sliding the hands from one location to the next in a smooth _____.

MULTIPLE CHOICE

66. Generally, when performing a foot massage, the foot should be gently grasped _____.

    A) just above the ankle   C) between the thumb and the fingers

    B) by the heel   D) just below the toes

67. Foot massage induces a high degree of relaxation and _____.

    A) slows blood flow   C) stimulates blood flow

    B) promotes exfoliation   D) is moisturizing

68. Never allow your _____ to touch the skin when performing a pedicure foot massage.

    A) palms   C) fingernails

    B) fingertips   D) gloves

SHORT ANSWER

69. What is the role of feathering in foot and leg massage?

    _____

    _____

    _____

70. Below are the typical steps of a foot massage. Put them in the correct order, from 1 to 9, beginning to end.

_____ Rest the client's heel on a footrest or stool

_____ Perform figure eights on each toe

_____ Move one thumb in a firm circular movement from one side of the foot above the heel, below the toes, and back to its original position

_____ Repeat thumb movements three to five times

_____ Put on a fresh pair of gloves

_____ Perform friction movement to the bottom of the foot

_____ Slide your hands so that thumbs are on the foot's plantar side while fingers hold the foot's dorsal side

_____ Perform effleurage movement

_____ Place both feet onto the footrest and firmly and slowly pressure the tops of the feet three times for two seconds each

SHORT ANSWER

71. Describe three ways to interact with your clients so that they can relax and feel pampered during their pedicure treatment.

_____

_____

_____

72. What is reflexology?

_____

_____

_____

73. List the two reasons that professional, hands-on training is essential in reflexology.

_____

_____

_____

MULTIPLE CHOICE

74. If your client drifts off to sleep during service, you should _____.

    A) gently wake them

    B) stop your service

    C) allow them to rest, pause your discussion, and continue your service

    D) charge them an additional fee

75. Which of the following discussion topics is acceptable when interacting with your client?

    A) the results of current political elections

    B) the argument you had with your in-laws

    C) a cute story about your dog

    D) details about the previous client's pedicure

76. During the procedure, you should consider talking about your client's foot health, a(n) _____ they may enjoy, and the products needed to maintain the pedicure between salon visits.

    A) movie   C) upgrade

    B) recipe   D) book

77. Reflexology is a unique method of applying pressure with the thumb and index fingers to the hands and feet and promotes _____.

    A) healing of chronic illness   C) control of foot pain

    B) healing of back pain   D) health benefits

78. A salon that offers reflexology services typically employs staff who have undergone authentic reflexology training and certification from a highly recommended reflexologist certified by _____.

A) the National Holistic Institute

B) the Reflexology Association of America

C) a member school in the Healing Arts Network

D) the Therapeutic Reflexology Studies Program

Clients with Health Considerations

FILL IN THE BLANK

79. Fill in the missing information in the table below about client accommodations

HEALTH CONSIDERATION	ACCOMMODATIONS
Limited mobility	
	Ensure the entire leg is supported during the pedicure service, including behind the knees and ankles
Visual impairment	
	Do not put pressure or manipulate the joints during the massage; instead, apply gentle pressure
Caregivers	
	Do not use sharp tools, cut their tissues, or push back their eponychium
Diabetes or circulatory diseases	

SHORT ANSWER

80. What are two accommodations you can give clients with limited mobility when performing a pedicure service?

_____

_____

_____

81. For what client is it important to check between their toes for lesions or infection before a pedicure service?

_____

_____

_____

82. List three reasons you need to take extra care when giving a pedicure service to an older client.

_____

_____

_____

RESEARCH

83. In addition to the special considerations described in your text, what are some other situations that might require you to demonstrate extra sensitivity during a pedicure? You may want to think about clients with sensory disorders (like autism spectrum disorder [ASD]), muscle disorders (like muscular dystrophies), or mental health issues like anxiety and depression. Do some research online and think about the special considerations some clients will need. How do you plan to accommodate them?

_____

_____

_____

Cleaning and Disinfecting Footbaths

SEQUENCE

84. Put the general steps for disinfecting a basic foot basin or tub in order, from beginning to end.

_____ Record the disinfection information in the salon's logbook if required by state law or salon policy.

_____ Rinse footbath with clean water and drain.

_____ Drain, rinse with clean water, and wipe dry with clean paper towel.

_____ Refill footbath with clean water and add disinfectant. Measure the correct amount of EPA-registered hospital disinfectant (as indicated on the label) and add to footbath's water. Leave this disinfectant solution in footbath for 10 minutes or the time recommended by manufacturer.

_____ Put on gloves and safety glasses then drain all water from footbath.

_____ Scrub all inside surfaces of footbath to remove all visible residue with clean disinfected brush, liquid soap, and clean water.

MULTIPLE CHOICE

85. Salons must always use an EPA-registered hospital disinfectant that is labeled as a broad-spectrum _____, viricide, and fungicide.

    A) bactericide   C) germicide

    B) tuberculocide   D) antibiotic

86. How often should cosmetologists clean and disinfect footbaths?

    A) after each client and, depending on how many clients used the footbath, once at the end of the week

    B) after each client, at the end of the day, and at least once a week

    C) at the end of each day

    D) at least three times a week

87. What is the last step of any cleaning and disinfecting procedure for footbaths?

    A) rinse and thoroughly dry the footbath

    B) spray the footbath basin with a fungicide

    C) record the disinfection information into the salon's logbook if required by state law or salon policy

    D) place a strip of paper across the basin that states, "Sanitized for your protection"

88. At the end of each day, it is recommended that cosmetologists circulate a(n) _____ detergent through the foot spas to break down stubborn films and help remove pedicure product residues.

    A) industrial strength   C) chemical

    B) chelating   D) commercial

89. The word bank below includes the three types of footbaths. Match each type of footbath from the word bank with the feature, function, or characteristic listed below. (*Hint:* Items in the word bank will be used more than once.)

Word bank: whirlpool footbath, air-jet footbath, pipeless footbath

Type of Footbath	Feature, Function, or Characteristic
_____	Creates an overall bubbling massage
_____	Also called a piped footbath
_____	Considered the new industry standard
_____	Creates a massaging effect by recirculating water through built-in pipes and jets
_____	Uses a pump's rotating blade (impellers) to circulate water
_____	Uses a blower to force air through small holes in an air channel and creates an overall bubbling massage
_____	Easily cleaned and disinfected
_____	Does not circulate water through its air channels
_____	Slowly being discontinued because disease-causing microorganisms can grow inside its pipes despite the disinfecting process

TRUE OR FALSE

Indicate whether each statement is true or false. For any false statements, explain why they are false.

90. It is considered mandatory to clean and disinfect all equipment that contains water for pedicures after every pedicure and enter the information into a logbook.

    T   F   _____

91. In footbaths that have disposable plastic liners, there is no need to disinfect the footbath after each client because the client's feet never touch the actual basin.

    T   F   _____

92. Only one state requires salons to record the time and date of every disinfecting procedure.

    T   F   _____

DISCOVERIES AND ACCOMPLISHMENTS

In the space below, write notes about key concepts discussed in this chapter. Share your discoveries with some of the other students in your class and ask them if your notes are helpful. You may want to revise your notes based on good ideas shared by your peers.

Discoveries:

_____

_____

_____

_____

_____

_____

_____

_____

List at least three things you have accomplished since you decided to enroll in school.

Accomplishments:

_____

_____

_____

_____

_____

_____

_____

_____

1. Identify a cosmetic service performed on the feet by a licensed cosmetologist or nail technician.

   A) threading   C) tweezing

   B) a pedicure   D) a manicure

2. Which of the following does a pedicure usually include?

   A) electrolysis   C) leg waxing

   B) microdermabrasion   D) callus reduction

3. Which of the following is a necessary pedicuring equipment that includes a comfortable chair with an armrest and footrest for the client and an ergonomic chair for the cosmetologist?

   A) a paraffin bath   C) a pedicure cart

   B) a pedicure station   D) a pedicure footbath

4. Which of the following is an advantage of using foot mitts during a pedicure?

   A) They remove and round off any sharp points on the sides of the free edges of nails.

   B) They reduce and smooth thick calluses on the heel and the ball of the foot.

   C) They enable the paraffin's conditioning agents to penetrate the skin more effectively.

   D) They allow for the efficient removal of debris from the eponychium and hyponychium areas.

5. A(n) _____ is a pedicuring implement with a small, scoop-shaped end that allows for the efficient removal of debris from the nail folds and eponychium and hyponychium areas.

   A) curette   C) nail rasp

   B) wooden pusher   D) autoclave

6. A _____ works best for shaping toenails.

   A) file with more than 240 grit

   B) fine-grit file

   C) file with less than 100 grit

   D) medium-grit file

continued

7. Which of the following is a disposable or single-use pedicure implement rather than a multiuse pedicure implement?

A) tweezers

C) gloves

B) toenail clippers

D) metal pushers

8. Which of the following are disposable foam rubber or cotton materials used to keep the toes apart while polishing the nails?

A) toenail nippers

C) toe separators

B) wooden pushers

D) pedicure slippers

9. Which of the following statements is true of pedicure slippers?

A) They keep the toes apart while a technician polishes the nails.

B) They are specially designed not to touch the nails while worn.

C) They are multiuse pedicuring implements.

D) They are also known as pedicure paddles.

10. A(n) _____ is a water-based lotion that contains a mild, gritty abrasive and moisturizers to help remove dry, flaky skin and reduce calluses.

A) exfoliating scrub

C) lacquer

B) foot soak

D) varnish

11. A(n) _____ is a concentrated treatment product often composed of mineral clays, moisturizing agents, skin softeners, aromatherapy oils, botanical extracts, and other beneficial ingredients to cleanse, exfoliate, tighten, tone, hydrate, and nourish the skin.

A) enamel

C) foot soak

B) mask

D) lacquer

12. Which of the following is the only chemical that has been approved by the Food and Drug Administration (FDA) to be marketed as a callus "remover"?

A) benzoyl peroxide

C) salicylic acid

B) potassium hydroxide

D) urea

continued

13. Which of the following should cosmetologists do as part of the client consultation before a pedicure?

    A) They should check if the client has the means to pay for the pedicure service.

    B) They should discuss dryness, calluses, red spots, or any markings of concern on the client's feet and legs.

    C) They should record all information on a hold harmless form.

    D) They should diagnose a disease or disorder.

14. If a client's feet have calluses or extreme dryness, the best option for a cosmetologist is to _____.

    A) conduct a client consultation and eventually refuse the service to the client citing the reason of unhealthy feet

    B) direct the client to a podiatrist for medical treatment

    C) work as long as necessary to get the feet in optimal condition in only one service

    D) sell the client home- care products to improve the condition and schedule a series of services one or two weeks apart

15. Identify a difference between a basic pedicure and a spa pedicure.

    A) A basic pedicure only includes toenail trimming and shaping, whereas a spa pedicure includes toenail trimming, shaping, and polishing.

    B) A spa pedicure includes callus reduction, whereas a basic pedicure does not.

    C) Exfoliation is usually part of a basic pedicure, but it is not part of a spa pedicure.

    D) In a basic pedicure, the massage is performed on only the foot, whereas in a spa pedicure, the massage is performed on the foot and lower leg.

16. Which of the following services is typically part of a basic pedicure?

    A) a foot soak   C) a leg mask

    B) nail repair   D) nail art

continued

17. Which of the following guidelines should you follow when performing a foot massage?

   A) Maintain a touch connection with the client only when required and not throughout the massage.

   B) Hold the foot lightly or loosely to avoid causing a ticklish sensation.

   C) Begin the massage with feathering to induce relaxation.

   D) Grasp the foot between the thumb and fingers at the mid-tarsal area with a gentle but firm grip.

18. Which of the following is most likely a technique that is generally used to signal the end of the massage and provide a gentle release?

   A) percussion   C) feathering

   B) effleurage   D) friction

19. Which of the following is a benefit of reflexology?

   A) It is used at the end of a massage to signal to experienced clients that the massage is ending.

   B) It involves the automatic manipulation of the reflex points in the body by a massaging machine and does not require a massage technician.

   C) It can reflect positive energy and increase blood flow to the reflex points in the feet and hands.

   D) It is based on scientific principles rather than on pseudoscience such as acupressure and acupuncture.

20. In the context of special client considerations, if a client cannot physically move into a pedicure chair, you should most likely _____.

   A) refuse to give the client a pedicure

   B) have a portable footbath with warm/cool water available

   C) avoid giving a foot/leg massage to the client

   D) avoid performing a dry massage

continued

21. When performing a pedicure service, which of the following guidelines should you follow if you have a client with diabetes or circulatory diseases?

    A) Use sharp implements during the service.

    B) Use vigorous or strong techniques when using a foot paddle during callus removal.

    C) Do not perform a pedicure without the permission of the client's physician.

    D) Ensure the toenails are long and sharp at the edges.

22. Which of the following is the most important reason to clean and disinfect pedicure footbaths?

    A) to create work for the salon employees

    B) to keep clients safe

    C) to maintain their polished look

    D) to gain word-of-mouth publicity via clients

23. Whirlpool footbaths have been slowly discontinued in the industry because _____.

    A) disease-causing microorganisms tend to grow inside their built-in pipes despite the disinfecting process

    B) water does not circulate through the air channels present in these footbaths

    C) they fail to create a massaging effect

    D) it is difficult to clean and disinfect the impellers that are used to circulate water in these footbaths

24. Which of the following types of pedicure footbaths is the new industry standard?

    A) piped footbaths   C) pipeless footbaths

    B) whirlpool footbaths   D) air-jet footbaths

25. Which of the following should you do as part of the salon disinfection protocol?

    A) Use a piped footbath rather than a pipeless footbath to adhere to the industry standard.

    B) Clean and disinfect all equipment that contains water for pedicures after every alternative pedicure.

    C) Avoid using disposable plastic liners in footbaths.

    D) Display visible pedicure cleaning and disinfecting procedures in employee areas for easy reference.

finished!

Practical Skills   Self-Evaluation Checklist

Regular self-assessment helps you to improve your technical skills and achieve success. After performing each procedure, review the procedure steps in the textbook and rate yourself as "Competent" or "Needs Work," and write in comments on how you were successful or where you can improve. Rating yourself helps you identify your strengths and weaknesses and develop your own plan for improvement.

CRITERIA	COMPETENT	NEEDS WORK	COMMENTS
PROCEDURE 21-1 PERFORMING THE BASIC PEDICURE			
Preparation			
Procedure			
Post-Service			
Timing			
PROCEDURE 21-2 FOOT AND LEG MASSAGE			
Preparation			
Procedure			
Post-Service			
Timing			
PROCEDURE 21-3 CLEANING AND DISINFECTING WHIRLPOOL, AIR-JET, AND PIPELESS FOOTBATHS			
Preparation			
Procedure after each client			
Procedure at the end of each day			
Procedure performed at least once each week			
Timing			
PROCEDURE 21-4 CLEANING AND DISINFECTING BASIC FOOTBATHS			
Preparation			
Procedure			
Timing			

TRACK MY PROGRESS!

Use this simple tracker to record your progress as you work through the activities in each learning objective.

COMPLETED	# OF CORRECT ANSWERS	OBJECTIVE
☐	_____/10	**LO 1** - Explain why cosmetologists should learn about nail extensions and resin systems.
☐	_____/7	**LO 2** - Explain how to prepare natural nails for a nail enhancement service.
☐	_____/20	**LO 3** - Describe different nail tip types.
☐	_____/8	**LO 4** - List the advantages of using nail forms.
☐	_____/7	**LO 5** - Name the eight most commonly requested nail extension shapes.
☐	_____/5	**LO 6** - Identify the qualities of a properly structured nail enhancement.
☐	_____/4	**LO 7** - Define nail resin and nail resin systems.
☐	_____/8	**LO 8** - Describe how nail wraps strengthen nails.
☐	_____/14	**LO 9** - Outline the advantages of applying a dip system.

Why Study Nail Extensions and Resin Systems?

SHORT ANSWER

1. Describe the difference between a nail enhancement and a nail extension.

   _____

   _____

   _____

2. Why do clients want your professional advice on altering or enhancing their nails—one of the most popular services you can offer?

_____

_____

_____

3. What are the five main reasons for having a thorough understanding of nail tips and wraps?

_____

_____

_____

TRUE OR FALSE

Indicate whether the statements below are true or false. For any false statements, explain why they are false.

4. Nail resin systems are a new addition to cosmetology services, made possible by recent technological and chemical advances.

   T   F   _____

5. Fabric wraps are one of the most common resin systems and have been a salon staple for decades.

   T   F   _____

6. Nail resin systems are one of the easier and faster nail enhancement systems to apply.

   T   F   _____

7. Tip applications are sufficiently strong on their own and require no overlay with a nail enhancement product.

   T   F   _____

8. Nail enhancement products include wraps, dip systems, liquids and powders, hard gels, soak-off gels, and polymer gels.

   T   F   _____

9. Dip systems have decreased in popularity in recent years.

   T   F   _____

10. Nail resin systems are a great option for overlaying or extending the natural nail.

T   F   _____

Preparing the Natural Nail for Nail Enhancements

11. Why must the natural nail be prepared before you start any nail extension services?

_____

_____

_____

12. What is a dry manicure, and when is it used?

_____

_____

_____

13. What is the purpose of buffing the cuticle area and the nail's sides down to the lateral folds during the dry manicure process?

_____

_____

_____

14. After the nails have been prepared and the nail dehydrator has been applied, what are two actions that must be avoided before performing nail enhancement service in order to prevent lifting?

_____

_____

_____

15. Number these first six steps of a dry manicure in order, from beginning to end. Then, for each step, write a brief description of that step (one or two sentences). The first step has been completed to get you started.

NUMBER	STEP	DESCRIPTION
	Push back cuticle.	
	Brush then scrub nails	
1	Remove polish.	Starting with pinky on client's left hand, remove any existing nail polish with acetone or polish remover. Repeat on right hand.
	File free edge.	
	Remove dried cuticle.	
	Buff nails.	

MATCHING

16. Match the terms in the word bank with their descriptions.

    a. Nail cleanser   b. Nail dehydrator

Term   **Description**

_____ Commonly made from isobutyl alcohol

_____ Commonly made from a chemical called butyl acetate

_____ Used on nails to temporarily stop them from producing moisture and natural oil

_____ Removes surface debris, moisture, and tiny amounts of oil on the natural nail plate, all of which can block adhesion

_____ Effect typically lasts about 10 minutes; then the natural nail oils will resurface

_____ Used to scrub the nail once it has been prepared for enhancement services

_____ Completely safe for the nail, so can be reapplied if needed

_____ Only appropriate for use on the natural nail plate; avoid skin contact

_____ Usually applied to a lint-free wipe, which is used to scrub the nail's surface and lateral folds to remove the dust after buffing.

17. What are the last two steps of the dry manicure?

_____

_____

_____

Nail Tip Types

MATCHING

18. Match each term to its description.

    Word bank: Well-less tip, Nail adhesive, Partial-well tip, French tip, Overlay, Nail tip, Full-well tip, Well, Full-coverage tip, ABS, Position stop

Term	Description
_____	Plastic pre-molded nail
_____	Tough plastic used to make nail tips
_____	Layer of nail enhancement product that covers surface of nail
_____	Shallow depression found in many nail tips
_____	Thin resin applied into well area that adheres tip to natural nail
_____	Point where free edge of natural nail meets the well
_____	Covers entire apex area; usually covers more than half of nail plate
_____	Usually altered at the well line to show more of the natural nail
_____	Can be attached to natural nail wherever it fits best; has no well and no position stop
_____	Covers the entire nail to cuticle; creates a very temporary nail extension
_____	Can be partial or well-less; meant to be applied without blending

Complete the following sentences about important points to consider when working with nail tips.

19. Always point the opening of a(n) _____ container away from your face and your client's face when opening.

20. Make sure that the tips you choose cover your client's nail plate from _____ to _____.

21. If you use a tip that is not _____ enough to fit the natural nail, it can be uneven at the sides and may eventually split or crack.

22. Nail professionals should wear _____ protection when working with nail tip adhesives.

23. It is better to apply a(n) _____ amount of adhesive to the nail than a(n) _____ amount because a _____ amount will provide a faster set to the natural nail.

24. _____ will create potential pockets for dirt or debris and can affect the overall strength of the nail enhancement.

25. Make sure to use _____ that are specifically designed not to put pressure on the nail tip when it is being cut.

26. If fingernail or toenail clippers are used to cut nail tips, the nail tips may weaken or crease, and the plastic may _____.

LABELING

27. Identify each type of nail tip depicted below.

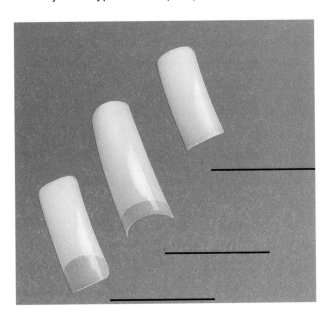

28. Describe how you know when you've selected the best, most appropriate fit with a nail tip.

_____

_____

_____

29. What should you do if the natural nail is between nail tip sizes?

_____

_____

_____

30. When shopping for nail tips to use in the salon, what size container should you choose and how should the tips be packaged?

_____

_____

_____

31. What are two advantages of trimming and/or reducing the well area with an abrasive before applying the tip to the nail?

_____

_____

_____

32. How should you fix a nail tip that has been applied crookedly?

_____

_____

_____

33. How are nail adhesives typically packaged?

_____

_____

_____

34. Once the nail tips are applied, what tool should be used to ensure that no visible line appears where the natural nail stops and the tip begins? What is the best way to use this tool to avoid damaging the natural nail?

_____

_____

_____

35. Why are professional tip cutters, not fingernail or toenail clippers, recommended for use on nail tips after they have been applied?

_____

_____

_____

FILL IN THE BLANK

36. Complete the sentences below using words from the word bank. (*Note:* Not all words will be used.)

   Word bank: air bubbles, large, heat, cold, free edge, small, tip, 5, 10, 30, 45, position stop, faster, slower, well, natural

   If you use a _____ amount of adhesive, setting the nail tip to the natural nail will

   take longer, while using a _____ amount will provide a _____ set due to the

   _____ of the _____ nail. For more time to work with the nail tip, apply adhesive

   into the tip's _____ by lining up the natural nail's _____ against the tip's

   _____. Gently press out any visible _____, and hold the tip for _____

   to _____ seconds, until it is fully attached.

37. Use the Internet or catalogues from a beauty supply store to conduct research on tools and materials related to applying nail tips. Follow the link or use the table below and find the three options for each item listed. Complete the table with your findings.

   Review the results of your research and, for each type of item, select the one you would be most likely to purchase for use in your salon and write a few sentences explaining why. (Try to avoid basing your choices on consumer reviews—instead, focus on what you've studied and imagine yourself actually using these items.) If the decision was difficult for any of the items you examined, explain how you weighed the advantages and disadvantages of your choices.

> **+ BONUS**
>
> **Visit:** bonus.milady.com/cos-wb/toc

TOOLS AND MATERIALS	BRAND NAME	COST (INCLUDE PACKAGE SIZES)	SOURCE (STORE OR WEBSITE)	PRODUCT DESCRIPTION (FEATURES AND DETAILS)
1. Professional tip cutters				
2. Professional tip cutters				
3. Professional tip cutters				
1. Nail tips				
2. Nail tips				
3. Nail tips				
1. Nail adhesives				
2. Nail adhesives				
3. Nail adhesives				

Advantages of Nail Forms

SHORT ANSWER

38. What are nail forms? How are they used?

_____

_____

_____

39. What are three advantages of mastering the use of nail forms?

_____

_____

_____

REFLECTION

40. For this activity, you will first pair up with a classmate and practice applying disposable nail forms on each other, using the method described in your textbook (Procedure 22-4). If there is time, also practice holding reusable nail forms, as you would in a nail enhancement service. Finally, describe your experience, including what was difficult about the procedure, what you liked about performing the procedure, and any aspects of your performance that you'd like to improve. In your reflection, also state whether you think you would prefer using disposable or reusable forms with your clients, and explain why.

_____

_____

_____

41. Match each type of nail form with its description. Each type of nail form will be used more than once.

a. Both   b. Reusable   c. Disposable

Type of Nail Form   **Description**

_____ Alternative to nail tips

_____ Peel the form from its backing

_____ Used as a guide to extend nail enhancement

_____ Pre-shaped plastic

_____ Usually sold in packs of 100 or 500

_____ Paper

_____ Resemble stickers on a roll

_____ Pre-shaped aluminum

_____ Placed under the edge of the natural nail

_____ Usually sold in packs of 10

_____ More difficult to keep in place

_____ Adhere to the client's fingers

_____ Provides a natural-looking nail extension

_____ Mylar

_____ Can save time not having to size, shape, and blend tips

TRUE OR FALSE

Indicate whether each statement below is true or false. For any false statements, explain why they are false.

42. For disposable forms, you can check if the form is straight by ensuring that the form's bottom line is lined up with the nail plate's center.

T   F   _____

43. Disposable nail forms are made of pre-shaped plastic or aluminum and can be cleaned and disinfected between clients.

   T   F   _____

44. A disposable form is perfectly positioned when there is no gap between the free edge and the nail form.

   T   F   _____

45. When working with disposable forms, always position the form's edge the same way, regardless of the desired extension shape.

   T   F   _____

Common Nail Extension Shapes

LABELING

46. Label each image below with its nail shape.

   Word bank: square, squoval, round, oval, pointed, almond, stiletto, ballerina

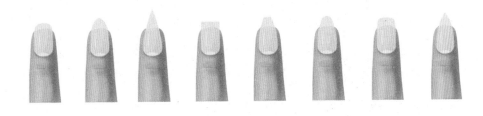

   _____ _____ _____ _____ _____ _____ _____ _____

REFLECTION

47. Of the eight nail shapes covered in this chapter, which one would you feel most comfortable creating for a client? Which one seems the most challenging to create for a client? Next, think about which nail shape you would like for your own nails, and which you find the least appealing. Why did you answer that way? Did you consider style or function? In what ways do you think your response will affect how you shape your clients' nails?

   _____

   _____

   _____

48. What are the five basic nail shapes for shorter nails?

_____

_____

_____

49. In addition to the five basic shapes for shorter nails, what are three shapes commonly requested when performing nail extension services?

_____

_____

_____

50. At what point in the service for nail extensions should you discuss nail shape with your client? Why?

_____

_____

_____

51. After applying the nail tips, should you file the basic shape before or after blending the well (or contact area)? Why?

_____

_____

_____

52. Compare the way a form should be used to create square, squoval, or round nails with the way it should be used to create oval, pointed, almond, stiletto, or ballerina nails.

_____

_____

_____

Properly Structured Nail Enhancements

53. Match each nail part with its description. Each nail part will be used more than once.

a. Stress area   c. Sidewall   e. C-curve

b. Apex   d. Nail extension underside

Nail Part   **Description**

_____ The highest point in the nail; visible no matter where you view the nail

_____ Another side of the nail extension that might either jut straight out or dip, depending on the nail style

_____ The lines of this area should come straight off the lateral folds of the nail, as if the extension naturally grew off the finger

_____ Needs extra product and strength to support the artificial extension

_____ Having the majority of the product in this area adds the necessary strength to allow the nail's tip to be thin while leaving the nail strong enough to resist breaking

_____ Shape or arch when looking at the nail from the tip down the barrel

_____ Also known as the arch

_____ Provides strength in a nail, like the curve in a bridge or an egg

_____ Where the natural nail grows beyond the finger and becomes the free edge

_____ Located on the side where the nail plate grows free of its natural attachment to the nail fold

_____ Oval-shaped and located in the center of the nail

_____ Should be even and match in length from nail to nail on all fingers

54. What are the two overall criteria for determining the quality of a nail enhancement that you completed for your client?

_____

_____

_____

55. How can you ensure that the lengths of the nail extensions and enhancements are appropriate and even?

_____

_____

_____

56. Describe how thick or thin a nail enhancement should be and explain how you can judge that quality in specific areas of the nail.

_____

_____

_____

LABELING

57. Label the part of the nail with the correct term.

    Word Bank: apex, c-curve, edge thickness, extension underside, sidewalls

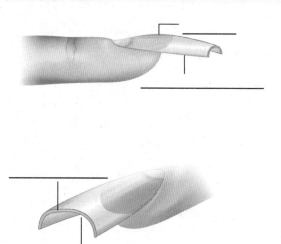

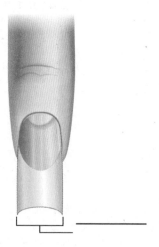

Nail Resin and Nail Resin Systems

58. Match each term with its description. Some terms will be used more than once.

a. Nail resin systems   c. Resin accelerator   e. Nail glue
b. Nail resins   d. Building resins

Term   **Description**

_____ Made from cyanoacrylate, a colorless liquid acrylate monomer easily cured and used as a powerful, fast-acting adhesive

_____ Groups of products that include nail resin to build strength and structure over a natural nail or nail tip

_____ Very thin version of nail resin; also known as tip adhesive

_____ Comes in forms such as brush-on, pump spray, and aerosol and can be used before or after the resin

_____ Provide adhesion to the natural nail and are also known to have great durability when partnered with a flexible product to overlay nails

_____ Assists in speeding up the resin's dry time

_____ In addition to nail resins, may include fabric, paper, cotton materials, or polymer powders

_____ Also known as a resin activator

_____ Thicker version of nail resin

_____ Can be used over natural nails or in conjunction with a nail tip application to add additional length to the nails

59. How do you remove nail resin systems for a client? What is the advantage of this method from the perspective of the client?

_____

_____

_____

60. Complete the sentences below using the words from the word bank. Some words will be used more than once.

    Word bank: thicker, resin, cyanoacrylates, resin, viscosity, thinner, resin

    _____ vary in viscosity. The _____ the viscosity, the better the adhesion

    and the faster the cure time. With a _____ viscosity, _____ are referred to

    as _____ or building _____. _____-viscosity resins are usually

    used as a base; _____-viscosity resins are used to build or are applied as a top coat.

    _____ refers to the thickness or flow-ability of liquids.

RESEARCH

61. Use the Internet or a catalogue from a beauty supply store to research and compare the variety of nail resin systems available on the market today. Follow the link or use the table below; find one system in each price range and complete the table.

    After you've completed your table, partner with a classmate and compare notes on your findings—for example, discuss what you learned during your research, share the best (and worst) systems that you discovered, and check out each other's findings to see if you agree with your partner's decision to buy or not buy.

+ BONUS
Visit: bonus.milady.com/cos-wb/toc

	UNDER $20	$21–$30	$31–$40	$41–$50	OVER $50
Brand Name of Nail Resin System					
Cost					
Contents (and Amounts)					
What's Missing from the System?					
What's Not Necessary in the System?					
For Use by Professionals? (Yes or No)					
Store or Website Selling the System					
Would You Buy This System for Use in Your Salon? (Yes or No)					
Reason(s) to Buy or Not Buy					

Strengthening with Nail Wraps

MATCHING

62. Match the equipment and materials used in nail wrap applications to their names.

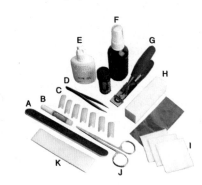

_____ nail glue   _____ tweezers

_____ scissors   _____ nail file

_____ nail wipes   _____ resin

_____ nail tips   _____ nail tip clippers

_____ fiberglass/   _____ buffer block
silk linen strips

_____ resin activator spray

63. Match each type of wrap with its description. Some types will be used more than once.

   a. Silk wrap   b. Fiberglass wrap   c. Both

Type of Wrap	Description
_____	Becomes transparent when wrap resin is applied
_____	Easy to use and allows the wrap resin to penetrate, which improves adhesion and clarity
_____	Very popular nail wrap type
_____	Lightweight with a smooth, translucent appearance when applied to the nail
_____	Made from a thin, natural material with a tight weave
_____	Made from a very thin synthetic mesh with a loose weave

64. What are nail wraps, and why are they used?

_____

_____

_____

65. Which type of absorbent material is most commonly used for nail wraps?

_____

_____

_____

66. Describe in detail why and how you would use stress strips when performing a nail wrap.

_____

_____

_____

67. For the maintenance service, what is the difference between a fill (or backfill) and a rebalance?

_____

_____

_____

68. What maintenance is performed two weeks after the nail enhancement is applied?

_____

_____

_____

69. What kind of maintenance is performed four weeks after the nail enhancement is applied?

_____

_____

_____

Dip System Advantages

70. What is unique about dip systems? How does this benefit both the client and cosmetologist?

_____

_____

_____

71. What is the best option to get an even color while avoiding dipping multiple clients' hands in the same powder container?

_____

_____

_____

72. List the five typical materials used in dip systems.

_____

_____

_____

73. What should you do if the application brush hardens?

_____

_____

_____

74. What are two possible consequences of getting resin on the skin?

_____

_____

_____

75. What is the purpose of the first layer of top resin? The second layer?

_____

_____

_____

76. Why should you avoid nipping off product that has lifted from a client's nail?

_____

_____

_____

77. Why is doing a clear dip powder extension different from a standard color application?

_____

_____

_____

78. List the four implements and materials needed for the resin system removal procedure (in addition to the basic materials already on your manicuring table).

_____

_____

_____

79. How should you use the wooden pusher stick in the nail resin system removal procedure?

_____

_____

_____

80. How is acetone used in the nail resin system removal procedure?

_____

_____

_____

81. Number the followings steps for performing a one-color application using the dip system, from 1 to 19, from beginning to end. Some steps have been provided for you.

NUMBER	STEP
	Polish the resin base coat onto nail's entire surface as close as you can get to the skin without touching it.
	Pull out your dust collector when beginning to file. Wear your NIOSH (National Institute for Occupational Safety and Health)-approved respirator mask.
8	Repeat on remaining nails. Dust away excess powder with soft makeup brush.
5	Repeat steps 3 and 4 on the remaining nails. Dust away excess powder with soft makeup brush.
	Apply activator to all 10 nails. Clean the surface with lint-free wipe to ensure there is no excess activator.
	Pour preferred powder color into dappen dish. Add more powder throughout service as needed.
	Apply second base resin coat on the nail, ensuring you capped the free edge. Wipe resin applicator brush on lint-free towel and put it back in the bottle.
	Apply resin activator over all 10 nails.
17	Repeat for a second coat. Let stand for about eight minutes until dry.
	Quickly dip nail into powder dappen dish. Hold for one to two seconds and pull it out. Gently tap the finger to remove excess powder.
	Smooth nail's surface with medium-grit buffer.
	Present the finished look to your client.
	Apply base resin over nail. Wipe resin applicator brush on lint-free towel and put it back in the bottle. Because of the activator, the base should dry very quickly.
	Use medium-grit abrasive to shape the nails, if needed.
1	Apply nail tips, if desired.
	Quickly dip nail into powder dappen dish. Hold for one to two seconds and pull it out. Gently tap finger to remove excess powder. Wipe resin applicator brush on lint-free towel and put it back in the bottle.
	Apply cuticle oil then hand lotion and massage them in.
	Apply top resin over entire nail, keeping product off the skin. Wipe resin applicator brush on a lint-free towel and put it back in the bottle.
	Remove dust with clean, dry disinfected nail brush.

FILL IN THE BLANK

82. Complete the sentences below using words from the word bank. Some words will not be used.

Word bank: smile line, stress area, entire, tip, apex, white, French, pink, clear, half-moon

To create a _____ manicure look, simply dip only the nail's _____ at an angle

into _____ powder to create a perfect _____. To complete the look, tap off

excess power and dip the _____ nail into a sheer _____ powder.

DRAW

83. Think about the various ways that you can use dip systems, powders, colors, nail shapes, and nail extensions (or tips) to create some signature designs. For example, how would you adapt the French manicure look to reflect your client's personality or a special event they might be attending? Draw and give a name to your signature designs here. Be creative and bold, and be sure to list any details, extra steps, or materials that you might need to implement your ideas.

DISCOVERIES AND ACCOMPLISHMENTS

In the space below, write notes about key concepts discussed in this chapter. Share your discoveries with some of the other students in your class and ask them if your notes are helpful. You may want to revise your notes based on good ideas shared by your peers.

Discoveries:

_____

_____

_____

_____

_____

_____

_____

List at least three things you have accomplished since you decided to enroll in school.

Accomplishments:

_____

_____

_____

_____

_____

_____

_____

1. Cosmetologists should have a thorough understanding of nail extensions and resin systems because _____.

   A) this knowledge helps perform colored dip systems, which are a very popular service

   B) this knowledge helps perform resin systems, which are ideal for clients wanting to extend their nails permanently

   C) they learn that most fabric wraps causes a crack or break in the natural nail

   D) they learn that properly prepared natural nails reduce the life of nail extensions

2. When clients request a nail extension service without scheduling a manicure service, first perform a(n) _____.

   A) basic manicure using water and nail cleanser

   C) dry manicure without using water

   B) spa manicure without using a nail cleanser

   D) antiaging manicure using water

3. A nail cleanser _____.

   A) blocks adhesion

   B) is commonly made from acetone

   C) temporarily stops the nails from producing moisture and natural oil

   D) removes surface debris, moisture, and tiny amounts of oil from the natural nail plate

4. Which of the following statements is accurate about nail dehydrators?

   A) They permanently stop the nails from producing moisture and natural oil.

   B) They are completely safe for the nail and can be reapplied if needed.

   C) They are commonly made from isobutyl alcohol.

   D) They typically last about one to two hours.

5. After applying a nail dehydrator, _____.

   A) do not apply product within 10 minutes

   B) touch the nail plates

   C) do not let makeup or moisturizer get on the prepped nail plates

   D) allow clients to rest their hands against their faces

continued

6. Which of the following statements associated with a nail overlay is accurate?

    A) Nail tips without an overlay do not easily lose adhesion.

    B) Nail tips without an overlay are not strong enough to wear alone.

    C) Nail wraps, which serve as an overlay, typically damage natural nails.

    D) Nail tips should be worn without an additional nail overlay.

7. A _____ nail tip covers the entire apex area and usually covers more than half of the nail plate.

    A) French   C) partial-well

    B) full-well   B) well-less

8. Identify a characteristic of French nail tips.

    A) They are cut like a smile line at the contact point.

    B) They cover the entire nail up to the cuticle.

    C) They are usually altered at the well line to expose more of the natural nail.

    D) They cover the entire apex area and usually cover more than half of the nail plate.

9. Which of the following is a guideline to follow when using a nail tip?

    A) Do not use fingernail or toenail clippers to cut the nail tip.

    B) Do not reduce the well or contact area between the nail tip and the natural nail with a medium-grit abrasive.

    C) When filing the contact area between the nail tip and the natural nail, hold the file at an angle.

    D) Continue filing for five minutes after the nail tip's well is flush with the natural nail.

10. Identify a true statement about nail forms.

    A) They are also known as nail tips.

    B) They are placed above the natural nail's free edge.

    C) They are metal tools specifically designed to cut tips without pressure.

    D) They are used as a guide to extend the nail enhancement product beyond the fingertip.

continued

11. Disposable nail forms are _____.

   A) made of pre-shaped plastic or aluminum and can be cleaned and disinfected between clients

   B) often made of paper or a strong, thin polyester film called mylar

   C) usually sold in a 10-piece container

   D) more difficult to keep in place than are reusable nail forms

12. Which of the following is one of the steps in using a nail form?

   A) looking at the nail from the side to ensure that the form comes straight out from the natural nail and is not tilted down

   B) checking if the form is straight by ensuring that the form's center line is lined up with the nail's free edges

   C) leaving the end tab of the nail form open to form a large circle at the edge for tapered nails, such as oval or stiletto

   D) ensuring that there is a small gap between the nail's free edge and the nail form

13. Reusable nail forms _____.

   A) are made of paper or a strong, thin polyester film called mylar

   B) are usually sold in 100- or 500-count containers

   C) can be cleaned and disinfected between clients

   D) need to be applied to two fingers at a time as you work

14. In the context of nail shapes for nail extensions, almond nails are _____.

   A) similar to a square shape

   C) similar to stiletto nails

   B) very tapered

   D) also known as stiletto nails

15. In the context of nail shapes for nail extensions, stiletto nails _____.

   A) resemble a long, skinny carrot

   B) are short

   C) are seldom tapered

   D) have edges that are square-shaped

continued

16. In the context of nail shapes for nail extensions, ballerina nails _____.

    A) resemble almond nails

    B) are short

    C) are extremely tapered

    D) have edges that come to a sharp point

17. In the context of nail shapes for nail extensions, the edge of a(n) _____ nail is square.

    A) ballerina   C) almond

    B) stiletto   D) eggshell

18. When sculpting square, soft square, or round nails using a nail form, the _____.

    A) end of the form should open into a pinhole circle

    B) form should come to a point at the end

    C) extension edge of the nail should be excessively filed

    D) form sides should come straight out from the natural nail grooves

19. The _____ is where the natural nail grows beyond the finger and becomes the free edge.

    A) stress area   C) C-curve

    B) sidewall   D) apex

20. The highest point in the nail is referred to as the _____.

    A) sidewall   C) apex

    B) C-curve   D) underside

21. For a client to wear a nail enhancement comfortably, _____.

    A) the cuticle area should graduate seamlessly and feel smooth without any glitches

    B) its thickness should be increased

    C) the surface, from the cuticle area to the end of the nail extension, should have at least two dips

    D) the sidewalls and tip's edge should be at least 2 inches thick

continued

22. Identify a true statement about the C-curve of a nail.

   A) A nail enhancement's C-curve is independent of the natural nail's C-curve.

   B) A 75 percent C-curve is considered average.

   C) It reduces the nail's strength and leads to breaking.

   D) It is the nail's arch when looking at the nail from the tip down the barrel.

23. Thicker cyanoacrylates are referred to as _____.

   A) nail glues

   B) tip adhesives

   C) nail cleansers

   D) building resins

24 A silk nail wrap _____.

   A) is made from a thin, natural material with a tight weave

   B) is made from a very thin synthetic mesh with a loose weave

   C) has a rough appearance when applied to the nail

   D) allows the wrap resin to penetrate easier than a fiberglass wrap does and is heavy

25. Which of the following statements related to dip systems is accurate?

   A) The polymer powders used in dip systems are the same as the polymer powders used in liquid and powder nail services.

   B) Using nail resins along with dip systems helps save time for both the client and the cosmetologist.

   C) Most dip powders can be used with a liquid monomer to create a nail.

   D) Dip systems provide a color service that lasts 21 days with an LED or UV lamp.

finished!

Practical Skills   Self-Evaluation Checklist

Regular self-assessment helps you to improve your technical skills and achieve success. After performing each procedure, review the procedure steps in the textbook and rate yourself as "Competent" or "Needs Work," and write in comments on how you were successful or where you can improve. Rating yourself helps you identify your strengths and weaknesses and develop your own plan for improvement.

CRITERIA	COMPETENT	NEEDS WORK	COMMENTS
PROCEDURE 22-1 DRY MANICURE			
Preparation			
Procedure			
Post-Service			
Timing			
PROCEDURE 22-2 NAIL TIP APPLICATION			
Preparation			
Procedure			
Post-Service			
Timing			
PROCEDURE 22-3 NAIL TIP REMOVAL			
Preparation			
Procedure			
Post-Service			
Timing			
PROCEDURE 22-4 DISPOSABLE NAIL FORM APPLICATION			
Preparation			
Procedure			
Post-Service			
Timing			
PROCEDURE 22-5 DIP SYSTEM ONE-COLOR APPLICATION			
Preparation			
Procedure			
Post-Service			
Timing			
PROCEDURE 22-6 RESIN SYSTEM REMOVAL			
Preparation			
Procedure			
Post-Service			
Timing			

Ch. 23: Liquid and Powder Nail Enhancements

Why Study Liquid and Powder Nail Enhancements?

SHORT ANSWER

1. What is a common term for nail enhancements that are based on mixing monomer liquids and polymer powders?

_____

_____

_____

2. How does your text refer to the two-part monomer liquid and polymer powder enhancement systems?

_____

_____

_____

3. How may industry literature and product marketing refer to the two-part monomer liquid and polymer powder enhancement systems?

_____

_____

_____

4. List the three reasons that you should study and thoroughly understand liquid and powder nail enhancements

_____

_____

_____

5. Why are liquid and powder nail enhancements so popular?

_____

_____

_____

Chemistry of Liquid and Powder Nail Enhancements

SHORT ANSWER

6. How are liquid and powder nail enhancements created?

_____

_____

_____

7. Define *monomer* and *polymer* using the meanings of the two parts of each word.

   _____

   _____

   _____

8. Explain what an SDS is and describe what type of information is provided in it.

   _____

   _____

   _____

FILL IN THE BLANK

Complete the following sentences about the chemistry of liquid and powder nail enhancements.

9. The best type of brush for applying liquid and powder nail enhancements is made of

   _____.

10. The liquid that is *not* recommended for use—and is illegal in most states—is

    _____ (MMA).

11. Liquid and powder products can be used as a _____ on the natural nail, as a

    _____ of the nail tip, on a _____ to create an extension, or to

    create nail art on top or inside of a nail enhancement.

12. _____ are additives that speed up chemical reactions in polymers and monomers.

13. In the polymerization process, _____ in polymers cause monomer molecules to

    permanently link together into long chains.

14. _____ is the initiator added to polymer powder that starts the

    _____ process of the nail enhancement.

15. Monomer liquid is absorbed into the brush, then touched to the polymer powder, and creates a

    small _____ of product that is then molded and shaped into the enhancement.

16. A _____ liquid mixed with a _____ powder forms the liquid and powder nail enhancement.

17. The three types of monomer liquid are _____ methacrylate, methyl _____, and odorless.

18. Using the wrong polymer powder for the monomer liquid you are using can cause the enhancements not to _____ properly.

19. The _____ has said not to use MMA, and the American Beauty Association and the _____ have taken this same stance.

MATCHING

20. Match each type of liquid and powder product its description. Some descriptions may have more than one answer.

   a. Ethyl methacrylate monomer (EMA)

   b. Methyl methacrylate monomer (MMA)

   c. Odorless

TYPE OF LIQUID AND POWDER PRODUCT	DESCRIPTION
_____	Have an inhibition layer when hardening
_____	Contain monomers that are used as customizing additives
_____	Banned for use by FDA and most states
_____	Industry standard
_____	Has a slight odor
_____	Use has been linked to onycholysis (nails detaching from the nail bed)
_____	Polymer powder made mostly from this liquid mixed with PMMA
_____	Must be used with a dry mix ratio

Complete the following sentences about odorless monomer liquid and polymer powder products.

21. Rewetting your brush with monomer liquid will _____.

22. Odorless products will have a tacky layer on top as they harden, called the _____

     layer.

23. Odorless liquid and powder products do not use _____ but instead rely on

     monomers that have minimal odor.

24. A dry mix ratio produces a bead that looks _____ on the brush; however, once

     pressed onto the nail, it will slowly form in a firm, _____ bead that will then be

     pressed and smoothed with a nail brush.

25. Odorless products harden more _____ than ethyl methacrylate products.

TRUE OR FALSE

Indicate whether the following statements about odorless monomer liquid and polymer powder are true or false. If a statement is false, explain why it is false.

26. Odorless monomer liquid and polymer powder products have the same chemistry as other monomer liquid and polymer powder products.

     T   F   _____

27. If an odorless product is too wet when it is applied, the client may experience skin irritation.

     T   F   _____

28. An inhibition layer must be removed from the nail using a special acetone solution.

     T   F   _____

Liquid and Powder Nail Enhancement Service Supplies

DOUBLE PUZZLE

29. Unscramble the words using the clues provided and write them in the squares. You'll see a number underneath some of the squares. Find the numbered square below and write that letter into that square to reveal the secret message!

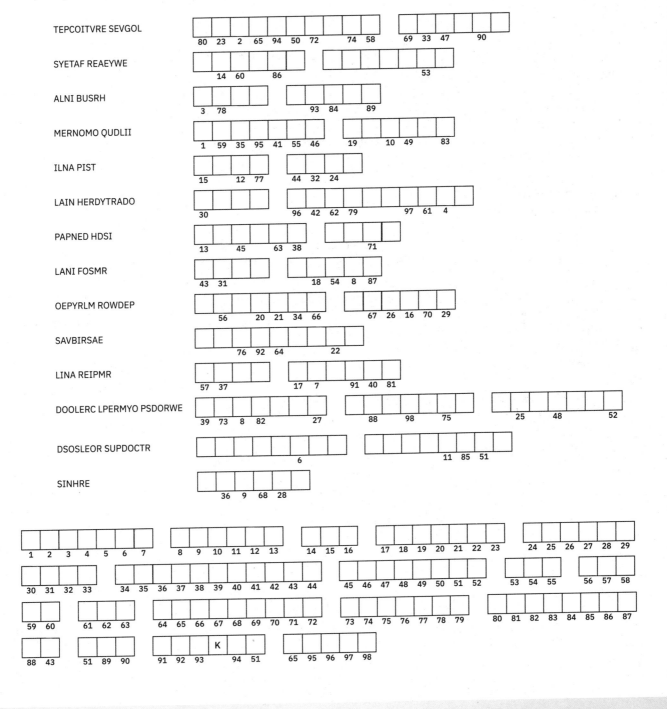

TEPCOITVRE SEVGOL

SYETAF REAEYWE

ALNI BUSRH

MERNOMO QUDLII

ILNA PIST

LAIN HERDYTRADO

PAPNED HDSI

LANI FOSMR

OEPYRLM ROWDEP

SAVBIRSAE

LINA REIPMR

DOOLERC LPERMYO PSDORWE

DSOSLEOR SUPDOCTR

SINHRE

30. Match each type of bead mix ratio with its description. Some types will be used more than once.

   a. Wet   b. Dry   c. Medium

   Type of Bead Mix Ratio   **Description**

   _____ Usually contains many air bubbles

   _____ Uses twice as much liquid as powder to create the bead

   _____ Can be difficult to press into place

   _____ Generally, the ideal mix ratio when working with monomer
                            liquids and polymer powders

   _____ Contains 1½:1 mix ratio of liquid to powder

   _____ Created with equal amounts of liquid and powder

SHORT ANSWER

31. List the six main types of supplies (in addition to the basic manicuring supplies and dry manicure
   procedure products) that you need to perform liquid and powder nail enhancement services.

   _____

   _____

   _____

32. Explain how the analogy about the role of flour in making cookie dough applies to mixing monomer
   liquids and polymer powders.

   _____

   _____

   _____

33. List three precautions you should always take when working with monomer liquids and polymer powders.

_____

_____

_____

34. If you find that the manufacturer's directions for working with liquid monomers and polymer powders differ from the information in your text, what should you do?

_____

_____

_____

Indicate whether the statements below are true or false. For any false statements, explain why they are false.

35. Nail professionals should never alter the traditional pink and white French manicure combinations.

    T   F   _____

36. Nail artistry with colored polymer powder is limited only by your imagination.

    T   F   _____

37. It's a good idea to maintain recipe cards for custom polymer powder colors that you create for your clients.

    T   F   _____

38. Use caution when creating and offering custom colors with polymer powders because clients are not willing to pay more for these customized services.

    T   F   _____

39. Polymer powders are only available in pink, white, natural, and clear.

    T   F   _____

40. An acid-free version of a nail primer creates a chemical bond between the nail and the enhancement.

    T   F   _____

41. Methacrylic acid primers are considered the industry standard.

    T   F   _____

42. When primer dries incorrectly, it will appear to be a chalky white color; when it dries properly, it will be shiny and sticky.

    T   F   _____

43. Nail primers are available in acid-free and acid-based versions.

    T   F   _____

44. Nail primers can be applied to the natural nail as many times as the nail technician deems necessary.

    T   F   _____

45. When nail primers are used, the nail technician must be sure to use just enough on each nail, and must be sure to prevent nail debris contamination in the bottle between applications.

    T   F   _____

46. When put on nail tips, nail primers do not damage them or their adhesive in any way.

    T   F   _____

SHORT ANSWER

47. What is the term used to describe nail files and buffers?

_____

_____

_____

48. What does the grit number tell you about how aggressive an abrasive is?

_____

_____

_____

49. What is a shiner?

_____

_____

_____

50. Why should you score your abrasives before using them? How do you score them?

_____

_____

_____

51. Where are nail forms placed? How do they aid in applying liquid and powder?

_____

_____

_____

SEQUENCE

52. The chart below includes the steps for applying nail primer. Fill in the missing information for steps 1–5.

1	
	Using a dotting action, dab the brush tip to the prepared natural nail and completely cover the nail plate with primer.
5	
	Touch the brush tip to the edge of the bottle's neck to release excess primer.
4	

53. Match the abrasive type to the corresponding description of its function or detail. Terms will be used more than once.

a. Buffer

b. Coarse-grit

c. Fine-grit

d. Medium-grit

e. Shiner

Abrasive Type	Description
_____	Creates high shine on nail (natural or enhancement)
_____	Prepares enhancement for a refill/rebalance
_____	240 grit or higher
_____	Should be avoided on freshly applied enhancements
_____	Removes scratches on nail surface
_____	A type of buffer
_____	Used for initial shaping of perimeter of nail
_____	100 grit or lower
_____	Usually comes in two- or three-sided form
_____	Can smooth the enhancement before buffing
_____	Strong enough to thin enhancement product
_____	Usually comes in 400; 1,000; and 4,000 grit
_____	Can shape the entire nail, as long as product is not too thick
_____	Shapes free edge of natural nail
_____	150 to 180 grit
_____	Can come in grit ranging from 100 to 400
_____	Refines and finishes filing
_____	After filing is complete, start with low grit and move to higher grit for desired smoothness
_____	Used for refining overall surface shape of enhancement
_____	Can create brilliance similar to top coat

Indicate whether the statements below are true or false. For statements that are false, explain why they are false.

54. Certain models of drills made for filing wood and metal will work just as well as e-files made for filing nail enhancements.

    T   F   _____

55. Electric files can be an expensive investment.

    T   F   _____

56. It's a good idea to purchase an e-file from a company that offers training.

    T   F   _____

FILL IN THE BLANK

57. Complete the sentences below using words from the word bank.

    Word bank: evaporation, cork, glass, monomer, cover, small, contamination, minimize, lid, plastic

    Dappen dishes are small _____ or _____ containers that hold the amount

    of product needed for one service use. These dishes usually have a _____ opening to

    _____ liquid _____. To prevent evaporation and _____ by dust and

    debris, and to help reduce _____ odors, a dappen dish should have a _____ or a

    _____ to _____ the product when not in use.

SHORT ANSWER

58. What should you do with unused monomer liquid after a service?

    _____

    _____

    _____

59. What technique is recommended for creating uniform beads with monomer liquid? What is another benefit of using this technique?

_____

_____

_____

60. What is the most commonly used brush (size and shape) for monomer liquid and polymer powder?

_____

_____

_____

61. Why should you avoid using overly large brushes?

_____

_____

_____

62. What is the best type of liquid and powder enhancement nail brush?

_____

_____

_____

63. Why are synthetic or less expensive brushes less desirable than natural hair versions?

_____

_____

_____

64. What should you do when product starts to stick to your brush?

_____

_____

_____

65. What's the best way to store your brush?

_____

_____

_____

66. The following table contains the procedure for a one-color liquid and powder overlay, steps 1–16. Put them in order from start to finish. Steps 1 and 10 are given.

_____ Press brush tip into polymer powder to pick up a bead wide enough to cover the free edge.

_____ Tap the product up and toward each sidewall, then smooth to blend with free edge.

_____ Present the finished look to your client.

_____ Pour monomer liquid and polymer powder into separate dappen dishes.

_____ Clean all nail enhancements with alcohol, then finish with polish or gel color.

__10__ Pick up a small wet bead of polymer powder with brush and place just above the center of the nail plate. Tap product up toward the cuticle and smooth to blend with the rest of the enhancement.

_____ Place bead toward edge of nail, then wipe on a disposable towel to remove excess product.

_____ Dip brush into monomer liquid.

_____ Pick up another medium bead and place it on the center of the nail.

_____ Buff the enhancement with medium- to coarse-grit buffer until entire surface is smooth.

__1__ Apply the nail dehydrator.

_____ Ask client to wash hands with soap and water. Dry thoroughly.

_____ Use brush's middle portion ("belly") to press and smooth product to cover the free edge.

_____ Massage cuticle oil into the surrounding skin and rub hand cream into the client's hands.

_____ Shape the nail with a medium-grit abrasive to remove any large imperfections. Refine surface with 180-grit abrasive.

_____ Apply nail primer sparingly on natural nail.

67. For each statement about storing and disposing of monomer liquid and polymer product, indicate whether it's a Do or a Don't.

DO OR DON'T?	STORING AND DISPOSING OF MONOMER LIQUIDS
_____	Store monomer liquid products separate from polymer powders in covered containers in a cool, dark area
_____	Leave items soiled with enhancement products on your manicuring station after you complete a service
_____	Check with your instructor or state board for chemical-based nail product storage laws
_____	Discard used materials after a service
_____	Save used monomer liquid removed from the original container
_____	Pour small amounts of leftover monomer liquid onto a very absorbent paper towel and place it in a plastic bag to dispose of it
_____	Avoid skin contact with the monomer liquid
_____	Pour the small amounts of leftover monomer liquid directly into a plastic bag
_____	Seal all used materials in a plastic bag and discard the bag in a closed waste receptacle
_____	Remove all items soiled with enhancement products from your manicuring station after each client, in accordance with local rules and regulations

Liquid and Powder Nail Art

Indicate whether each statement is true or false. For any false statements, explain why they are false.

68. You can apply 3-D art directly over wet nail polish.

    T   F   _____

69. Liquid and powder nail art holds very well on a clean, natural nail.

    T   F   _____

70. Using monomer liquid and polymer powder to create nail art can be challenging to master, but it also has the most versatile results.

    T   F   _____

71. When first working in this medium, it's best to try a variety of the brushes and tools available to apply and mold the liquid and powder to nail tips and overlays.

T   F   _____

72. When working on top of a polished nail, it's important to avoid stroking the polish's surface too many times with a brush wet with monomer liquid because you might ruin the polish.

T   F   _____

CREATE

73. With so many ways to use liquid monomers and powder polymers, you can see every nail as an opportunity to express yourself as an artist—and to help your clients express their personality. Creating unique nail art is also an opportunity to showcase your professional skills and build client loyalty.

    For this activity, pair up with a classmate and find out about an event happening in their life, such as a birthday, holiday, vacation, or date, that you want to create a unique nail design for. How does the atmosphere of the event inspire your design? Then plan and sketch two different designs (each for 10 nails) for your classmate: one that includes 3-D art and another that includes inlaid art (or mix and match if you'd like!).

    Next, describe how you will use the liquid monomer and polymer powder techniques to execute each design, including the tools needed. Did you find that you need to know more about the capabilities of the monomer–polymer combinations to execute your design?

    Even if you need to adjust your design, you probably realized that the more you understand the capabilities of those materials and tools, the more possibilities for creativity—and client loyalty—you will have.

SHORT ANSWER

74. What is one way to describe the difference between 3-D and inlaid nail art?

    _____

    _____

    _____

75. Describe how your bead and brush techniques for creating a 3-D flower would be modified to create an inlaid version of the same image.

    _____

    _____

    _____

76. How can you achieve a matte finish on a nail that will have 3-D art applied to it? How can you create a glossy finish?

_____

_____

_____

Liquid and Powder Nail Enhancement Maintenance and Removal

SHORT ANSWER

77. Why is regular maintenance of liquid and powder nail enhancements important?

_____

_____

_____

78. How is a backfill different from the initial application of liquid and powder nail enhancements?

_____

_____

_____

79. What causes lifting of the product and how is it remedied?

_____

_____

_____

80. What is meant by the rule of thumb about lifting—"If you can see it now, you will see it later"?

_____

_____

_____

DOUBLE PUZZLE

81. Unscramble the words using the clues provided and write them in the squares. You'll see a number underneath some of the squares. Find the numbered square below and write that letter into that square to reveal the secret message!

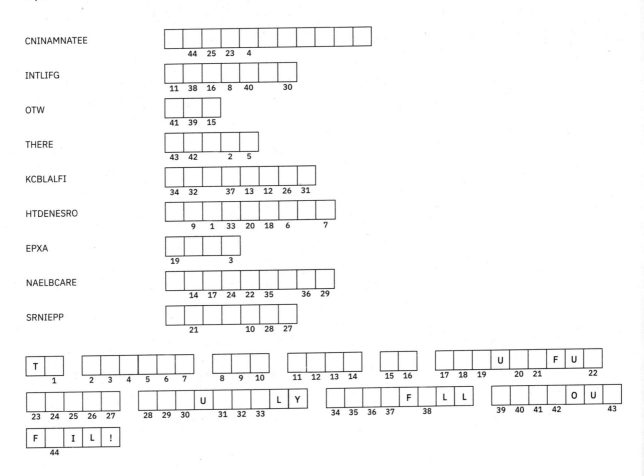

CNINAMNATEE   44 25 23 4

INTLIFG   11 38 16 8 40 30

OTW   41 39 15

THERE   43 42 2 5

KCBLALFI   34 32 37 13 12 26 31

HTDENESRO   9 1 33 20 18 6 7

EPXA   19 3

NAELBCARE   14 17 24 22 35 36 29

SRNIEPP   21 10 28 27

T _ | _ _ _ _ _ _ | _ _ _ | _ _ _ _ | _ _ | _ _ _ U _ _ F U _
1   2 3 4 5 6 7   8 9 10   11 12 13 14   15 16   17 18 19   20 21   22

_ _ _ _ _ | _ _ _ U _ _ L Y | _ _ _ _ F _ L L | _ _ _ _ O U _
23 24 25 26 27   28 29 30   31 32 33   34 35 36 37   38   39 40 41 42   43

F _ I L !
44

82. Place the steps for a liquid and powder nail repair in order from 1 to 14.

_____ Shape the nail enhancement with a medium-grit abrasive.

_____ Apply a nail form.

_____ Prepare the monomer liquid and polymer powder. Use your brush to wet the existing product with a monomer. Pick up a small wet bead of product and apply it to the cracked area.

_____ Apply nail primer to any exposed natural nail.

_____ Apply an additional bead, if needed, to reinforce the rest of the nail.

_____ Present the finished look to your client.

_____ Clean nail enhancements with alcohol and finish with clear polish or gel.

_____ When the product is cured, remove the form.

_____ Remove the existing polish, then use a medium-grit abrasive to file the area around the crack or break flush to the nail. Gently file over entire enhancement. Remove dust with a nylon brush.

_____ Buff the natural nail enhancement with a coarse-grit or higher buffer until the entire surface is smooth.

_____ Ask the client to wash their hands with soap and water or use a nail brush to clean the nails over a fingerbowl. Rinse with clean water and dry thoroughly with a clean disposable towel.

_____ Apply nail dehydrator to any exposed natural nail.

_____ Press and smooth the bead to fill the crack. Be careful not to let the product seep under the form.

_____ Massage cuticle oil into the surrounding skin. Apply hand cream and massage the hand and arm.

83. Why must the nail technician purchase acetone from a beauty supply store instead of a hardware store?

_____

_____

_____

84. What is the key idea to ensure safe removal of liquid and powder nail enhancements?

_____

_____

_____

85. What is an alternative to immersing a client's fingers in acetone for long periods?

_____

_____

_____

86. Explain why nail plates may appear thinner after enhancements are removed.

_____

_____

_____

87. Place the steps for a liquid and power enhancement removal in order from 1 to 7.

_____ Remove polish. Soak the client's nail enhancements for 20 to 30 minutes, or as long as needed to remove the enhancement product.

_____ Fill the glass bowl with enough acetone or product remover to cover 1/2" (1.27 cm) higher than the client's enhancements. Place the bowl inside another bowl of hot water to heat the acetone safely.

_____ If needed, use a fine grit buffer to remove any remaining product or to smooth the natural nail.

_____ Have the client wash their hands or use a nail brush to clean the nails over a fingerbowl. Rinse with clean water and dry thoroughly with a clean disposable towel.

_____ Using a wooden pusher, gently push off the softened enhancement. Repeat until all enhancements have dissolved and then use a plastic-backed cotton pad to remove the remaining product.

_____ Massage cuticle oil into the surrounding skin, then apply hand cream and massage the hand and arm. If the client wants a basic manicure (which the technician should recommend), this should be done now.

_____ Present the finished look to your client.

In the space below, write notes about key concepts discussed in this chapter. Share your discoveries with some of the other students in your class and ask them if your notes are helpful. You may want to revise your notes based on good ideas shared by your peers.

Discoveries:

_____

_____

_____

_____

_____

_____

_____

List at least three things you have accomplished since you decided to enroll in school.

Accomplishments:

_____

_____

_____

_____

_____

_____

_____

1. Nail enhancements created by mixing monomer liquids and polymer powders are commonly referred to as _____.

   A) wet nails   C) nail tips

   B) acrylic nails   D) nail rasps

2. Cosmetologists benefit from having a detailed understanding of liquid and powder nail enhancements because _____.

   A) they are licensed to diagnose, treat, prescribe, or work on unhealthy nails and perform any service required in the process

   B) nail enhancement services are medical procedures and cosmetologists are required to perform procedures that are listed under any medical license

   C) knowing how to properly work with enhancement materials and understanding their chemical makeup allow them to perform services safely for themselves and their clients

   D) learning about nail enhancements is essential in order to tell a client that a specific nail or skin disease or disorder is present and to suggest ways to treat it

3. Liquid and powder nail enhancements are created by _____.

   A) combining polymer liquids with polymer powders to form the nail enhancements

   B) combining polymer liquids with monomer powders to form the nail enhancements

   C) combining monomer liquids with monomer powders to form the nail enhancements

   D) combining monomer liquids with polymer powders to form the nail enhancements

4. Identify a way in which liquid and powder products are used.

   A) to create the lunula

   B) on the natural nail as a protective overlay

   C) to create the nail bed

   D) under a nail tip as reinforcement

continued

5. Identify the chemical process that causes monomers to join to create very long chains.

   A) lanthionization

   B) depilation

   C) polymerization

   D) keratinization

6. _____ are additives designed to energize and activate initiators and are added to monomers to start or speed up the chemical reaction.

   A) Boosters

   B) Chemical relaxers

   C) Catalysts

   D) Activators

7. Which of the following is an initiator added to polymer powder to start the chain reaction that leads to curing (hardening)?

   A) ethanol

   B) calcium hydroxide

   C) methyl methacrylate

   D) benzoyl peroxide

8. Identify a true statement about odorless monomer liquid and polymer powder products.

   A) They harden faster than other monomer liquid and polymer powder products.

   B) They create a tacky layer on top of the nail called the inhibition layer.

   C) They invariably have the same chemistry as other monomer liquid and polymer powder products.

   D) They must generally use a wet mix ratio.

9. The amount of monomer liquid and polymer powder used to create a bead is called the _____.

   A) bead level

   B) viscosity ratio

   C) mix ratio

   D) grit number

10. In general, _____ beads have the ideal mix ratio when working with monomer liquids and polymer powders.

    A) dry

    B) solid

    C) medium

    D) wet

continued

11. Which of the following products is used on the natural nail before product application to prepare it for liquid and powder nail enhancements and to assist in adhesion?

A) nail primer

C) a shiner

B) benzoyl peroxide

D) a nail buffer

12. Which of the following guidelines should be followed when applying acid-based and acid-free nail primers?

A) Apply the nail primer at least twice to each natural nail.

B) Apply the nail enhancement product only over wet nail primer.

C) Avoid putting the nail primer on plastic nail tips.

D) Never wipe the brush on a lint-free towel before dipping it back into the container.

13. Which of the following indicates the number of grains or particles per square inch of a file?

A) nail buffers

C) viscosity

B) a grit number

D) the mix ratio

14. Which of the following occurs when artificial products pull away from the nail?

A) lanthionization

C) lifting

B) epilation

D) depilation

15. A(n) _____ is a buffer (usually three sided with 400/1,000/4,000 grits) that creates a high gloss on the natural nail or the nail enhancement when no polish is worn.

A) nail primer

C) autoclave

B) shiner

D) curette

16. In the context of liquid and powder nail enhancement service supplies, a(n) _____ is a small plastic or glass container that holds a minimal amount of product for one service use.

A) dappen dish

C) nail rasp

B) curette

D) autoclave

continued

17. The best liquid and powder enhancement nail brush is _____.

    A) a boar-bristle brush or a vent brush

    B) a natural hair brush that is either composed of sable or kolinsky or offers a sable or red sable blend

    C) a synthetic hair brush composed of Kanekalon®

    D) a brush composed of the hair of animals such as alpaca, yak, and angora

18. Identify a guideline you should follow to care for your nail brush.

    A) Store the brush top down or in a vertical position.

    B) Soak the brush in acetone for at least 10 minutes if the product hardens on the hairs.

    C) Wipe the brush rapidly back and forth against a table towel.

    D) Use a brush cover to protect the hairs from contamination or bending.

19. Which of the following terms refers to any art that protrudes from the nail?

    A) airbrush nail art   C) balayage

    B) inlaid design   D) 3-D nail art

20. _____ are designs inside a nail enhancement created by sandwiching nail art between two product layers while the nail enhancement is formed.

    A) Inlaid designs   C) Balayage designs

    B) Airbrush designs   D) Dotted designs

21. Which of the following statements is true of liquid and powder nail art?

    A) It holds well on a clean, natural nail that has not been prepped and primed.

    B) It lacks versatility in terms of design.

    C) It can be used over polish or any other hardened nail enhancement surface.

    D) It can only be used with a vent brush.

continued

22. In the context of liquid and powder nail enhancement maintenance, _____ is a two- to three-week maintenance service to infuse new growth areas with new product, rebalance the nail's shape, perform needed repairs, and restore the enhancement's original beauty.

   A) slicing   C) glaze

   B) a fill   D) the foil technique

23. In the context of liquid and powder nail enhancement maintenance, which of the following is most likely responsible for the product lifting around the cuticle and sidewalls?

   A) leaving a gap between the liquid and powder and the skin

   B) the use of a medium-grit file

   C) poor natural nail preparation

   D) leaving the product too thin around the cuticle and sidewalls

24. Which of the following guidelines should you follow to remove lifting?

   A) You should use nippers to clip the lifted product.

   B) You should hold a 180-grit file flat against the lifted area and file until it is so thin that the lifted piece flakes away.

   C) You should remove lifting after applying the new product.

   D) You should use coarse, low-grit abrasives on freshly applied enhancement products to remove lifting.

25. Nail plates may appear thinner after enhancements are removed because _____.

   A) the onyx becomes weak after the application and removal of nail enhancements

   B) the nail plates lose keratin, which is responsible for the hard texture of the plates, after nail enhancements are removed

   C) there is generally more moisture in the natural nail plates after soaking them for 30 minutes, making them more flexible

   D) the nail enhancements weaken the nail plates

finished!

Practical Skills
Self-Evaluation Checklist

Regular self-assessment helps you to improve your technical skills and achieve success. After performing each procedure, review the procedure steps in the textbook and rate yourself as "Competent" or "Needs Work," and write in comments on how you were successful or where you can improve. Rating yourself helps you identify your strengths and weaknesses and develop your own plan for improvement.

CRITERIA	COMPETENT	NEEDS WORK	COMMENTS
PROCEDURE 23-1 ONE-COLOR LIQUID AND POWDER OVERLAY			
Preparation			
Procedure			
Post-Service			
Timing			
PROCEDURE 23-2 TWO-COLOR LIQUID AND POWDER NAIL ENHANCEMENTS USING FORMS			
Preparation			
Procedure			
Post-Service			
Timing			
PROCEDURE 23-3 ONE-COLOR LIQUID AND POWDER MAINTENANCE			
Preparation			
Procedure			
Post-Service			
Timing			
PROCEDURE 23-4 LIQUID AND POWDER NAIL ENHANCEMENT REMOVAL			
Preparation			
Procedure			
Post-Service			
Timing			

⚐ TRACK MY PROGRESS!

Use this simple tracker to record your progress as you work through the activities in each learning objective.

COMPLETED	# OF CORRECT ANSWERS	OBJECTIVE
☐	_____/6	**LO 1** - Explain why cosmetologists should learn about light-cured gels.
☐	_____/4	**LO 2** - Discuss light-cured gel chemistry.
☐	_____/14	**LO 3** - Explain the difference between LED and UV light used to cure gels.
☐	_____/27	**LO 4** - Distinguish between different nail service gel types.
☐	_____/1	**LO 5** - List gel application supplies.
☐	_____/15	**LO 6** - Describe how to store, use, and remove gels.
☐	_____/6	**LO 7** - Recognize when to choose gel services.

Why Study Light-Cured Gels?

TRUE OR FALSE

Indicate whether each statement below is true or false. For any false statements, explain why they are false.

1. The 2000s brought significant changes and expansions to gels.

   T   F   _____

2. Light-cured gels are longer lasting than traditional lacquers but are very difficult and time-intensive to apply.

   T   F   _____

3. Light-cured gels dry and cure harder than standard liquid and powder enhancements.

   T   F   _____

4. Light-cured gels are named because they harden (cure) when exposed to a specific type of light, such as LED or UV, among others.

   T   F   _____

SHORT ANSWER

5. Explain what a light-cured gel is.

   _____

   _____

   _____

6. What are the five reasons that cosmetologists should have a thorough understanding of light-cured gels, including their features, advantages, and benefits?

   _____

   _____

   _____

Gel Chemistry

DOUBLE PUZZLE

7. Unscramble the words using the clues provided and write them in the squares. You'll see a number underneath some of the squares. Find the numbered squares below and write that letter into that square to reveal the secret message!

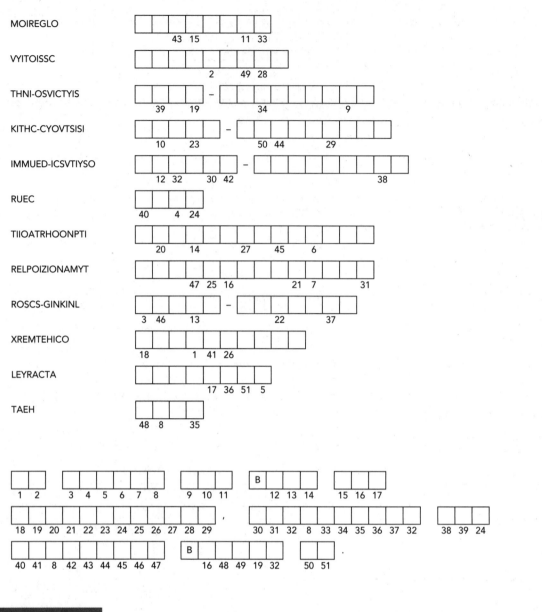

MOIREGLO ☐☐☐☐☐☐☐☐
43 15   11 33

VYITOISSC ☐☐☐☐☐☐☐☐
2   49 28

THNI-OSVICTYIS ☐☐☐☐ – ☐☐☐☐☐☐☐☐☐
39   19   34   9

KITHC-CYOVTSISI ☐☐☐☐ – ☐☐☐☐☐☐☐☐
10   23   50 44   29

IMMUED-ICSVTIYSO ☐☐☐☐☐☐ – ☐☐☐☐☐☐☐☐☐
12 32 30 42   38

RUEC ☐☐☐☐
40 4 24

TIIOATRHOONPTI ☐☐☐☐☐☐☐☐☐☐☐☐
20 14   27 45 6

RELPOIZIONAMYT ☐☐☐☐☐☐☐☐☐☐☐☐
47 25 16   21 7   31

ROSCS-GINKINL ☐☐☐☐☐ – ☐☐☐☐☐☐
3 46 13   22   37

XREMTEHICO ☐☐☐☐☐☐☐☐☐
18   1 41 26

LEYRACTA ☐☐☐☐☐☐☐
17 36 51 5

TAEH ☐☐☐☐
48 8 35

☐☐ ☐☐☐☐☐☐ ☐☐☐ [B]☐☐☐ ☐☐☐
1 2   3 4 5 6 7 8 9 10 11   12 13 14 15 16 17

☐☐☐☐☐☐☐☐☐☐☐☐ , ☐☐☐☐☐☐☐☐☐☐ ☐☐☐
18 19 20 21 22 23 24 25 26 27 28 29   30 31 32 8 33 34 35 36 37 32 38 39 24

☐☐☐☐☐☐☐☐ [B]☐☐☐☐☐ ☐☐ .
40 41 8 42 43 44 45 46 47   16 48 49 19 32 50 51

SHORT ANSWER

8. To successfully and easily soak off the gel polish, how much acetone should be in the polish remover used for gels?

_____

_____

_____

9. What is the difference between the color layer and the top coat, in terms of their cross-linking, when using gel polish?

_____

_____

_____

10. In addition to applying and curing a thin first layer of gel polish or applying multiple small (instead of large) beads to control the heat spike, what are two other methods you can use?

_____

_____

_____

UV and LED Light

TRUE OR FALSE

Indicate whether each statement is true or false. For each statement that is false, explain why it is false.

11. There is only one type of curing lamp that should be used in salons that provide gel services.

    T   F   _____

12. A curing lamp is specially designed for use in nail salons to cure gel enhancements.

    T   F   _____

13. Violet light cures gel enhancements in LED bulbs.

    T   F   _____

14. The size of bulbs in curing lamps impacts the power of the lamp.

    T   F   _____

15. Nanometer is the unit of measure indicating how much electricity a lamp consumes.

    T   F   _____

16. Gel-curing lamps use either LED or UV fluorescent bulbs.

    T   F   _____

17. UV fluorescent lamps are the most common type of curing lamp in modern salons.

    T   F   _____

SHORT ANSWER

18. What does LED stand for? What does UV stand for?

    _____

    _____

    _____

19. How often should you change a UV bulb inside a curing lamp, according to manufacturers'
    recommendations? Why is this important for you as a cosmetologist and for your clients?

    _____

    _____

    _____

20. What are three features of a curing lamp that can affect its curing power?

    _____

    _____

    _____

21. How is the curing power of a lamp determined? What is the curing power of a lamp that has four
    8-watt bulbs?

    _____

    _____

    _____

22. Even though they initially cost the same, what are three main reasons that LED lamps are now more common in salons than UV lamps are?

_____

_____

_____

23. Why don't gel products start to cure as soon as they are exposed to the light of the salon?

_____

_____

_____

MATCHING

24. Match each type of bulb/light with its description. Both bulb types might apply to a description.

    a. LED   b. UV

Type of Bulb/Light	Description
_____	Produces wavelengths of optical light from about 365 to 405 nanometers (nm)
_____	Radiates light in ranges from about 320 to 400 nanometers (nm)
_____	Bulb lasts about 5 years or 50,000 hours
_____	Harnesses the violet color and its intensity
_____	Radiates light inside the lamp so that all nails are equally exposed
_____	Creates a direct light that must shine directly on the gel for it to cure
_____	Cure times usually range from 5 to 60 seconds for each gel layer
_____	Cure times usually range from one to two minutes for each gel layer
_____	Should be changed every six months

Gel Types

25. Complete the table by filling in each type of gel for the corresponding detail.

Type of Gel	Description
_____	Soak-off gels
_____	Used to build nail extensions
_____	Strong with nonporous surface
_____	Formulated to overlay the natural nail
_____	Easily removed with acetone
_____	Traditional gels
_____	Low odor

Indicate whether each statement below is true or false. For any false statements, explain why they are false.

26. There are six basic types of gel systems used in salons.

    T   F   _____

27. Hard gels are generally thought of as traditional gels.

    T   F   _____

28. Soft gels are best for adding significant length to nails.

    T   F   _____

29. Soak-off gels, otherwise known as soft gels, are a great alternative for traditional nail polish.

    T   F   _____

30. What are bonding gels used for in a light-cured gel system?

_____

_____

_____

31. Are bonding gels applied thickly or thinly to the nail?

_____

_____

_____

32. What is an effective alternative to curing bonding gels with a lamp?

_____

_____

_____

33. How are building gels typically packaged and applied?

_____

_____

_____

34. What are three advantages of working with a polymer gel?

_____

_____

_____

35. How are polymer gels maintained and removed?

_____

_____

_____

36. Order the steps for completing a one-color hard gel overlay, steps 1–14. Steps 4 and 7 are given.

_____ Float a small bead of gel on the apex of the nail to create a slight arch. Cure and repeat on every nail.

_____ Ask client to wash their hands with soap and water and dry thoroughly.

_____ Massage the hand and arm.

_____ Remove sticky inhibition layer with alcohol or nail cleaner on a lint-free wipe.

_____ Massage cuticle oil into nail area, then apply hand cream.

___4___ Properly position hand in gel-curing lamp. Cure. Repeat on each nail until curing is complete.

_____ Applying bonding gel or primer. Cure if necessary.

_____ Buff surface with coarse-grit buffer to smooth and refine shape.

_____ Remove finishing gel inhibition layer, if required.

___7___ Use a medium- or fine-grit abrasive to refine the surface contour. Check free-edge thickness and even out imperfections.

_____ Present the finished look to your client.

_____ Pick up a medium bead of building gel with a gel brush

_____ If gel polish is not requested, apply finishing gel and cure.

_____ Apply the bead, starting with left pinky. Place gel on center of nail and gently float it over entire nail's surface, including the free edge.

CASE STUDY

37. Use the Internet or a beauty supply catalogue to identify and compare the features of two different bonding gels, building gels, and polymer gels. Follow the link or use the table provided to record your findings.

+ BONUS

Visit: bonus.milady.com/cos-wb/toc

FEATURES	BONDING GEL #1	BONDING GEL #2	BUILDING GEL #1	BUILDING GEL #2	POLYMER GEL #1	POLYMER GEL #2
Name/Brand						
Packaging						
Colors Available						
Curing Method						
Specifics	Viscosity:	Viscosity:	Self-leveling? (Y/N)	Self-leveling? (Y/N)	Includes shaping liquid? (Y/N)	Includes shaping liquid? (Y/N)
Recommended Nail Prep Products?						
Cost						
Size/Amount						
Source (store/website)						
Other Features, if Any						

Review the results of your research and state which of each gel you would consider purchasing. Also, identify one gel of the six above that you would not purchase. In a few short sentences, explain why you made these choices.

Finally, partner with a classmate and compare notes on your findings. Discuss whether you agree or disagree with each other's purchasing choices. What did you learn about new products?

FILL IN THE BLANK

38. _____ are thick-viscosity gels that allow you to build an arch or _____.

39. A _____ gel has a very _____ viscosity and can leave the nail bumpy. A

_____ gel is more fluid and leaves the nail _____.

40. _____ gels are a mixture of polymer _____ and _____ gels.

These gels often come with a _____ that keeps the application brush

_____ so that it does not stick to the _____.

41. Another name for a bonding gel is _____.

MATCHING

42. Match each type of gel to the corresponding detail. All terms will be used more than once.

Word bank: a. Bonding   b. Building   c. Polymer

Type of Gel   **Description**

_____ Varies in viscosity

_____ Used to add thickness to an enhancement or build an extension

_____ Also known as polygel or acrygel

_____ A mixture of polymer powder and hard gel

_____ Usually hard gel, but can be soak-off/soft as well

_____ Most come in a tube, like toothpaste

_____ Does not always need to be cured with a curing lamp

_____ Allows for more control during sculpting due to viscosity

_____ Usually sold in a small pot container

_____ Often used in 3-D art

_____ Will be used with another type of gel to complete service

_____ Can be either self-leveling or non-self-leveling

_____ Usually used with nonacid primer or bonding gel to prep nail

43. Complete the sentences below using the word bank. Some words will not be used.

    Word bank: natural, bonding, soft, inlaid, polish, paint, tube, synthetic, can, cannot, thin, encapsulated, hard, pot, pigment, building, art, thick

    Pigmented gels contain color _____. Most are sold in a small _____. They are

    usually _____ gels and _____ be soaked off. Some manufacturers create gel

    with very _____ viscosity and call it a gel _____, which is used for detailed nail

    _____. Sometimes _____ gels are used over the design to create an _____

    look. Other pigmented gels are used like _____ and are painted over nails with a

    _____ brush.

44. What are soak-off gels an alternative to?

    _____

    _____

    _____

45. With an array of colors available, what options do soak-off gel polishes provide, for both the cosmetologist and the client?

    _____

    _____

    _____

46. Although soak-off gel polishes can vary in opacity and viscosity, what do they all have in common?

    _____

    _____

    _____

47. Number the steps of the procedure for applying soak-off gel polish over nail enhancements, from beginning to end. The fourth step in this sequence has been provided for you.

_____ Massage cuticle oil into nail and surrounding skin then apply hand cream and massage the hand and arm.

___4___ Repeat steps 2 and 3 with a second coat of gel polish.

_____ Apply thin coat of soak-off gel polish in client's preferred color over the enhancement's entire surface with a brushing technique. Apply small amount of gel polish to fingernail's free edge to cap the end and create an even and consistent appearance.

_____ Cure top coat and remove inhibition layer with alcohol or cleansing solution on lint-free wipe if required.

_____ Place hand inside gel-curing lamp in proper location and cure for recommended time.

_____ After nail enhancement application and filing are complete, remove dust and filings with clean, disinfected nylon brush.

_____ Polish each nail with soak-off gel top coat.

_____ Clean the nails.

_____ Present the finished look to your client.

SHORT ANSWER

48. Why should you use a soak-off gel top coat when finishing a soak-off polish?

_____

_____

_____

49. What is finishing gel used for?

_____

_____

_____

50. What is the inhibition layer? How is it removed?

_____

_____

_____

MATCHING

51. Match each type of gel to its description. All types of gel will be used more than once.

   Word bank: a. Pigmented   b. Soak-off   c. Finishing

Type of Gel	**Description**
_____	Can be removed with an acetone soak (or other product remover)
_____	Used with building gel to create artistic encapsulated look
_____	Used to create high shine
_____	Cures in one of two ways: tack-free or sticky, requiring cleaning of the inhibition layer
_____	Usually hard gel that cannot be soaked off
_____	Some can be used like polish that is painted over nails
_____	An alternative to traditional lacquer
_____	Comes in a wide variety of colors and finishes
_____	Sometimes used as a last step with dip nails

Gel Application Supplies

DOUBLE PUZZLE

52. Unscramble the words using the clues provided and write them in the squares. You'll see a number underneath some of the squares. Find the numbered square below and write that letter into that square to reveal the secret message.

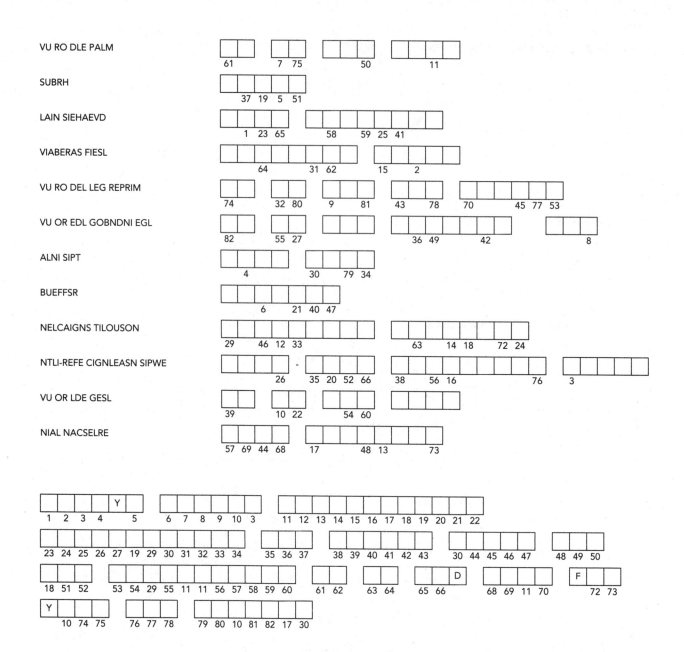

Storing, Using, and Removing Gels

Indicate whether the statements below are true or false. For each false statement, explain why it is false.

53. Gel products are light cured.

    T   F   _____

54. To protect them from moisture, dust, and light, gel products must be stored in a cabinet when not in use.

T   F   _____

55. During the service, keep all gels away from sunlight, gel lamps, and full-spectrum table lamps to prevent the gel from hardening; these factors don't affect the brushes.

T   F   _____

56. If gel cures in your brush, the brush is ruined and cannot be repaired.

T   F   _____

57. Gel enhancements must be maintained every four to six weeks, depending on how fast the client's nails grow.

T   F   _____

58. Hard gels cannot be removed with acetone or product remover.

T   F   _____

59. Hard gels must be filed off using an electric or hand file. It is best to file off all of the product.

T   F   _____

SHORT ANSWER

60. What is one way to help your clients choose gel colors while protecting your gel products in a cabinet?

_____

_____

_____

61. Why is it recommended that you cure each finger immediately after applying gel?

_____

_____

_____

62. How does temperature affect a gel's viscosity?

_____

_____

_____

63. How can you help decrease a client's risk of skin irritation and sensitivity when applying gel products?

_____

_____

_____

64. Describe how to use your brush to apply beads of gel to (1) cover the entire nail surface and (2) fill low spots.

_____

_____

_____

65. What are two different ways to remove soft gels and soak-off gels?

_____

_____

_____

66. What are three benefits of wrapping nails when removing gel products?

_____

_____

_____

67. Number the steps of the procedure for removing hard gels and polymer gels, from beginning to end. The first step has been provided to get you started.

_____ Present the finished look to your client.

_____ Massage cuticle oil into nail and surrounding skin then apply hand cream and massage hand and arm.

_____ Use medium-grit file to further reduce thickness of the enhancement. Do not file into natural nail.

___1___ Remove polish if present.

_____ Use medium-grit nail buffer to smooth enhancement. Talk with client about how to allow the enhancements to grow out and off the fingernails.

_____ Use coarse-grit file to thin the gel by 60 percent.

_____ Clean the nails. Ask client to wash hands with soap and water at hand-washing station or use nail brush to clean nails over fingerbowl. Rinse with clean water and dry thoroughly with clean disposable towel.

When to Choose Gel Services

TRUE OR FALSE

Indicate which statements below are true or false. For statements that are false, explain why they are false.

68. If a client is looking for a relatively long-term solution to weak nails or a more consistent colored polish, gels are a good option.

    T   F   _____

69. If a client likes to change polish colors regularly (more than once every two weeks or so), gels are the best option.

    T   F   _____

70. If a client complains of other types of enhancements lifting, gels could possibly be a good solution.

T   F   _____

71. Clients with short nails who prefer very long nails should consider soft gels for added length.

T   F   _____

72. Clients looking for short-term enhancements for a special occasion are good candidates for gels.

T   F   _____

ROLE PLAY

73. Partner with a classmate to practice making recommendations for gel polish services. Take turns being the nail technician and client. As the nail technician, ask a series of questions similar to those found in your text (or create your own questions) and make recommendations to the client based on their responses. As the client, provide truthful answers or challenge your partner by inventing some of your answers. Engage in a discussion about each other's recommendations and ultimately come to an agreement about the best option for each of you. Use the space below for some notes, such as questions you might ask or responses you would give as a client.

DISCOVERIES AND ACCOMPLISHMENTS

In the space below, write notes about key concepts discussed in this chapter. Share your discoveries with some of the other students in your class and ask them if your notes are helpful. You may want to revise your notes based on good ideas shared by your peers.

Discoveries:

_____

_____

_____

_____

_____

_____

List at least three things you have accomplished since you decided to enroll in school.

Accomplishments:

_____

_____

_____

_____

_____

_____

1. As a cosmetologist, you should have a thorough understanding of light-cured gels because _____.

   A) learning about gel products' chemistry helps choose the best products to use on each client by considering their safety and suitability

   B) gel polish services are popular as gels are very thin, making it very easy for them to dry on their own

   C) cosmetologists are required to identify gels by their odor, and most gels have a very appealing odor, which makes them popular among clients

   D) light-cured gels, invented in the 2010s, are a new addition to the nail industry

2. Most gels use a(n) _____ oligomer, which has excellent adhesion and a lower sensitivity risk.

   A) urethane methacrylate

   B) polyester

   C) epoxy siloxane

   D) polycaprolactone

3. Thick-viscosity gels are _____.

   A) either monomers or polymers

   B) brush-on formulas

   C) sometimes referred to as self-leveling gels

   D) used for building or sculpting nail extensions

4. Polymerization, also known as cross-linking, is the process by which _____.

   A) a solid substance is transformed into a liquid substance

   B) oligomers link into a solid chemical-resistant material

   C) a photoinitiator creates a reaction when exposed to UV or visible light

   D) polymers are converted to monomers

5. Which of the following statements related to gel chemistry is accurate?

   A) An exothermic reaction occurs as each bond of a polymer is created.

   B) The more bonds formed when a gel cures, the less heat is generated.

   C) The more bonds created when a gel polymerizes, the weaker the nail enhancement.

   D) Gels need photoinitiators to help them transform from a solid to a liquid.

continued

6. A way to control the heat spike when using a light-cured gel on the nail is to _____.

   A) start with a thick application over the natural nail and cure

   B) apply and cure multiple large, instead of small, beads of gel

   C) remove the hand from the light for 5 to 10 seconds if the client feels the increase in heat

   D) generate less heat by avoiding exposing the gel directly to the source of light

7. Identify a characteristic of LED bulbs.

   A) Usually, an LED bulb lasts about 10 years.

   B) Cure times of light-cured gels with an LED lamp usually range from one to two minutes for each gel layer.

   C) LED bulbs used to cure light-cured gels produce wavelengths of optical light from about 150 to 180 nanometers (nm).

   D) LED bulbs create a light that must shine directly on a light-cured gel for it to cure.

8. On the visible light spectrum scale, the _____.

   A) green light needed to cure light-cured gels is produced at around the 200 nm mark

   B) violet light needed to cure light-cured gels is produced at around the 400 nm mark

   C) violet light needed to cure light-cured gels is produced at around the 600 nm mark

   D) green light needed to cure light-cured gels is produced at around the 500 nm mark

9. Identify an accurate statement about ultraviolet (UV) florescent bulbs used in a curing lamp.

   A) UV florescent bulbs radiate light inside the lamp so all nails are equally exposed in ranges from about 320 to 400 nm.

   B) The range of UV florescent bulbs is wider than that of LED bulbs.

   C) UV florescent bulbs typically stop glowing after six months of use.

   D) Most manufacturers recommend changing the UV florescent bulbs inside a curing lamp every year.

10. Which of the followings shows an accurate comparison between ultraviolet (UV) florescent bulbs and LED bulbs used in a curing lamp?

    A) Some clients feel more comfortable with gel services using LED bulbs than with UV bulbs because of reduced light exposure.

    B) UV bulbs last approximately 10 times longer than LED bulbs.

    C) LED lamps cure slower than do UV bulbs, and this results in fitting less clients into a cosmetologist's schedule.

    D) The range of ultraviolet UV bulbs is wider than that of LED bulbs.

continued

11. Which of the following is an accurate statement about hard gels?

A) They are strong enough to build nail extensions.

B) They are also known as soak-off gels.

C) They have a porous surface that acetone can penetrate.

D) They have a strong odor and are made with pigment.

12. Identify a characteristic of soft gels.

A) Soft gels cannot be easily removed with acetone.

B) Most soft gels have a crystal-clear appearance.

C) Most soft gels do not replace traditional polishes.

D) Soft gels are formulated to overlay the natural nail.

13. Bonding or base gels _____.

A) are often applied with a primer

B) vary in viscosity

C) are applied with a thick coat to the nail

D) reduce adhesion to the natural nail plate

14. Building gels _____.

A) allow you to build an arch or extension

B) are thin-viscosity gels

C) reduce thickness of nail enhancements

D) are also known as base gels

15. A characteristic of a non-self-leveling gel is that it _____.

A) is more fluid than a self-leveling gel

B) typically leaves the nail smooth, unlike a self-leveling gel

C) adds more thickness to the fingernail than does a self-leveling gel

D) is a type of base gel or bonding gel

continued

16. Identify a true statement about polymer gels.

    A) They are advantageous because they do not soften until the technician pushes them or brushes them into place.

    B) They are usually very difficult to file.

    C) They move or lose shape before curing.

    D) They are thin-viscosity bonding gels and harden without a curing lamp.

17. Which of the following shows a characteristic of pigmented gels?

    A) Most pigmented gels are sold in a large pot.

    B) Generally, pigmented gels can be soaked off.

    C) Pigmented gels are also known as polygel or acrygel.

    D) Pigmented gels are usually hard gels.

18. Which of the following most likely consists of uncured gel and/or leftover solvents that create a tacky surface on a nail after a gel cures?

    A) an overlay   C) a position stop

    B) an inhibition layer   D) a backfill

19. Finishing gel, a hard clear gel with a high-gloss or matte finish, is used _____.

    A) to complete the gel service

    B) as a base coat

    C) to overlay the natural nail and create an arch or an extension

    D) to improve gel adhesion to the natural nail plate

20. A nail cleanser is used _____.

    A) after applying primer on the nail

    B) to add an inhibition layer to the nail before filing the cured gel in order to increase the gel's durability

    C) to remove surface moisture and tiny amounts of oil left on the natural nail plate that can impair a gel's adhesion

    D) as a top coat or when color is not desired

continued

21. Abrasive files and buffers with a medium-grit buffer are primarily used _____.

    A) for natural nail preparation, including contouring and shaping

    B) to remove surface moisture and tiny amounts of oil left on the natural nail plate

    C) to prevent nail enhancement lifting

    D) as tools to remove residue or fibers on the nail surface after the desired service

22. Identify a guideline related to the use of gels.

    A) When not in use, store gel products in an open container to expose them to natural heat and light.

    B) During a service, keep gels next to a full-spectrum table lamp.

    C) When applying beads of gel, start at the nail's free edge and float them toward the cuticle.

    D) When a service is complete, cover your gel application brush from all light sources.

23. Which of the following should be kept in mind when removing gels from nails?

    A) Hard gels can be removed with acetone or product remover.

    B) Hard gels must be filed off using an electric or hand file.

    C) When removing soft or soak-off gels, the nails should not be soaked in acetone or product remover.

    D) When removing soak soft or soak-off gels, the nails should not be wrapped with cotton and foil.

24. Which of the following points should be kept in mind when discussing hard gel extensions with a client?

    A) Since gels can only be filed off, they are not the best option for a short-term extension service.

    B) If the extension edge will be shorter than the nail bed, it is best to choose a stronger product, such as liquid and powder.

    C) Gel services have weak adhesion, making them the last option for clients whose nails lift easily.

    D) Hard gel extensions can be easily removed with acetone or product remover.

25. Identify a point that should be kept in mind when discussing gel polishes with a client.

    A) If changing the polish color often is preferred, gel polish is preferred over traditional polish.

    B) Traditional polish is stronger than gel polish because traditional polish provides extra strength to the natural nail.

    C) Gel polish hardens immediately, so one can resume daily tasks right after the service.

    D) If wearing the same color for longer periods is preferred, traditional polish is the right fit because it remains chip-free for two weeks.

finished!

Practical Skills

Self-Evaluation Checklist

Regular self-assessment helps you to improve your technical skills and achieve success. After performing each procedure, review the procedure steps in the textbook and rate yourself as "Competent" or "Needs Work," and write in comments on how you were successful or where you can improve. Rating yourself helps you identify your strengths and weaknesses and develop your own plan for improvement.

CRITERIA	COMPETENT	NEEDS WORK	COMMENTS
PROCEDURE 24-1 ONE-COLOR HARD-GEL OVERLAY			
Preparation			
Procedure			
Post-Service			
Timing			
PROCEDURE 24-2 TWO-COLOR HARD-GEL OVERLAY			
Preparation			
Procedure			
Post-Service			
Timing			
PROCEDURE 24-3 ONE-COLOR HARD-GEL SCULPTURE EXTENSIONS			
Preparation			
Procedure			
Post-Service			
Timing			
PROCEDURE 24-4 ONE-COLOR POLYMER GEL OVERLAY			
Preparation			
Procedure			
Post-Service			
Timing			
PROCEDURE 24-5 HARD-GEL MAINTENANCE			
Preparation			
Procedure			
Post-Service			
Timing			
PROCEDURE 24-6 SOAK-OFF GEL POLISH OVER NAIL ENHANCEMENTS			
Preparation			
Procedure			
Post-Service			
Timing			
PROCEDURE 24-7 SOAK-OFF GEL POLISH ON NATURAL NAILS			
Preparation			
Procedure			
Post-Service			
Timing			

Practical Skills Self-Evaluation Checklist

CRITERIA	COMPETENT	NEEDS WORK	COMMENTS
PROCEDURE 24-8 HARD GEL AND POLYMER GEL REMOVAL			
Preparation			
Procedure			
Post-Service			
Timing			
PROCEDURE 24-9 SOAK-OFF GEL OR GEL POLISH REMOVAL			
Preparation			
Procedure			
Post-Service			
Timing			

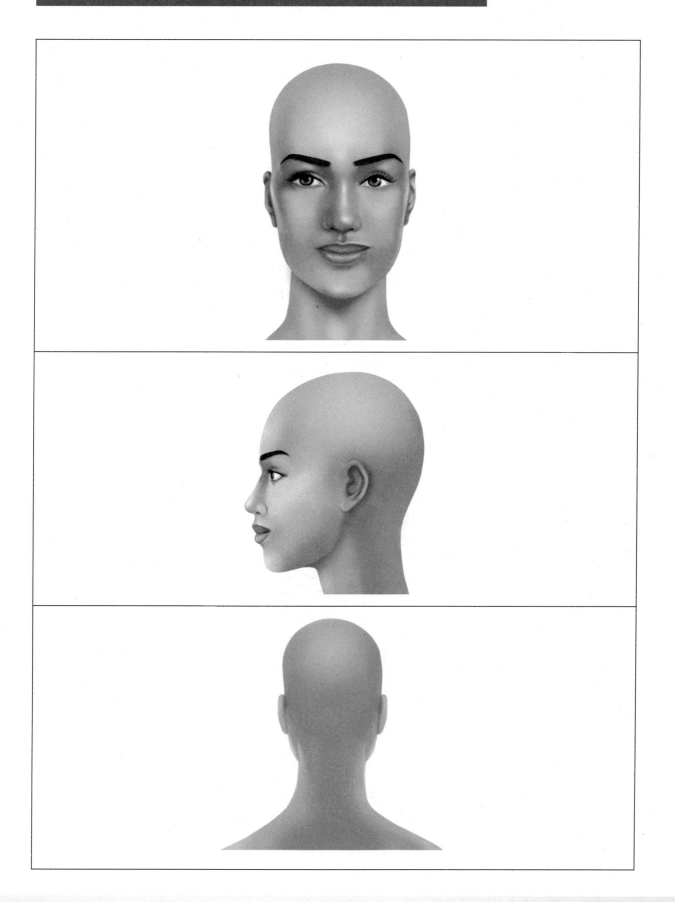

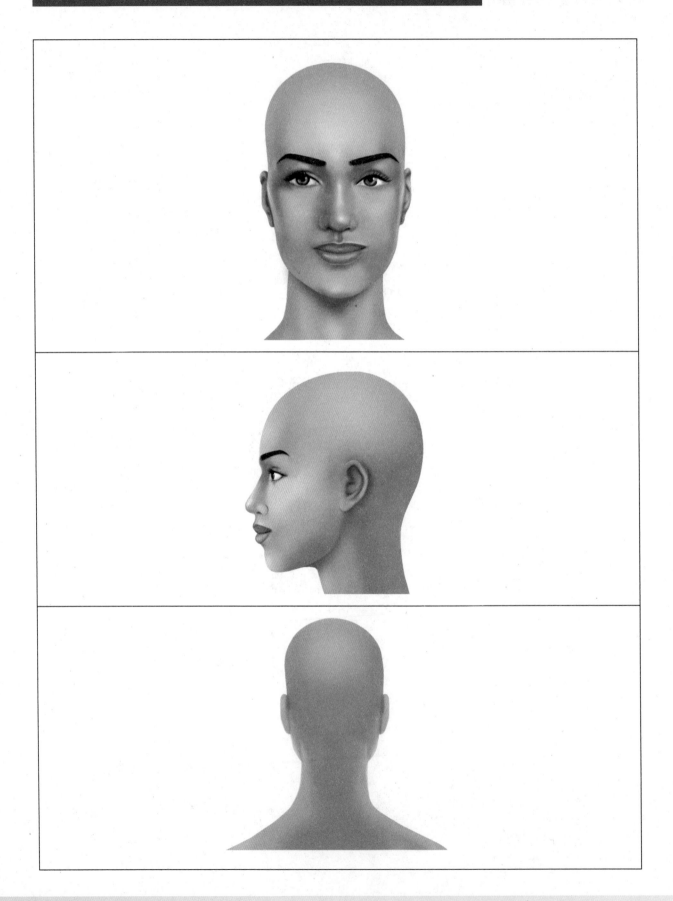

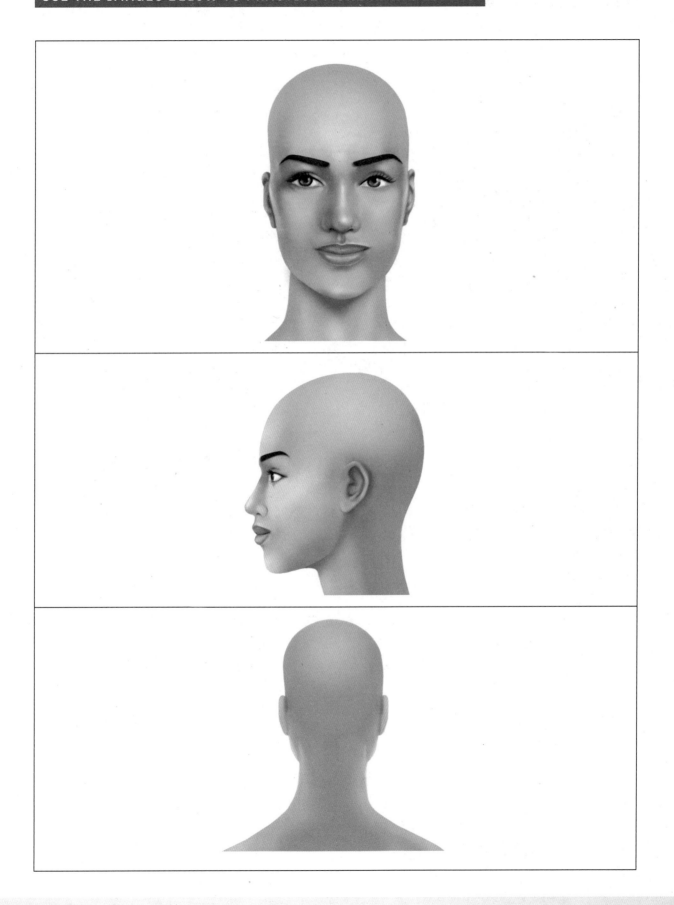